STEM CELL ONCOLOGY

PROCEEDINGS OF THE INTERNATIONAL STEM CELL AND ONCOLOGY CONFERENCE (ISCOC 2017), 1–2 DECEMBER, 2017, MEDAN, INDONESIA

Stem Cell Oncology

Editor

Adeya Cut Adella
Universitas Sumatera Utara, Medan, Indonesia

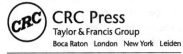

CRC Press
Taylor & Francis Group
Boca Raton London New York Leiden

CRC Press is an imprint of the
Taylor & Francis Group, an **informa** business

A BALKEMA BOOK

CRC Press/Balkema is an imprint of the Taylor & Francis Group, an informa business

© 2018 Taylor & Francis Group, London, UK

Typeset by V Publishing Solutions Pvt Ltd., Chennai, India

Although all care is taken to ensure integrity and the quality of this publication and the information herein, no responsibility is assumed by the publishers nor the author for any damage to the property or persons as a result of operation or use of this publication and/or the information contained herein.

Published by: CRC Press/Balkema

      Schipholweg 107C, 2316 XC Leiden, The Netherlands
      e-mail: Pub.NL@taylorandfrancis.com
      www.crcpress.com – www.taylorandfrancis.com

ISBN: 978-0-8153-9272-9 (Hbk)
ISBN: 978-1-351-19015-2 (eBook)

Table of contents

vii

Preface

Stem cell research is one of the fascinating areas of contemporary biology, but, as with many expanding fields of scientific inquiry, research on stem cells raises scientific questions as rapidly as it generates discoveries. Research on stem cell treatment continues to advance knowledge about how an organism develops from a single cell and how healthy cells replace damaged cells in adult organisms. The most important potential application of human stem cells is the generation of cells and tissues that could be used for cell-based therapies, especially oncology.

The Faculty of Medicine, Universitas Sumatera Utara, collaborated with the center of excellence and innovation (Pusat Unggulan Inovasi /PUI). The Stem Cell center of the Universitas Sumatera Utara (USU) organized an International Conference. The International Stem Cell and Oncology Conference (ISCOC) 2017 was an comprehensive academic conference in the field of stem cell and oncology research and also tropical medicine and related scientific topics.

We expect this conference will benefit academics and practitioners in the field of health sciences in Indonesia. During the two day conference, researchers presented the most recent discoveries in stem cell and oncology and also general medical topics, and served as well in establishing networking for joint researchers and collaboration among participants.

The editors and the scientific committee would like to thank the participants and express their gratitude to Faculty of Medicine of the Universitas Sumatera Utara for their support to ISCOC 2017. Lastly, we are most indebted for the generous support given by Universitas Sumatera Utara, Medan, Sumatera Utara, Indonesia.

February 2018
Editors
Prof. Dr. dr. Delfitri Munir, Sp.T.H.T.KL(K)

Organizing committee

CHAIRMAN

Prof. Dr. dr. Delfitri Munir, Sp.T.H.T.KL(K)

FIRST CO-CHAIRMAN

dr. Kamal Basri Siregar, Sp.B, K.Onk

SECRETARY

dr. Cut Adeya Adella, Sp.OG(K)

VICE SECRETARY

dr. Lokot Donna Lubis, Sp.PA

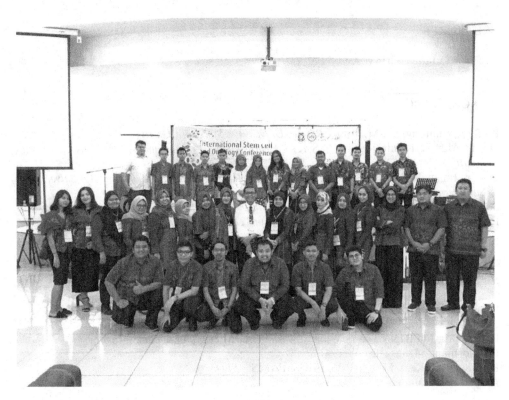

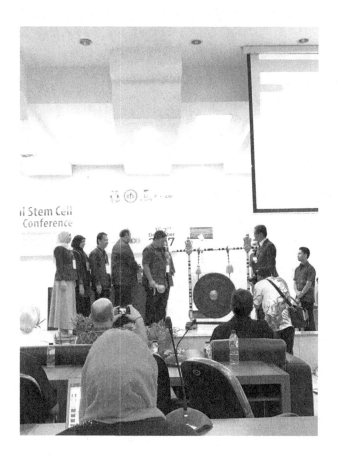

TREASURER

dr. Mutiara Indah Sari, M.Kes

HONORARY BOARD

Prof. Dr. Runtung, SH.M.Hum – *Rector, Universitas Sumatera Utara*
Dr. dr. Aldy Safruddin Rambe, SpS(K) – *Dean, Faculty of Medicine, Universitas Sumatera Utara*
Dr. dr. Imam Budi Putra, MHA. Sp.KK(K) – *Dean 1, Faculty of Medicine, Universitas Sumatera Utara*
dr. Zaimah Z. Tala, MS. Sp.GK – *Dean 2, Faculty of Medicine, Universitas Sumatera Utara*
Dr. dr. Dina Keumala Sari, MG. Sp.GK – *Dean 3, Faculty of Medicine, Universitas Sumatera Utara*

SCIENTIFIC COMMITTEE

Hans Vrielink, MD, Ph.D – *The Netherlands*
drg. Ferry Sandra, Ph.D. LFIBA. CIPM. MIPM – *Indonesia*
Prof. Dr. dr. Ida Bagus Tjakra Wibawa Manuaba, MPH. Sp.B(K) Onk – *Indonesia*
Dr. Normando Iznaga-Escobar – *Cuba*
Prof. Siow Jin Keat, MD. MBBS. FRCS. FAMS – *Singapore*
Ahmad R Utomo, Ph.D – *Indonesia*

xiv

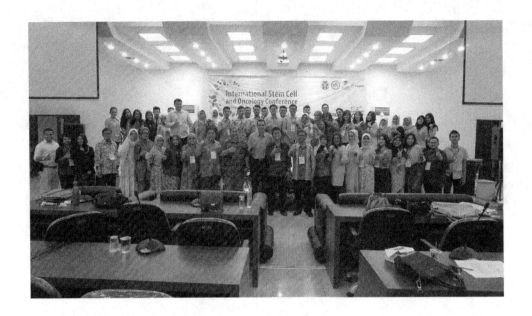

Prof. dr. Aznan Lelo, Ph.D – *Indonesia*
Prof. Dr. dr. Nur Indrawati Lipoeto, SpGK – *Indonesia*

EDITOR

Prof. Dr. dr. Delfitri Munir, Sp.T.H.T.KL(K)

MEMBERS

Prof. Dr. dr. Iskandar Japardi, Sp.BS(K)
dr. Deri Edianto, Sp.OG(K)
Prof. Dr. dr. M. Fidel Ganis Siregar, M.Ked(OG), Sp.OG(K)
dr. M. Rusda Harahap, M.Ked, Sp.OG(K)
dr. Selvi Nafianti, M.Ked, Sp.A(K)
dr. Sarah Dina, Sp.OG(K)
dr. Dewi Masyithah Darlan, DAP & E.MPH.Sp.ParK
dr. Feby yanti Harahap, Sp.PA
dr. Triwidyawati, Msi, Ph.D

Stem Cell Oncology – Adella (Ed.)
© *2018 Taylor & Francis Group, London, ISBN 978-0-8153-9272-9*

Association of the Anal Position Index (API) with constipation

H.A. Sinuhaji, E. Azlin, Supriatmo, A. Rahmad, A. Sinuhaji & A.B. Sinuhaji
*Department of Child Health, Faculty of Medicine, Universitas Sumatera Utara, Medan,
North Sumatera, Indonesia*

ABSTRACT: Constipation is one of the most common chronic disorders of childhood. Anterior displacement of the anus is one of the organic causes of constipation. Reisner et al. proposed an objective method to determine the normal position of the anus using the Anal Position Index (API). An API of less than 0.46 in boys and less than 0.36 in girls indicates anterior displacement of the anus. A cross-sectional study of 66 children was conducted. Subjects were chosen using consecutive sampling. Study data were collected by conducting demographic data and by using the API. The API, which is the ratio of anus-scrotum distance in boys and anus-fourchette in girls between the coccyx and fourchette/scrotum, was calculated in this study. Girls were more likely to develop constipation than boys. There was no relationship between the API and constipation (PR 0.825; 95% CI 0.201 to 3.394).

Keywords: anal position index, anterior displacement anus, constipation

1 INTRODUCTION

Constipation is one of the most common chronic disorders of childhood, affecting 1% to 30% of children worldwide. Constipation is responsible for 3% of all primary care visits for children and 10% to 25% of paediatric gastroenterology visits (Nurko & Zimmerman, 2014). Constipation is a symptom rather than a disease (Karami & Shokohi, 2013).

According to the aetiology, constipation can be classified into two categories: functional and organic. The functional type is also called idiopathic, as there is no identified pathology, and organic aetiology. In the organic type, constipation is part of the symptoms of an underlying pathology or disease (Hammo et al., 2012).

Although most constipation is functional, congenital anatomic malformations in an anorectal area may be responsible in some of these cases. Similar to many other abnormalities, congenital anorectal malformations occur in a wide spectrum of severity. Slight anterior displacement of the anus is the less severe form of anorectal malformation. These abnormalities in the neonate are easily diagnosed at birth by a simple inspection, yet ectopic anterior anus is very difficult to diagnose without using diagnostic measurement tools (Davari & Nazem, 2004).

Today, despite controversies, many researchers believe that anterior anus gives rise to up to one-third of childhood chronic constipations and the diagnosis of it remains uncertain. In 1978, Leape and Ramenofsky stated that the usual anal position is midway between the vaginal fourchette and coccyx. Reisner et al. (1984) presented a simple method, the Anal Position Index (API), to define the normal position of the anus in a neonate (Davari & Nazem, 2004). The aim of the present study is to determine the association of the API with anterior displacement of the anus.

2 METHODS

A cross-sectional study of children under four years of age was conducted in Simalingkar community healthcare centre, Medan, Indonesian. Subjects were chosen using consecutive sampling. Subjects with warning signs (delayed passage of meconium, failure to thrive, bloody stools, severe abdominal distention, perianal fistula, absent anal wink, sacral dimple), congenital anomalies or syndromes, and taking medical treatment that affects constipation were excluded from this study. Study data were collected by conducting demographic data and by using the API. The child was held in the lithotomy position, and adhesive transparent tapes were used on the longitudinal axis of the mid-perineum. The fourchette/scrotum, anus centre and lower margin of the coccyx were marked on it. The strip was removed and flattened out onto a flat surface, and the distances were measured using a flexible measuring tape. The API, which is the ratio of anus-scrotum distance in boys and anus-fourchette in girls between the coccyx and fourchette/scrotum, was calculated. The association of the API and demographic data with constipation were tested. Results were considered to be statistically significant for P values <0.05. This study was approved by the Ethics Committee of the Faculty of Medicine at the Universitas Sumatera Utara.

3 RESULTS

Sixty-six children were included in this study, of which 34 were males and 32 were females. The incidence of constipation in this study was 16.7%. Demographic characteristics are detailed in Table 1.

Based on the API, there were 14 subjects with an anterior anus and two subjects with a normal anus.

Table 1. Demographic characteristics.

Characteristic	Constipated N = 11	Not constipated N = 55	P	CI 95%
Age, months (SD)	25.7 (13.39)	16.5 (12.88)	0.040*	
Body weight, kg (SD)	8.48 (5.37)	6.98 (4.05)	0.042*	
Height, cm (SD)	84.6 (11.89)	75.1 (13.6)	0.036**	0.651–18.330
API, cm (SD)				
Male	0.56 (0.02)	0.52 (0.05)	0.248*	−0.035–0.133
Female	0.36 (0.05)	0.35 (0.05)	0.969*	−0.044–0.446
Gender, n (%)				
Female	9 (81.8)	23 (41.8)	0.015***	1.235–31.737
Male	2 (18.2)	32 (58.2)		
Feeding, n (%)				
Breast milk	0 (0.0)	14 (25.5)	0.089****	
Formula	1 (9.1)	4 (7.2)		
Others	10 (90.9)	37 (67.3)		

*Mann-Whitney test; **T independent test; ***Chi-squared; ****Kruskal–Wallis test.

Table 2. Association of anterior anus and constipation.

	Constipation		P	PR	CI 95%
	Yes	No			
Anterior anus	2 (18.2)	12 (21.8)	0.574	0.825	0.201–3.394
Normal anus	9 (81.8)	43 (78.2)			

4 DISCUSSION

A systematic review conducted in 2011, resulting from 19 articles, investigated the prevalence of constipation in children. The median value rate was 12% (Mugie et al., 2011). A review article from China found that the mean value of prevalence rate in the paediatric population was 18.8% (Chu et al., 2014). In this study, the incidence of constipation was 16.7%.

The peak age of the onset of childhood constipation and the age category in which constipation is most common could not be assessed with certainty. Possibly, constipation in different age categories has various aetiologies. Approximately half of the affected children developed constipation within the first year of life. The transition from breast to formula feeding was considered to be a possible cause of constipation in this age group. Also, constipation was found to be significantly more prevalent in children between 2 and 4–5 years old. On the other hand, Olaru et al. (2016) found that the average age of the onset of constipation was 26.39 months. These prevalence data suggest the highest prevalence to be around the preschool age. The time of toilet training is thought to be a critical period in which constipation may occur. Difficulties with toilet training are associated with childhood constipation. It is, however, unclear whether difficulties with toilet training are the result or the cause of constipation (Berg et al., 2006; Olaru et al., 2016).

Conflicting data about the gender ratio in the occurrence of constipation have been reported. Some outcome studies have reported a higher number of constipated boys compared with girls. A study in children younger than four years found a 1:1 ratio (Berg et al., 2006). In this study, we found that girls were more likely to develop constipation than boys.

The aetiology of constipation in childhood may be multifactorial. In most children, constipation is functional, without objective evidence of a pathological condition. Otherwise, the congenital abnormality of the anus position was considered to be a possible cause of constipation, especially in infancy and early childhood. In previous studies, the diagnosis of an anterior anus has usually relied on inspection; therefore, the incidences vary widely, according to the experience of the physician. However, in less severe cases, slight anterior displacement was very difficult to diagnose without using diagnostic measurement tools. The quantitative measurement to define the normal position of the anus was first proposed in 1984. Reisner et al. presented a simple method using the API, which is the ratio of anal-fourchette distance to coccyx-fourchette distance for females and the ratio of anal-scrotum distance to coccyx-scrotum distance for males, to define the normal position of the anus in the newborn. They suggested that an API of less than 0.46 in boys and less than 0.34 in girls was indicative of an anterior displacement of the anus (Rerksuppaphol, 2010; Shahin & Abdelsalam, 2011).

The association between an anterior displacement of the anal opening and constipation is still controversial. In a large case study involving 134 patients with ADA, nearly all of the patients had constipation from birth or from the time of weaning from breastfeeding and required surgical correction. A comparative study in two European healthcare centres found that 31% of newborns with anterior anus presented constipation in their first months of life. However, studies that are more recent do not describe any association between anal position and constipation (Shahin & Abdelsalam, 2011; Ramoz et al., 2011). In this study, we found that there was no association between API and constipation.

This study had some limitations. This was a cross-sectional study so we could not assess precisely the association between API and constipation. This was the first study in Indonesia that measured API in children. Further research should be done by considering the methods, whether case-control or cohort, grouping the age or gender, determining the centre of the anal, or using the digital calliper.

5 CONCLUSION

Although constipation in most children is functional, organic causes, such as anterior displacement of the anus, might be considered in children with constipation. API is a simple method of defining anterior displacement of the anus in children. We should consider measuring the API in children with constipation. Based on this result, there is no association between the API and constipation.

REFERENCES

Berg, M.M., Benninga, M.A. & Di Lorenzo, C. (2006). Epidemiology of childhood constipation: A systematic review. *American Journal of Gastroenterology, 101*, 2401–2409.

Chu, H., Zhong, L., Li, H., Zhang, X., Zhang, J. & Hou, X. (2014). Epidemiology characteristics of constipation for a general population, pediatric population, and elderly population in China. *Gastroenterology Research and Practice, 2014*, 1–11.

Davari, H.A. & Nazem, M. (2004). The anal position index: A simple method to define the normal position of the anus in the neonate. *Journal of Research in Medical Sciences, 6*, 294–298.

Hammo, A.H., Wahab, A., Telmesani, A. & Nazer, H.M. (2012). Constipation. In A.Y. Elzouki, H.A. Harfi, H.M. Nazer, F.B. Stapleton, O.H. William & R.J. Whitley (Eds.), *Textbook of clinical paediatrics* (pp. 1763–1765). Springer.

Karami, H. & Shokohi, L. (2013). Management of childhood constipation. *Journal of Pediatrics Review, 1*, 45–51.

Mugie, S.M., Benninga, M.A. & Di Lorenzo, C. (2011). Epidemiology of constipation in children and adults. A systematic review. *Best Practice and Research Clinical Gastroenterology, 25*, 3–18.

Nurko, S. & Zimmerman, L.A. (2014). Evaluation and treatment of constipation in children and adolescents. *American Family Physician, 90*(2), 82–90.

Olaru, C., Diaconescu, S., Trandafir, L., Gimiga, N., Stefanescu, G., Ciubotariu, G. & Burlea, M. (2016). Some risk factors for chronic functional constipation identified in a pediatric population sample from Romania. *Gastroenterology Research and Practice, 2016*, 1–8.

Ramoz, R.N., Fabbro, M.A., Gonzalez, M., Nunez, R.N., Romanato, B., Vecchiato, L., ... Sanchez, E.B. (2011). Determination of the anal position in newborns and children with chronic constipation: Comparative study in two European healthcare centres. *Pediatric Surgery International, 27*, 1111–1115.

Rerksuppaphol, S. & Rerksuppaphol, L. (2008). Normal anal position index in Thai newborns. *Journal of the Medical Association of Thailand, 91*, 1839–1845.

Shahin, M. & Abdelsalam, M. (2011). The anal position index: A simple method to define the normal position of the anus and its significance in diagnosis constipation. *Al-Azhar Assiut Medical Journal, 9*(3), 374–384.

Stem Cell Oncology – Adella (Ed.)
© 2018 Taylor & Francis Group, London, ISBN 978-0-8153-9272-9

Comparison of thyroid hormone levels between severe and mild-moderate malnutrition

W. Mondana, T. Sembiring, Y. Dimyati, T. Faranita & W. Pratita
Department of Child Health, Faculty of Medicine, Universitas Sumatera Utara, Medan, North Sumatera, Indonesia

ABSTRACT: Malnutrition is one of the major health problems in developing countries and contributes to child mortality throughout the world. Thyroid hormones play a crucial role in the metabolism, which is used for growth and maturation. Objective: To understand the differences in thyroid hormone levels between severe and mild-moderate malnutrition. Methods: This was a cross-sectional study between April and May 2016 at the Adam Malik General Hospital, Medan. The subjects are 1–5 years old with severe and mild-moderate malnutrition. Children with hypothyroid/hyperthyroid who took medicine that could affect their thyroid hormone levels were excluded. Data were analysed using independent T and Mann-Whitney U tests with 95% CI. P value <0.05 were considered statistically significant. Result: The level of T3 was different between severe and mild-moderate malnutrition. The level of T3 was lower in cases of severe malnutrition than in cases of mild-moderate malnutrition (p < 0.001, 95% CI 0.29–1.00) but the T4 level was not lower (p 0.065, 95% CI −0.32–3.00). Conclusion: There was a significant difference in the T3 level between severe and mild-moderate malnutrition, where the T3 level was lower in cases of severe malnutrition.

Keywords: Malnutrition, Thyroid hormones, T3, T4, TSH

1 INTRODUCTION

Malnutrition remains a major health problem in developing countries and accounts for more than 54% of the mortality of children under five year of age and 10.8 million of the annual mortality rate (Susanto et al., 2011). Approximately 9% of children in sub-Saharan Africa and 15% in South Asia suffer from severe malnutrition and mild to moderate malnutrition. In developing countries, there are approximately 2% of children suffering from Severe Acute Malnutrition (SAM). In India, 2.8% of children under five years of age are severely wasted. In underdeveloped countries, such as Malawi, SAM remains the major cause for hospitalisation (Schaible et al., 2007). In Indonesia, based on basic health research *Riset kesehatandasar* (*Riskesdas*) for the year 2007, the number of children with severe malnutrition and mild to moderate malnutrition is still approximately 18.4, which is registered as third in the world for severe malnutrition (Lenters et al., 2013).

The thyroid hormone plays an important role in the regulation of lipid and carbohydrate metabolism for normal growth and maturation. Mild to moderate malnutrition correlates with a deficiency of iodine, vitamin A and iron, which can cause anaemia. In mild to moderate malnutrition, there are changes in the growth, development and decrement of all systems and organ functions, with impairment in metabolism and secretion of the thyroid hormone from the thyroid glands, therefore causing a reduction of thyroid gland activity, and a reduction of triiodothyronine (T3), thyroxine (T4) and Thyroid Stimulating Hormone (TSH) are noted. This entity will affect iodine metabolism and decrease protein circulation. This mechanism affects protein and energy malnutrition metabolism (Brinker et al., 2005).

The close association between thyroid hormone metabolism disorders with mild-moderate malnutrition and severe malnutrition has led to a growing number of studies on the use of thyroid hormones as biochemical markers in mortality rates in malnutrition patients (Brent, 2012). A study in India in January 2016 showed that 43% of malnourished children showed a decrease in the value of T3 and T4 without a decrease of TSH (Sandeep & Krishnamurthy, 2016). However, in Indonesia there has never been any similar research; therefore, we wanted to assess the relationship of severe malnutrition status and mild-moderate malnutrition to thyroid hormone levels in children aged 1–5 years.

2 METHODS

A cross-sectional study was conducted between April and May 2016 in the paediatrics ward at the Adam Malik Hospital, Medan, North Sumatera. Subjects were collected by consecutive sampling. The criteria for inclusion was children who were 1–5 years old with severe and mild-moderate malnutrition. Children with hypothyroid or hyperthyroid, or who took medicine that could affect their thyroid hormone levels, were excluded. Anthropometry was used to determine nutritional status. Blood samples were taken from all of the subjects to determine their thyroid hormone levels (T3, T4 and TSH). A physical examination was conducted on the children. Body Weight (BW) was measured using Camry scales with 0.1 kg precision. Body Height (BH) was measured using a microtome with 0.1 cm precision, with the children standing up straight, feet parallel, and heels, buttocks and the back of the head touching the wall. Nutritional status was assessed using the WHO growth chart. The nutritional status classification was based on body weight/body height (BW/BH). Blood samples were obtained from peripheral veins, and the serum levels of triiodothyronine (T3), thyroxine (T4) and Thyroid Stimulating Hormone (TSH) were measured by radioimmunoassay (RIA). A Mann-Whitney test and independent T-test were done to analyse the comparison of the thyroid hormone levels between severe and mild-moderate malnutrition in 1–5 year olds. The results were considered to be statistically significant for P values <0.05.

3 RESULTS

Two groups of children (severe malnutrition and mild-moderate malnutrition) were studied. Of the 64 children initially recruited, seven children were rejected for inclusion in this research and four children who took medicine that could affect their thyroid hormone levels were excluded. From the remaining 53 children, we found 38 children with severe malnutrition and 15 children with mild-moderate malnutrition (Figure 1).

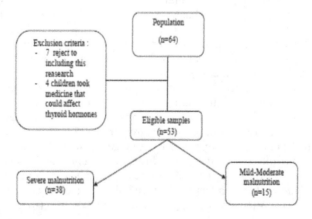

Figure 1. Consort diagram.

Table 1. Characteristics of subjects.

Characteristics	Severe malnutrition	Mild-moderate malnutrition
Age, years		
1–2 years	16	4
2–3 years	10	5
3–4 years	10	3
4–5 years	2	2
Co-morbid		
Leukaemia	18	5
Heart failure	7	0
Chronic kidney disease	5	0
CNS infection	4	2
HIV	3	2
Diarrhoea	1	1
Tuberculosis	0	3
Dengue	0	2
Sex		
Boys	20	7
Girls	18	8
Mean height, cm (SD)	78.1 (10.02)	86.8 (10.13)
Mean body weight kg, median (min–max)	8 (2.13–4)	10 (3.01–5)

Table 2. Characteristics of subjects.

	Severe malnutrition (N = 38)	Mild-moderate malnutrition (N = 15)	CI 95%	Mean difference	P
T3 median	1.4 (0.29–4.97)	0.67 (0.26–2.15)	0.29–1.00	0.65	<0.001**
T4 mean	7.21 ± 2.80	5.64 ± 0.48	−1.01–3.23	1.56	0.065***
TSH median	2.51 (0.61–12.76)	2.33 (0.07–7.16)	−0.32–3.00	1.34	0.17**

The subjects' characteristics are shown in Table 1. In 1–5 year olds, severe malnutrition was more commonly found than mild-moderate malnutrition. Leukaemia was more commonly found in severe malnutrition.

Table 2. There were significantly different levels of T3 between severe and mild-moderate malnutrition (P < 0.001). Meanwhile, T4 and TSH showed no significant difference between the two groups.

4 DISCUSSION

Severe and mild malnutrition are suffered by almost 20 million children worldwide. Most of them are in the preschool age group and live in African and South East Asian countries. Severe malnutrition has become a major contributor to mortality in under-fives (Sandeep & Krishnamurthy, 2016).

Thyroid hormones enhance the metabolism in almost all body tissues, including growth and development, oxygen consumption, energy formation, neural function, fat, carbohydrate, protein, nucleic acid, vitamin, and organic ions metabolism (Depkes, 2012). The mean metabolism velocity rate increases by 60% to 100% over its normal value when the thyroid hormone is secreted (Bone et al., 1992).

A study in India in 2001, which took 80 severely malnourished and mild-moderately mal-nourished children as subjects, found that there was a decreasing T3 value without a decline in the values of T4 and TSH (Abrol et al., 2001). Other studies in Bangladesh and Turkey obtained similar results (Klein & Delbert, 1981). Such results were also observed in this study, which found that in 38 severely malnourished children and 15 mild-moderately mal-nourished children, abnormalities in T3, T4 and TSH were observed, as shown in Table 2.

The decline of the value of T3 in severe and mild-moderate malnutrition patients is asso-ciated with the reduction of protein biosynthesis in the liver. After the decline of thyroid hormone values, there will be a decreasing free thyroxine level, which results in a decline in thyroid hormone values (Monig et al., 1995).

Another study in India in 2016 of 250 severely malnourished children aged 1–5 years, with 139 girls and 111 boys, found a T3 and T4 decline with $p < 0.001$ without a decline in the TSH level (Sandeep & Krishnamurthy, 2016). This study also took children of 1–5 years old as subjects and showed that boys with severe and mild-moderate malnutrition were more preva-lent than girls, which was 27 children. This study also found that there was a decline in the T3 hormone level. In the relationship analysis between the T3 level and malnutrition, there was a significant relationship between the T3 level and malnutrition (CI 95% 0.29–1.00) with a $p < 0.001$. The reason for the low T3 serum level is a diminished production or increased excretion. In this state, the body will always attempt to compensate by lowering the body's metabolism, so that the serum T3 level falls and a reverse T3 (rT3) level arises, thus energy becomes well balanced. With a progressive natural history of the disease, the serum T4 level is much more likely to be decreased.

Another study found that there was a non-thyroidal illness in critically ill patients, which included a condition where there was a decline in serum T3 levels when the TSH and T4 levels were normal. This condition is called the ESS type 1 or the low T3 syndrome. This study showed evidence of ESS type 1 or low T3 syndrome in the most critically ill patients and in chronic disease patients with slow progressivity and long continuity, such as leukae-mia, asthma, cerebral palsy, diabetes, heart failure, renal failure and HIV. This study also showed that patients with chronic diseases, such as heart failure, renal failure, HIV and cen-tral nervous system infection, were at a greater risk of a decline of thyroid hormone levels (Burmeister, 1995).

There are some limitations to the present study. The sample size is too small to properly evaluate the comparison of thyroid hormone levels between severe and mild-moderate mal-nutrition in children, the authors did not evaluate the antibodies of thyroid peroxidase or thyroglobulin and did not consider the family history of thyroid disease. Therefore, further evaluation of thyroid functions with larger sample sizes and long-term follow-up will be needed to address the influence of thyroid hormones.

5 CONCLUSION

There is a relationship between the decline of T3 levels in severe and mild-moderate malnu-trition without T4 and TSH disturbance. Children aged 1–3 years with chronic diseases are at risk of becoming malnourished and experience a decline in T3 level. Changes in thyroid hormone metabolism that occur probably represent adaptive changes to the illness; treat-ment with 1-thyroxine to restore serum thyroid concentrations to the normal range is not indicated.

REFERENCES

Abrol, P., Verma, A. & Hooda, H.S. (2001). Thyroid hormone status in protein energy malnutrition in Indian children. *Indian Journal of Clinical Biochemistry*, *16*(2), 221–223.
Brent, G.A. (2012). Mechanisms of thyroid hormone action. *Journal of Clinical Investigation*, *122*(9), 3035–3043.

Brinker, M., Joosten, K.F.M., Visser, T.J., Hop, W.C.J., Rijke, Y.B., Hazelzet, J.A., ... Hokken-Koe-lega, A.C.S. (2005). Euthyroid sick syndrome in meningococcal sepsis: The impact of peripheral thyroid hormone metabolism binding proteins. *Journal of Clinical Endocrinology and Metabolism*, *90*, 5613–5620.

Das, B.K., Agarwal, J.K., Agarwal, P.A. & Mishra, O.P. (2002). Serum cortisol and thyroid hormone levels in neonates with sepsis. *Indian Journal of Pediatrics*, *69*, 663–665.

Fisher, D.A. (2003). The thyroid. In C.D. Rudolph, A.M. Rudolph, M.K. Hostetter, G. Lister & N.J. Siegel (Eds.), *Rudolph's Pediatrics* (21st ed., pp. 2059–2066). New York, NY: McGraw-Hill.

Guyton, A.C. & Hall, J.E. (2010). Hormon metabolic tiroid. In A.C. Guyton & J.E. Hall (Eds.), *Buku ajar fisiologikedokteran* (9th ed., pp. 1188–1201). Jakarta, Indonesia: EGC.

Lenters, L.M., Wazny, K., Webb, P., Ahmed, T. & Bhutta, Z.A. (2013). Treatment of severe and moder-ate acute malnutrition in low- and middle-income settings: A systematic review, meta-analysis and Delphi process. *BMC Public Health*, *13*(3), 1–15.

Sandeep, M. & Krishnamurthy, B. (2016). Thyroid hormone status in children with protein energy mal-nutrition. *International Journal of Contemporary Pediatrics*, *3*(1), 193–199.

Schaible, U.E., Stefan, H. & Kaufmann, E. (2007). Malnutrition and infection: Complex mechanisms and global impacts. *PLOS Medicine*, *4*(5), 806–811.

Schalch, S.A. & Cree, T.C. (1985). Protein utilization in growth: Effect of calorie deficiency on serum growth hormone, somatomedins, total thyroxine (T4), and triiodothyronine, free T4 index and total cortisone. *Endocrinology*, *117*, 2307–2312.

Singer, M., Santis, V.D., Vitale, D. & Jeffcoate, W. (2004). Multiorgan failure is an adaptive, endocrine-mediated, metabolic response to overwhelming systemic inflammation. *Lancet*, *364*, 545–548.

Susanto, J.C., Maria, M. & Sri, S.N. (2011). Malnutrisi Akut Beratdanterapinutrisiberbasiskomunitas. In *Buku Ajar Nutrisi Pediatrik Dan Penyakit Metabolik* (1st ed., pp. 128–146). Jakarta, Indonesia: Badan Penerbit IDAI.

Zargar, A.H., Ganie, M.A., Masoodi, S.R., Laway, B.A., Bashir, M.I. & Wani, A.I. (2004). Prevalence and pattern of sick euthyroid syndrome in acute and chronic non-thyroidal illness: Its relationship with severity and outcome of the disorder. *Journal of Association of Physicians of India*, *52*, 27–31.

Stem Cell Oncology – Adella (Ed.)
© 2018 Taylor & Francis Group, London, ISBN 978-0-8153-9272-9

Identification of HPV types 6 and 11 in skin tags using PCR

J. Karayana, N.K. Jusuf & I.B. Putra
Department of Dermatovenereology, Faculty of Medicine, Universitas Sumatera Utara, Medan, North Sumatera, Indonesia

ABSTRACT: The Human Papilloma Virus (HPV) infection is suspected to be one of the causes of skin tag lesions. In order to identify HPV types 6 and 11 in skin tag lesions using the Polymerase Chain Reaction (PCR) technique, this study is a descriptive study with a cross-sectional design involving 30 skin tag lesions. PCR examination of skin tag lesions was performed to identify HPV types 6 and 11. The collected data was processed and presented descriptively. In this study we found that eight (26.7%) skin tag lesions identified with HPV type 6, and six (20%) skin tag lesions identified with HPV type 11. From a total of 30 skin tag lesions that were examined using the PCR technique, 14 (46.7%) of the lesions identified with HPV types 6 and 11.

Keywords: skin tag, HPV, polymerase chain reaction

1 INTRODUCTION

A skin tag is a benign lesion composed of loose fibrous tissue that occurs mainly on the neck and major flexures as a small, soft, pedunculated protrusion (Quinn & Perkins, 2010). Skin tags may present singly or as multiple lesions, they tend to grow progressively and they do not involute spontaneously. These lesions are commonly found in the adult population over 40 years of age, and increase in incidence in the elderly (Tamega et al., 2010). Skin tags can manifest clinically as three types: multiple small papules, single or multiple filiform, and bag-like pedunculated growths (Shashikala et al., 2014). Histological findings show epidermis slight acanthosis and papillomatosis with a fibrovascular connective tissue core (Heenan, 2005; Ko, 2012).

To date, the aetiology or pathogenesis of skin tags is still unclear. Obesity, ageing, dyslipidemia, diabetes mellitus, pregnancy and Human Papilloma Virus (HPV) have been proposed as a potential aetiological or associated factor of the skin tag (Tamega et al., 2010; Erkek et al., 2011). The HPV infection has been suggested to be one of the factors involved in the pathogenesis of skin tags, and the first study to correlate this theory was conducted by Dianzani et al. in 1998. Dianzani and his colleagues were able to detect HPV DNA 6 and 11 in 88% of the samples of skin tags by using the Polymerase Chain Reaction (PCR) technique (Dianzani et al., 1998).

HPV is a small non-enveloped virus (50–55 nm) that contains a double-stranded closed circular DNA genome associated with histone-like proteins and protected by a capsid formed by two late proteins, L1 and L2 (Fermandes, 2012). Over 100 HPV types have been identified to date. HPV is an epitheliotropic virus that can induce squamous epithelial tumours (benign cutaneous and mucosal lesions) in many different associated anatomical localisations, which produces cytopathic effects in infected keratinocytes (Dianzani et al., 1998; Morshed et al., 2014).

HPV DNA can be detected in biopsy specimens by various methods, such as hybridisation procedures and PCR. PCR is the most widely used method for amplification of nucleic acids, and has a high sensitivy and specifity (Moljin et al., 2005). In this study, PCR was used to detect HPV DNA types 6 and 11 genomes in skin tag lesions.

2 METHOD

This study aimed to detect HPV DNA in skin tags by using the PCR technique. This study was performed on skin tag patients with a clinical and anamnesis diagnosis. Thirty skin tag biopsy specimens were obtained under local anaesthesia from body sites (colli, axillaris, auricularis, and femoralis). The specimens were preserved at below –20°C, and DNA was then extracted from the skin tag samples using a commercial DNA isolation kit from tissue (GeneAid®) according to the manufacturer's instructions.

All of the samples were subjected to PCR, using primers specific to the HPV genome. The presence of HPV type 6 was investigated by PCR amplification of 258–361 bp (base pairs) target from the locus control region (LCR) using the sequence forward primer 5'-TAG-GGGACGG TCCTCTATTC-3' and reverse primer 5'-GCAACAGCCTCTGA GTCACA-3'. The presence of HPV type 11 was investigated by PCR amplification of 356 bp target from the L1 region using the sequence forward primer 5'-GAATACATGCGCCATGTGGA-3' and reverse primer 5'-AGCAG ACGTCCGTCCTC GAT-3'. The reaction was carried out in a volume of 20 µl containing 12 ul PCR fast ready mix (KAPA 2G®), 2.5 µl forward primer, 2.5 µl reverse primer, and 5 ul DNA isolate. The amplification cycles comprised 1 min at 95°C for initial denaturation, 15 seconds at 95°C for denaturation, 15 seconds at 55–65°C for annealing, 5 seconds/kb at 72°C for extension, and 10 mins at 72°C for the final extension using a thermocycler (Applied Biosynthesis™ Veriti 384®).

For analysis of the PCR product, 5–7 µl amplification product were electrophoresed on 2.5% agarose gel (Bioron®) in Tris Acetate EDTA (TAE) buffer with 1 ul ethidium bromide (Invitrogen®). Gel was visualised on an ultraviolet transilluminator; visualising the 258–361 bp fragment was interpreted as a positive result for HPV type 6 and visualising the 356 bp fragment was interpreted as a positive result for HPV type 11. Precautions to avoid cross-contamination and false-positive results were taken in every assay.

3 RESULT

In this study, 30 samples of skin tag lesions were obtained from 16 skin tag patients (6 men and 10 women), who were in the age group 20 to 60 years. Samples from patients were taken from the following areas: 20 (66.7%) samples from the colli region, 7 (23.3%) samples from the axilla region, 2 samples (6.6%) from the auricularis region, and 1 (3.3%) sample from the femoralis region.

Analysis of the presence of HPV DNA by PCR showed that 14 (46.7%) of the 30 positive samples contained HPV DNA, 8 (26.7%) of the positive samples contained HPV type 6 with restriction band level at 258 bp (Figure 1), and 6 (20%) of the positive samples contained HPV type 11 with restriction band level at 356 bp (Figure 2).

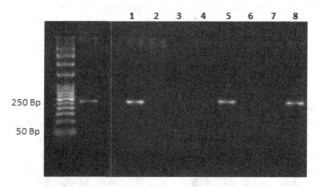

Figure 1.   Gel electrophoresis PCR with HPV type 6. Line 1 weight marker 50 bp ladder, line 2 is positive control, line 3 is negative control. Sample nos. 1, 5 and 8 showed a positive band (258 bp).

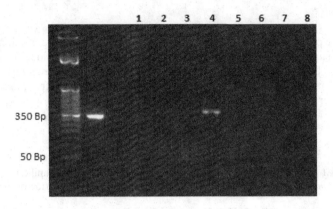

Figure 2.   Gel electrophoresis PCR with HPV type 11. Line 1 weight marker 50 bp ladder, line 2 is positive control, line 3 is negative control. Sample no. 4 showed a positive band (356 bp).

4   DISCUSSION

HPV is epitheliotropic and host-specific, with infection across the species being uncommon (Androphy & Kirnbauer, 2012). HPV infection occurs through inoculation of the virus into a viable epidermis through breaks in the epithelial barrier. Maceration of the skin is probably an important predisposing factor. Animal models using HPV virions demonstrate that attachment to heparan sulfate proteoglycans on the basement membrane is a required initial step in natural infection. A furin protease then cleaves L2, inducing a conformation change that allows binding to an unidentified basal cell receptor. This experimental model explains how PV reserva indection for and specifically target epithelial basal cells (Androphy & Kirnbauer, 2012).

Suzuki and his co-workers demonstrated the high association between the presence of HPV DNA types and other benign tumours, such as laryngeal papillomas (Al-Shaiji & Al-Buainian, 2005). The clinical condition of skin tags is closely similar to that of mucocutaneous papillomatosis and their clinical behaviour may be reminiscent of that of laryngeal papillomas, which might raise the suggestion of a common aetiology. Since HPV has been detected in many papillomas, they may consequently be responsible for the development of skin tags (Sallam et al., 2003)

The result of this study was in accordance with a study by Gupta et al. (2008), who previously reported the presence of HPV 6/11 DNA in 48.6% of biopsies; however, the results of this study were lower in comparison with the study conducted by Dianzani et al. (1998), who reported the presence of HPV type 6/11 in 88% of skin tag samples, and the study by Sallam et al. (2003), who reported that 23 (76.6%) out of 30 positive samples contained HPV DNA type 6/11.

The finding of HPV DNA types 6 and 11 in biopsies of the skin tag lesions suggests that this virus may be involved in the pathogenesis of these cutaneous lesions. It has been known that skin tags or fibroepithelial polyps are developed in areas of skin that are prone to rubbing or friction (Pezeshkpoor et al., 2012) and can lead to disruption of the skin, which might serve as a route of entry for the virus. The presence of HPV DNA and mechanical friction seem to be significant co-factors in the pathogenesis of skin tags (Shashikala et al., 2014).

It has been postulated that HPV infection begins with the inoculation of the virus into the interrupted epithelium and the interaction with a putative specific cellular receptor (Gupta et al., 2008). HPV infection involves squamous epithelium and can cause growth stimulation, cell proliferation and the formation of pathologic cells (Morshed et al., 2014) through the role of E5 oncoprotein, which can activate growth factor receptors, epithelial hyperplasia, papillomatosis, hyperkeratosis and koilocytic change that are regarded as cytopathic effects of HPV (Shashikala et al., 2014).

5 CONCLUSION

In this study the presence of HPV types 6 and 11 genomes in the skin tag lesions from different sites could support the viral aetiology theory, but cannot be considered as proof of the aetiological role, because the results of this study are not of a high percentage. The presence of HPV DNA that can affect cellular differentiation and mechanical friction seem to be significant co-factors in the pathogenesis of skin tags.

REFERENCES

Al-Shaiji, A. & Al-Buainian, H. (2005). Skin tags in relation with Human Papilloma Virus. *The Gulf Journal of Dermatology*, *12*(2), 31–33. Retrieved from http://www.gulfdermajournal.net/pdf/2005-10/3.pdf.

Androphy, E.J. & Kirnbauer, R. (2012). Human Papilloma Virus infections. In L.A. Goldsmith, S.I. Katz, B.A. Gilchrest, A.S. Paller, D.J. Leffel, & K. Wolff (Eds.), *Fitzpatrick's dermatology in general medicine* (8th ed., pp. 2421–2433). New York, NY: McGraw-Hill.

Dianzani, C., Calvieri, S., Pierangeli, A., Imperi, M., Bucci, M. & Degener, A.M. (1998). The detection of human papillomavirus DNA in skin tags. *British Journal of Dermatology*, *138*, 649–651.

Erkek, E., Kasi, U., Bagci, Y. & Sezikli, H. (2011). Leptin resistance and genetic predisposition as potential mechanism in the development of skin tag. *Hong Kong Journal of Dermatology and Venereology*, *19*, 108–114.

Fernandes, J.V. & Fernandes, T.A.A. (2012). Human Papillomavirus: Biology and pathogenesis. In D.V. Broeck (Ed.), *Human Papillomavirus and related diseases—From bench to bedside – A clinical perspective* (pp. 1–40). Rijeka, Croatia: In Tech Europe.

Gupta, S., Aggarwal, R., Gupta, S. & Arora, S.K. (2008). Human papillomavirus and skin tags: Is there any association? *Indian Journal of Dermatology, Venereology and Leprology*, *74*, 222–225.

Heenan, P.J. (2005). Tumors of fibrous tissue involving the skin. In D.E. Elder (Ed.), *Lever's histopathology of the skin* (pp. 980–1013). Philadelphia, PA: Lippincott Williams & Wilkins.

Ko, C.J. (2012). Dermal hypertrophies and benign fibroblastic/myofibroblastic tumors. In L.A. Goldsmith, S.I. Katz, B.A. Gilchrest, A.S. Paller, D.J. Leffel, & K. Wolff (Eds.), *Fitzpatrick's dermatology in general medicine* (8th ed., pp. 1174–1188). New York, NY: McGraw-Hill.

Molijn, A., Kleter, B., Quint, W. & Van Doorn, L.J. (2005). Molecular diagnosis of human papillomavirus (HPV) infection. *Journal of Clinical Virology*, *32*(1), 43–51.

Morshed, K., Polz-Gruszka, D., Szymanski, M. & Polz-Dacewiz, M. (2014). Human Papillomavirus (HPV): Structure, epidemiology and pathogenesis. *Otolaryngologia Polska*, *68*(5), 1–7.

Pezeshkpoor, F., Jafarian, A.H., Ghazvini, K., Yazdanpanah, M.J., Sadeghian, A., … Shirdel, M. (2012). An association of Human Papillomaviruses low risk and high risk subtypes with skin tag. *Iranian Journal of Basic Medical Sciences*, *15*(3), 840–844.

Quinn, A.G. & Perkins, W. (2010). Non-melanoma skin cancer and other epidermal skin tumours. In T. Burns, S. Breathnach, N. Cox & C. Griffiths (Eds.), *Rook's textbook of dermatology* (8th ed., pp. 2613–2661). Oxford, UK: Wiley-Blackwell.

Sallam, M.A., Kamel, M.M., El Missiry, A.G. & Helal, M.F. (2003). Detection of Human Papilloma Virus DNA in skin tag. *The Scientific Journal of Al-Azhar Medical Faculty*, *24*(1), 311–317.

Shashikala, P., Nandyal, S.S. & Sawkar, S. (2014). Acrochordon infected with human papilloma virus. *Journal of Public Health and Medical Research*, *2*(1), 61–62.

Tamega, A.A., Aranha, A.M., Guiotoku, M.M., Miot, L.D. & Miot, H.A. (2010). Association between skin tags and insulin resistance. *Anais Brasileiros de Dermatologia*, *85*(1), 25–31.

Stem Cell Oncology – Adella (Ed.)
© *2018 Taylor & Francis Group, London, ISBN 978-0-8153-9272-9*

Ferritin levels after ferrous fumarate supplementation in the 2nd trimester of pregnancy

L.S. Lintang
Department of Obstetrics and Gynaecology, Faculty of Medicine, Universitas Sumatera Utara, Medan, North Sumatera, Indonesia

ABSTRACT: This study is to determine the comparison of ferritin levels after ferrous fumarate supplementation in the second trimester of pregnancy. This study was an experimental study with a pre-/post-test design. All of the subjects' ferritin serum levels were compared after one month of ferrous fumarate consumption. The study began in April 2015. Blood sampling was conducted on all mothers who met the inclusion criteria; they were given ferrous fumarate for one month and then they were re-examined. The mean rate of ferritin in maternal serum after iron supplementation measured after one month was 28.7689 ± 20.77 ng/ml higher than before treatment, that is, 17.5 ± 19.09 ng/ml. A Wilcoxon test gave p-value < 0.05. There is a significant increase in the serum levels of pregnant women's ferritin after iron supplementation.

Keywords: Ferritin, Ferrous Sumarate Supplementation, Pregnancy

1   INTRODUCTION

Anaemia during pregnancy is a risk factor for both the mother and the foetus. The serum concentrations of ferritin will continue to decline progressively during pregnancy, although erythropoiesis is increased (Cunningham, 2010). Haemoglobin (Hb) concentration and haematocrit (Ht) slightly decreased during normal pregnancy, resulting in the overall blood viscosity decreasing. Also, plasma concentrations of various substances decreased during pregnancy (Schmitt, 2005).

Examination for iron deficiency includes serum iron, red blood cells, serum total iron binding capacity, serum transferrin saturation, serum transferrin serum levels and serum ferritin levels. Several studies have shown that the test for serum ferritin is the best and most useful non-invasive test and gives a reliable index of iron storage during pregnancy with a low-grade interpretation that indicates iron deficiency (Pena-Rosas & Viteri, 2006).

Other examinations to prove the occurrence of iron deficiency include red blood cells, iron serum, total iron binding capacity serum, serum transferrin saturation, transferrin serum levels and ferritin serum levels. Microcytosis is a sensitive iron deficiency index whose value is limited by the physiologic increase in Mean Corpuscular Volume (MCV) that often occurs during pregnancy.

Transferrin-iron irradiance is often abnormal in pregnancy (Fai & Lao, 1999) The transferrin saturation is less sensitive with regards to day-to-day fluctuations to iron serum hours is less efficient than serum ferritin levels to diagnose iron deficiency (Mast, 2001). Several studies have proved that the test for serum ferritin is the best non-invasive test and it has the greatest benefits for the iron storage index, especially during pregnancy, with low levels indicating iron deficiency (Hou et al., 2000).

The best parameter for measuring maternal iron status is serum ferritin concentration. Ferritin is the largest iron storage protein, which is found not only in the lymph, liver and bone marrow, but also in the small intestinal mucosal cells, in the placenta, kidneys, testes, skeletal muscles and in the blood circulation. Prenatal minerals and vitamin supplementation in the first trimester will keep serum ferritin at higher concentrations (Cunningham, 2010). This study assessed whether, after supplementation of iron ferrous fumarate, there is an increase in ferritin in the second trimester of pregnancy after one month of supplementation therapy.

2 METHOD

This study was an experimental study with pre- and post-test design in which all of the subjects were compared with routine ferritin and blood tests before and after one month of ferrous fumarate consumption. This research was conducted in an outpatient clinic at RSUP H. Adam Malik, Medan, Department of Obstetrics & Gynaecology and at a specialist private office. The study was conducted from April 2015 until the number of samples was complete.

The target population in this research were pregnant women who came for antenatal care at polyclinic RS H. Adam Malik, Medan, and at the obstetrician's private office. The subjects of this study were pregnant women in the second trimester who met the acceptance criteria and were willing to participate in this study.

The inclusion criteria of this study were pregnant women 20–35 years old, in the second trimester of pregnancy, with a clear history of the first day of their last menstrual period or the presence of Crown-Rump Length (CRL) data in the first trimester, and who were willing to participate in this study. The exclusion criteria were pregnant woman with major congenital abnormalities, twin foetuses, pregnancy infections, placenta that implanted too deeply, pregnancy with chronic disease, smokers, and those who declined to join this study.

2.1 Research procedures

After obtaining approval from the ethics committee of the Faculty of Medicine, Universitas Sumatera Utara to conduct the research, research began with anamnesis, physical examination, gynaecological examination, and ultrasound.

After the diagnosis was established, the patients signed the informed consent. The data were collected for characteristic and demographic data, the physical diagnosis of vital signs (consciousness, blood pressure, pulse, respiratory rate and body temperature), general circumstances, localised status and genital status. All mothers who met the inclusion criteria were given serum tests of ferritin, then given ferrous fumarate for one month and then re-examined.

3 RESULTS

Research has been conducted on 70 pregnant women who visited the gynaecological outpatient clinic at RSUP H. Adam Malik, Medan, and the specialist practice.

Table 1 shows that the average amount of ferritin content in maternal serum (Ferritin 1) compared with ferritin serum after one month of treatment with iron supplementation (Ferritin 2), measured after one month, was 28.7689 ± 20.77 ng/ml higher than before treatment, that is, 17.5 ± 19.09 ng/ml.

Table 1. The average value of ferritin levels before and after iron supplementation.

Ferritin	N	Mean	SD	Min	Max	p*
Ferritin 1	70	17.5	19.094	2	99	0.001
Ferritin 2	70	28.7689	20.7717	4.4	99.9	

*Wilcoxon test.

Because the data is not normally distributed based on the Kolmogorov–Smirnov test, then the Wilcoxon statistical test was performed and got the p-value < 0.05. This suggests that there is a significant increase in serum levels of ferritin in pregnant women after iron supplementation.

4 DISCUSSION

Ferritin is a protein that is present in almost all cells. The water-soluble iron-containing protein comprises a protein (apoferritin) shell, which is a combination of ferric salts with proteins and inticristalin comprising thousands of ferrioxihydroxide molecules (Fleming & Bacon, 2005). Free iron is toxic, and the body is able to protect itself by binding the free iron. In the cells, iron is stored in bonded form with ferritin proteins. Ferritin serves to store iron in a dissolved and nontoxic form. The level of ferritin in blood serum is correlated with the total amount of body iron deposits. Ferritin contains about 23% iron; one ferritin complex can store ± 3,000–4,500 Fe3e + ions therein. Ferritin is stored and acquired in the liver, spleen, skeletal muscle and bone marrow (Wallace et al., 2005).

During pregnancy, iron is needed for foetal development, the placenta, and increasing maternal erythrocyte mass, as well as the normal daily requirements for non-pregnant women. The ability of pregnant women to provide for extrinsic needs will depend on what they eat, their efficiency of iron absorption and their levels of iron reserves. The absorption of iron increases during pregnancy. In theory, the mechanism should be able to accommodate all or most of the extra needs of pregnancy. However, the concentration of serum ferritin decreases progressively during pregnancy, and it is recognised that serum ferritin describes iron deposits in non-pregnant, progressive drop in concentrations during pregnancy suggests decreasing iron reserves. Conversely, plasma concentrations of many substances decrease during pregnancy, often reflecting physiologic regulation rather than efficiency (Svanberg et al., 1975).

Iron deficiency anaemia or sideropenic anaemia is usually caused by poor iron intake, pregnancy, parasite infection, menorrhagia, metrorrhagia, menstruation, premenopause, peptic ulcer, long-term use of drugs, and so on. If the body loses iron beyond its intake, then the body will disassemble and use iron stored in ferritin in the liver, spleen, muscle and bone marrow, which is the body's reserves. The reduced iron reserves cannot meet the needs for the formation of erythrocytes, and the resulting amount of erythrocytes results in fewer haemoglobin decreases and anaemia develops. The body will be compensated, and the bone marrow replaces iron deficiency by accelerating cell division and producing erythrocytes of a very small (microcytic) size, which is a characteristic of iron deficiency anaemia. During pregnancy, the need for iron is not always the same, and this affects the degree of iron absorption by pregnant women.

5 CONCLUSION

There was a significant increase in the levels of ferritin in pregnant women after the supplementation of ferrous iron.

Iron supplementation may be given to pregnant women in the second trimester to significantly increase levels of ferritin.

REFERENCES

Cunningham, F., Leveno, K.J., Bloom, S.L., Hauth, J.C., Rouse, D.J. & Spong, C.Y. (2010). Hematological disorders. In *Williams Obstetrics* (23rd ed., pp. 1079–1103). New York, NY: McGraw-Hill.
Fai, T.K. & Lao, T.T. (1999). Hemoglobin and red cells indices correlated with serum ferritin concentration in late pregnancy. *Obstetrics and Gynecology*, *93*, 427–431.
Fleming, R.E. & Bacon, B.R. (2005). Orchestration of iron homeostasis. *The New England Journal of Medicine, 325*, 17.

Hou, J., Cliver, S.P., Tamura, T., Johnston, K.E. & Goldenberg, R. (2000). Maternal serum ferritin and fetal growth. *Obstetrics and Gynecology, 95*, 447–452.

Mast, A. (2001). Peripheral blood tests in iron deficiency anemia. *Bloodline, 1*(2), 24–27.

Pena-Rosas, J.P. & Viteri, F. (2006). Effects of routine oral iron supplementation with or without folic acid for women during pregnancy. *Cochrane Database System Review, 3*, CD004736.

Schmitt, B., Golub, R.M. & Green, R. (2005). Screening primary care patients for hereditary hemo-chromatosis with transferrin saturation and serum ferritin level. Systematic review for the American College of Physicians. *Annals of Internal Medicine, 143*, 522–536.

Scholl, T.O., Hediger, M.L., Fischer, R.I. & Shearer, J.W. (1992). Anemia vs iron deficiency: Increased risk of preterm delivery in a prospective study. *American Journal of Clinical Nutrition, 55*, 985–988.

Svanberg, B., Arvidsson, B., Norrby, A., Rybo, G. & Solvell, L. (1975). Absorption of supplemental iron during pregnancy: A longitudinal study with repeated bone marrow studies and absorption measure-ments. *Acta Obstetricia et Gynecologica Scandinavica, 54*(Suppl48), 87–108.

Wallace, J.M., Regnault, T.R., Limesand, S.W., Hay, W.W. & Anthony, R.V. (2005). Investigating the causes of low birth weight in contrasting ovine paradigms. *Journal of Physiology, 565*(1), 19–26.

Stem Cell Oncology – Adella (Ed.)
© 2018 Taylor & Francis Group, London, ISBN 978-0-8153-9272-9

The relationship of HER2 overexpression to the histopathologic grading of breast cancer

S. Indriani, K. Siregar & Suyatno
Surgical Department, Faculty of Medicine, Universitas Sumatera Utara, Medan, North Sumatera, Indonesia

ABSTRACT: Human Epidermal Growth Factor Receptor 2 (HER2) has a close relationship with the histopathologic grading of breast cancer that is thought to be associated with prognosis and recurrence. The data was taken from 2011–2014 tissue histopathology, grading, and HER2 medical records data. An immunohistochemistry examination for HER2 with values of +1 or +2 is said to be negative (unexpressed), and for +3 is said to be overexpressed; the grades were grouped into low grade (grades 1 and 2) and high grade (grade 3). From this study, we obtained a prevalence ratio of 7.667. Thus it can be said that HER2 expression was eight times more likely to have a high grading when compared with negative HER2 results. There was a significant association between HER2/neu overexpression and the histopathologic grading of breast cancer.

Keywords: Breast cancer, HER2, Histopathologic grading

1 INTRODUCTION

Breast cancer is still the leading cause of death in woman to date, with as many as 522,000 deaths by 2012, and it is the most commonly diagnosed cancer in 184 countries around the world. In 2012, as many as 1.7 million women worldwide were diagnosed with breast cancer and there were 6.3 million women alive who had been diagnosed with breast cancer in the previous five years. Since 2008, the incidence of breast cancer has increased by more than 20%, while the mortality rate has increased by 14%. In Indonesia, there were an estimated 133.52 cases of cancer per 100,000 adults in 2012, and an estimated 299,673 cases in total (IARC, 2012).

Due to the high number of cases there is an urgent need for cancer control. Currently, it is necessary to develop an effective and affordable approach to early detection, diagnosis, and the treatment of breast cancer. With regards to breast cancer treatment approaches, a variety of predictive and prognostic factors of breast cancer were used. The most currently used examination is HER2, an Epidermal Growth Factor Receptor (EGFR) that acts in cell proliferation and differentiation. The overexpression of this protein in breast cancer tissue is associated with a lack of oestrogen receptors and increased histopathology grading. Other routine examinations are hormonal status through Oestrogen Receptor (ER) and Progesterone Receptor (PR), a body steroid receptor acting as a nuclear receptor in a suppressor gene and an oncogene transcription modulator against a targeted gene (Walf, 2013; Axilbund et al., 2011). Overexpression in HER2/neu is associated with histopathologic grading, where histopathologic grading itself is a classification of breast cancer representing the potential aggressiveness of the tumour. The low classes have a low aggressiveness compared to the high classes. In the case of overexpression of HER2, there is an increase in the proliferative activity of the cancer cells, so it has a very strong correlation with high-grade histopathology of breast cancer tumours (AJCC, 2012).

The breast cancer therapy approaches range from hormonal therapy to chemotherapy and, currently, hormone receptor therapy depends on hormonal expression and growth factors (ER/PR, HER2, EGFR), not only as therapeutic guidelines but also as a monitoring method to detect recurrences (Rakha et al., 2010).

Some researchers have suggested HER2/neu relationships with histopathologic grading, such as Fisher et al. (2004), Huang et al. (2005), Menard et al. (2004), Rile et al. (1991), Tsuda et al. (1990) and Hoff et al. (2002).

The strong association of HER2/neu overexpression with histopathologic grading gives meaning to the treatment and the prognostics associated with worsening, as well as with high rates of recurrence (Wood et al., 2005). Relevant to this, no studies have been done on the association of HER2/neu overexpression with the histopathologic grading of breast cancer patients at RSUP H. Adam Malik. For that reason, the author wanted to study the relationship of the HER2/neu protein with histopathologic grading in breast cancer patients.

2 RESEARCH METHODS

This research used descriptive analytic design with a cross-sectional approach. In this study, we did not provide treatment but only saw the results or expression of immunohistochemistry HER2/neu that existed in the medical records. This research was conducted in the Oncology Division of the Surgical Department of RSUP Haji Adam Malik in co-operation with the Anatomical Pathology Department of RSUP H. Adam Malik, Medan. Immunohistochemistry examinations for HER2 with values of +1, and +2 are said to be negative/unexpressed, and +3 is said to be overexpressed. The histopathologic grading was done according to the Nottingham Histologic Score system (Johns Hopkins University, 2012). However, the grades were grouped into low grade (grades 1 and 2) and high grade (grade 3). The data were then analysed to find the relationship between HER2 overexpression with the histopathologic grading of breast cancer.

3 RESULTS

From the results of the analysis, the mean age in this study was 50 years old. The highest age was 77 years old and the lowest was 30 years old. HER2 with a result of +1 was found in 50 people (55.6%), HER2 with a result of +2 was found in 13 people (14.4%), and HER2 with a result of +3 was found in 27 people (30.0%) (Table 1).

The frequency of the histopathologic grading of breast cancer in RSUP H. Adam Malik was: grade 1 in 40 patients (44.42%), grade 2 in 39 patients (43.3%), and grade 3 in 11 patients (12.2%) (Table 2). From this study, we obtained a prevalence ratio of 7.667. Thus it can be

Table 1. Frequency distribution of subjects' HER2/neu value.

HER2	Frequency	N = 90
+1	50	55.6
+2	13	14.4
+3	27	30.0

Table 2. Frequency distribution of subject's histopathologic grading.

Tumour grading	Frequency (N = 90)	%
1	40	44.4
2	39	43.3
3	11	12.2

said that HER2 expression was eight times more likely to have a high grading when compared with negative HER2 results.

4 DISCUSSION

In this study, the HER2/neu examination was done by immunohistochemistry staining on 90 breast carcinoma patients who came to RSUP H. Adam Malik between 1 June 2011 and 1 June 2014. The mean age of the patients was 50 years old. From the HER2/neu frequency that was obtained (Table 1), there were 50 (55.6%) patients with HER2 +1, 13 (14.4%) patients with HER2 +2 and 27 (30.0%) patients with HER2 +3. The number of breast cancer patients with negative HER2/neu was 63 (70.0%), and 27 patients (30.0%) had HER2 overexpression. This corresponds to the literature's incidence of HER2/neu overexpression in 10–30% of breast carcinomas.

In several studies at Surabaya Oncology Hospital from 2007 until 2010 with 844 patients, 216 (25.6%) patients with breast carcinoma were found to have an overexpression rate of HER2/neu. Other studies by Huang et al. (2005) obtained 149 (10.9%) patients with overexpression of HER2/neu out of 1,362 respondents. Another study conducted by Naqvi et al. (2002) reported an incidence rate of 33% of HER2/neu overexpression in patients with breast carcinoma (Naqvi et al., 2002).

Histopathologic grading was obtained from Elston–Ellis, which was modified from Scarff–Bloom–Richardson. This study obtained 29 (32.2%) grade 1, 47 (52.2%) grade 2 and 14 (15.6%) grade 3 patients (Table 2).

From the statistical analysis of this study, we found a significant relationship between HER2/neu overexpression with histopathologic grading of breast cancer patients, in which the prevalence ratio was 7.667 (Table 3), therefore it can be concluded that overexpression of HER2 was eight times more likely to have a high grading when compared to negative HER2. This is shown by the existing literature in several studies, both domestically and internationally. In their study, Bartlett et al. (2007) reported a significant association between HER2/neu overexpression and histopathologic grading as a predictor of breast carcinoma, where overexpression was found in high-grade breast tumours. These studies were reanalysed by Neven et al. (2008) and they reported a high recurrence rate in patients with overexpression of HER2.

In Indonesia, it was reported that there was a significant association of overexpression with histopathologic grading of breast carcinoma in which high HER2/neu overexpression was found, such as the research conducted at Surabaya Education Centre/Surabaya Oncology Hospital by Octovianus and Ariodjatmiko (2012), in a study involving 1,426 patients, which reported a significant association between HER2/neu overexpression and breast cancer histopathologic grading. In that study 34.6% overexpression of HER2/neu was present in grade 3, and the study also stated that grade 3 had 3.9 times more risk compared with grades 1 and 2 for the occurrence of HER2/neu expression.

The existence of the relationship of HER2 overexpression with histopathologic grading was a predictor factor and prognosis factor of breast cancer, in addition to therapy. Therefore, the examination should be able to follow the guidelines that have been agreed. False positives or false negatives may occur on HER2 examination with IHC or HER2 +2 equivalent results, requiring further examination with Fluorescent In Situ Hybridisation (FISH) as the gold standard (Prati et al., 2005). Similarly, the results of this study had many shortcomings, one of which is mentioned above.

Table 3. Prevalence ratio of HER2/neu with histopathologic grading of breast cancer.

HER2/neu	Histopathologic grading		Prevalence ratio (RP)	CI 95% Lower–upper	P
	Low grade	High grade			
Negative (no expression)	36	27	7.667	2.372–24.781	0.000
Positive (overexpression)	4	23			

5 CONCLUSION

There was a significant association between HER2/neu overexpression with histopathologic breast cancer grading. Overexpression of HER2/neu was eight times more likely to have a high grading when compared to unexpressed HER2.

REFERENCES

American Joint Committee on Cancer (AJCC). (2012). The University of Texas MD. Anderson cancer center. Houston. Texas. 473–481,505–509.

Axilbund, J.E., Gross, A.L. & Visvanathan, K. (2011). Genetics. In *Early diagnosis and treatment of cancer* (pp. 71–88). Philadelphia, PA: Saunders.

Bartlett, J.M.S, Ellis, I.O., Dowsett, M., Mallon, E.A., Cameron, D.A., ... Ellis, P. (2007). Human epidermal growth factor receptor 2 status correlates with lymph node involvement in patient with estrogen receptor (ER)-negative, but with grade in those with ER-positive early-stage breast cancer suitable for cytotoxic chemotherapy. *Journal of Clinical Oncology, 25,* 4423–4430.

Hoff, E.R., Tubbs, R.R., Myles, J.L. & Procop, G.W. (2002). HER2/neu amplification in breast cancer. Stratification by tumor type and grade. *American Journal of Clinical Pathology, 117*(6), 916–921.

Huang, H.J., Nevan, P., Drijkoningen, M., Parideans, R., Wildiers, H., Van Limbergen, E., ... Christiaens, M.R. (2005). Associated between tumor characteristic and HER2/neu by immunohistochemistry in 1362 women with primary operable breast cancer. *Journal of Clinical Pathology, 58*(6), 611–616.

International Agency for Research on Cancer (IARC). (2012). Estimated cancer incidence, mortality, and prevalence worldwide in 2012.

Johns Hopkins University. (2012). Pathology breast cancer and breast pathology. Overview of histologic grade: Nottingham histologic score (Elston grade).

Lal, P., Tan, L.K. & Chen, B. (2005). Correlation of Her2 status with estrogen and progesterone receptor and histologic feature in 3,655 invasive breast carcinomas. *American Journal of Clinical Pathology, 123*(4), 541–546.

Naqvi, Q.H., Jamal, Q., Zaidi, M.H., Mehmood, R.K. & Abbas, F. (2002). HER-2/neu overexpression: Immunohistochemical determination in invasive lobular carcinoma of breast. *Professional Medical Journal, 9,* 213–217.

Neven, P., Brouckaert, O., Van Belle, V., Vanden Bempt, I., Hendrickx, W., Cho, H., ... Christiaens, M.R. (2008). In early-stage breast cancer, the estrogen receptors interacts with correlation between human epidermal growth factor receptors 2 status and age at diagnosis, tumor grade and lymph node involvement. *Journal of Clinical Oncology, 26*(10), 1768–1769.

Octovianus, J. & Ariodjatmiko, S. (2012). Hubungan Faktor Usia dengan grading histopatologi, status reseptor hormonal, dan ekspresi HER-2/neu pada penderita karsinoma payudara di Rumah Sakit Onkologi Surabaya. *Indonesian Journal of Cancer.*

Patriet, N., Olivier, B. & Vanya, V.B. (2007). In early breast cancer the estrogen receptors interact with correlation between human epidermal growth factor receptors 2, status and age at diagnosis, tumor grade, and lymph node involvement. *Journal of Clinical Oncology.*

Prati, R., Apple, S.K., He, J., Gornbein, J.A. & Chang, H.R. (2005). Histopathologic characteristics predicting HER-2/neu amplification in breast cancer. *Breast Journal, 6,* 4333–4339.

Rakha, E.A., Reis-Filho, J.S., Baehner, F., Dabbs, D.J., Decker, T., Eusebi, V., Fox, S.B., ... Ellis, I.O. (2010). Breast cancer prognostic classification in the molecular era: The role of histological grade. *Breast Cancer Research, 12,* 207.

Tsuda, H., Hirohashi, S., Shimosato, Y., Hirota, T., Tsugane, S., Watanabe, S., ... Yamamoto, H. (1990). Correlation between histologic grade of malignancy and copy number of c-erbb-2 gene in breast cancer. A retrospective analysis of 176 cases. *Cancer, 65,* 1794–1800.

Wolff, A.C., Hammond, M.E., Hicks, D.G., Dowsett, M., McShane, L.M., Allison, K.H., ... College of American Pathologists. (2013). Recommendation for human epidermal growth factor receptors 2 testing in breast cancer: American Society of Clinical Oncology/College Of American Pathologists clinical practice guideline update. *Journal of Clinical Oncology, 31,* 3997–4013.

Wood, W.C., Muss, H.B., Solin, L.J., et al. (2005). Malignant tumors of the breast. In V.T. DeVita, S. Hellman, & S.A. Rosenberg (Eds.), *Cancer: Principles and practice of oncology* (pp. 1415–1477). Philadelphia, PA: Lippincott Williams & Wilkins.

Stem Cell Oncology – Adella (Ed.)
© *2018 Taylor & Francis Group, London, ISBN 978-0-8153-9272-9*

The association of the nicotine metabolite ratio with lung cancer among smokers

D. Afiani, N.N. Soeroso & E. Mutiara
Department of Pulmonology and Respiratory Medicine, Faculty of Medicine,
Universitas Sumatera Utara, North Sumatera, Indonesia

B.Y.M. Sinaga
Department of Biostatistics, Faculty of Public Health, Universitas Sumatera Utara,
North Sumatera, Indonesia

ABSTRACT: The ratio of trans-3′-hydroxicotinine (3′-OH) to cotinine (COT) is referred to as the Nicotine Metabolite Ratio (NMR). Faster metabolisers of nicotine increase the risk of lung cancer. The aim of this study was to identify the association between the urinary NMR and lung cancer patients. Consecutive sampling and case-control study were applied. All of the samples were men and were either smokers or ex-smokers. We investigated NMR by using the Liquid Chromatography Tandem Mass Spectrometry (LC-MS/MS) technique. Statistical analysis was performed by chi-squared analysis using SPSS. This study involved 46 samples, consisting of 23 cases of lung cancer and 23 healthy controls. There was a significant association between urinary NMR levels and lung cancer incidence ($p = 0.00$). Fast metabolisers were 0.115 times more susceptible to lung cancer incidence than the slow metaboliser group (95% Confidence Interval (CI): 0.03–0.5). There was a significant association between urinary NMR levels with lung cancer incidence among smokers.

Keywords: Nicotine, Nicotine Metabolite Ratio, Lung Cancer

1   INTRODUCTION

Lung cancer in the broad sense involves all of the malignant diseases in the lung, including malignancies originating from the inside of the lung and malignancies outside of the lung (Jusuf et al., 2011). The incidence of lung cancer is highly correlated with smoking, and about 10% of smokers will usually be diagnosed with lung cancer in the long term. Continually consuming tobacco is a major cause of lung cancer (Silvestri et al., 2015).

Nicotine is a psychoactive component in tobacco. The variant of genetics effect of the nicotine pharmacokinetics and pharmacodynamics is associated with cigerette consumption and lung cancer risk. The most widely used nicotine biomarkers are blood, urine, saliva, hair and nails (Yildiz, 2004).

Nicotine is primarily metabolised to cotinine (COT) and trans-3′-hydroxycotinine (3HC) by liver enzyme cytochrome p450 2A6 (CYP2A6). The Nicotine Metabolite Ratio (NMR) (3HC/COT) is commonly used as a biomarker of CYP2A6 enzymatic activity, the rate of nicotine metabolism and total nicotine clearance (Benowitz et al., 2010).

A faster nicotine metabolism (greater CYP2A6 activity) can lead to more smoking being necessary in order to maintain the desired level of nicotine in the body. This could lead to a greater intake of tobacco smoke and a high risk of tobacco-related diseases. The CYP2A6 activity is also associated with the bioactivity of tobacco-specific nitrosamine, which is a potent carcinogen that contributes to cigarette-related cancers (Pelkonen & Raounio, 1995; Yamazaki et al., 1992).

2 METHOD

2.1 *Subjects*

Forty-six subjects with a history of cigarette smoking were recruited in this study: 23 subjects with lung cancer as sample cases and 23 healthy people with a smoking habit as the control. All of the subjects were patients in Adam Malik General Hospital from October 2016 to March 2017. The inclusion criteria for this sample were lung cancer patients diagnosed by cytology/histopathology, aged between 25 and 75 and of male gender. The exclusion criteria in both groups were pulmonary tuberculosis patients who consumed antituberculosis drugs and dexamethasone, and mistakes of data collection (ravage from the beginning isolation). This study was approved by the Ethical Committee of Faculty of Medicine, Universitas Sumatera Utara, and obtained informed consent from each participant.

2.2 *Urine acquisition*

Before the sample was taken, the subjects should chew on nicotine gum (4 mg) for 10 minutes. Afterwards, the urine subject of 15 ml was collected in a standard container of urine. Samples taken can be stored in a refrigerator at a temperature of −70°C. Samples should be mixed well and placed in the appropriate vials (Corning 50 ml polypropylene tubes), and the tube should be sealed properly. The sample will be analysed by LC-MS/MS (Liquid Chromatography-Mass Spectrometry Tandem Mass Spectrometry).

2.3 *Statistical analysis*

The chi-squared test was used to compare NMR between the cases and control. The OR and 95% CI were calculated to determine the association between the variables and the risk of lung cancer with regards to the NMR in both the cases and control. Statistical analyses were conducted using the statistical software SPSS 17.0 and a p-value of < 0.05 was required for statistical significance.

3 RESULTS

The demographic characteristics of the subjects of this study, based on age, cigarette type, Brinkman index and Body Mass Index (BMI), are shown in Table 1. There were statistically significant differences in the age mean between the two groups ($p < 0.001$). The smoking

Table 1.   Demographic characteristics of the study subjects.

		Lung cancer		Healthy people		
		n	%	n	%	P-value
Age	<40	0	(0)	6	(26.1)	0.001
	40–49	2	(8.7)	9	(39.1)	
	50–59	10	(43.5)	4	(17.4)	
	≥60	11	(47.8)	4	(17.4)	
Brinkman index	Mild	1	(4.3)	2	(8.7)	0.523
	Moderate	9	(39.1)	11	(47.8)	
	Severe	13	(56.5)	10	(43.5)	
BMI	Under	2	(8.7)	0	(0)	0.01
	Normal	14	(60.9)	8	(34.8)	
	Over	2	(8.7)	5	(21.7)	
	Obese I	5	(21.7)	7	(30.4)	
	Obese II	0	(0)	3	(13.0)	

Table 2. Nicotine metabolite ratio of both groups.

	Lung cancer		Healthy people				
	n	%	n	%	p	OR	95% CI
Fast	3	13.0	13	56.5	0.002	0.115	0.027–0.500
Slow	20	87.0	10	43.5			

history of the samples and controls for this study was categorised according to the Brinkman index. There was no statistically significant difference between the Brinkman index of the two groups (p = 0.523). The nutritional status of the sample and control groups in this study was categorised according to the BMI. There was a significant difference in the BMI averages between the two groups (p = 0.01).

Nicotine metabolism rates in this study based on the NMR (cotinine and trans-3'-hydrox-icotinine ratio) were categorised into fast metabolism (≥0.51) and slow metabolism (0–0.50). The mean of NMR ± SD in the lung cancer group was 0.29 ± 0.28, while the control group obtained a mean of NMR ± SD of 0.85 ± 0.78 (Table 2). Based on statistical analysis using the Mann–Whitney test, it was found that there was a significant difference between the two groups related to NMR (p < 0.001).

Based on statistical analysis using the chi-square test method, it was shown that there was a significant relationship between NMR in urine and lung cancer incidence (p < 0.001). A fast metabolism was 0.115 times more susceptible to lung cancer incidence, compared with a slow metabolism (95% Confidence Interval (CI): 0.03–0.5).

From multivariate analysis it was found that significant variables, such as NMR, age and BMI (p = 0.03, p = 0.01, and p = 0.03, respectively), contributed to lung cancer incidence.

4 DISCUSSION

Based on statistical analysis, this study showed that there is a significant difference in the mean of age between the case and control groups. The case group (lung cancer) obtained the highest average at ≥ 60 years old (47.8%) with a smoking history. Thun et al. (1997) reported that among the male sex, mortality rates between the ages of 35 and 59 were three times higher in smokers than in non-smokers.

Based on statistical analysis, this study revealed a significant difference in the average BMI between the two groups. A previous study by Koh et al. (2010), showed that smoking and the number of years since quitting smoking, and low BMI were associated with a significantly increased risk of lung cancer.

In this study, the heaviest Brinkman index is the most common category of lung cancer (46.7%). Zhang et al. (2001) reported that most of the patients with Lung Cancer-Combined Pulmonary Fibrosis and Emphysema (LC-CPFE) were smokers and had an average Brinkman index of 1131.7 ± 490.8.

Based on statistical analysis, this study showed significant differences between the two groups in relation to NMR (p < 0.001). Statistical analysis showed that there is a significant association between NMR in urine and lung cancer incidences (p < 0.001). Fast metabolisers are 0.115 times more susceptible to lung cancer incidence than the slow metaboliser group (95% Confidence Interval (CI): 0.03–0.5). This is in contrast to the previous study undertaken by Strasser et al. (2011), which reported that a faster nicotine metaboliser based on NMR values showed a significant increase in total daily cigarette smoking volume and total NNAL (as a carcinogen biomarker). Ellard et al. (1995) reported that significant results were obtained that described the estimated capacity of nicotine metabolite with 12-hour urine samples to predict the risk of lung cancer. Park et al. (2017) evaluated the relationship between urinary biomarkers to nicotine consumed (Total Nicotine Equivalent/TNE) and CYP2A6 activity (NMR) with lung cancer risk in multi-ethnic smoker subjects. It was found that both TNE and CYP2A6 activities were associated with an increased risk of lung cancer.

5 CONCLUSION

This study consisted of case subjects and control subjects with a large total of 46 subjects, consisting of a case group, which was a group of lung cancer patients with a smoking history, and a control group, which was a group of smokers who did not have lung cancer. There are significant differences between NMR in urine and lung cancer incidence (p < 0.001). Fast metabolisers are 0.115 times more susceptible to lung cancer incidence than the slow metaboliser group (95% Confidence Interval (CI): 0.03–0.5).

ACKNOWLEDGEMENT

The authors thank all the supervisors who supported this study. There was no financial support from other parties.

REFERENCES

Benowitz, N.L., Hukkanen, J. & Jacob, P. (2010). Nicotine, chemistry, metabolism, kinetics and biomarkers. *National Institute of Health*, *192*, 29–60.

Ellard, G.A., de Waard, F. & Kemmeren, J.M. (1995). Urinary metabolite excretion and lung cancer risk in female cohort. *British Journal of Cancer*, *72*, 788–791.

Jusuf, A., Haryanto, A., Syahruddin, E., Endardjo, S., Mudjiantoro, S. & Sutandio, N. (2011). 'Kanker Paru', Perhimpunan Dokter Paru Indonesia Perhimpunan Onkologi Indonesia, 1–48.

Koh, W.P., Yuan, J.M., Wang, M., Lee, H.P. & Yu, M.C. (2010). Body mass index and smoking-related cancer risk in the Singapore Chinese health study. *British Journal of Cancer*, *102*, 610–614.

Park, S.L., Murphy, S.E., Wilkens, L.R., Stram, D.O., Hecht, S.S. & Marchand, L.L. (2017). Association of CYP2A6 activity with lung cancer incidence in smokers: The multiethnic cohort study. *PLOS One*, *12*(5), e0178435.

Pelkonen, O. & Raounio, H. (1995). Individual expression of carcinogen-metabolizing enzymes: Cytochrome P4502A. *Journal of Occupational and Environmental Medicine*, *37*(1), 19–24.

Silvestri, G.A., Vachani, A., Whitney, D., Elashoff, M., Smith, K.P., Ferguson, S., ... Aegis Study Team. (2015). Bronchial genomic classifier for the diagnostic evaluation of lung cancer. *The New England Journal of Medicine*, *373*(3), 243–251.

Strasser, A.A., Benowitz, N.L., Pinto, A.G., Tang, K.Z., Hecht, S.S., Carmella, S.G., ... Lerman, C.E. (2011). Nicotine metabolite ratio predicts smoking topography and carcinogen biomarker level. *Cancer Epidemiology*, *20*(2), 234–238.

Thun, M.J., Myers, D.G., Lally, C.D., Namboodiri, M.M., Calle, E.E., Flanders, W.D., ... Heath, C.W. (1997). Age and the exposure-responses relationships between cigarette smoking and premature death in cancer prevention study II. In *Smoking and tobacco control monograph 8* (pp. 383–413). Bethesda, MD: National Cancer Institute.

Yamazaki, H., Inui, Y., Yun, C.H., Guengerich, F.P. & Shimada, T. (1992). Cytochrome P450 2E1 and 2A6 enzymes as major catalysts for metabolic activation of N-nitrosodialkylamines and tobacco related nitrosamines in human liver microsomes. *Carcinogenesis*, *13*, 1789–1794.

Yildiz, D. (2004). Nicotine, its metabolism and an overview of its biological effects. *Toxicon*, *43*, 619–632.

Zhang, W., Kilicarslan, T., Tyndale, R.F. & Seller, E.M. (2001). Evaluation of methoxsalen, tranylcypromine, and tryptamine as specific and selective CYP2 A6 inhibitors in vitro. *Drug Metabolism and Disposition*, *29*, 897–902.

Stem Cell Oncology – Adella (Ed.)
© *2018 Taylor & Francis Group, London, ISBN 978-0-8153-9272-9*

Relationship between habitual snoring and primary enuresis in children

M.A. Mahara, O.R. Ramayani, E. Effendy, M.L.R.S. Siregar,
B. Siregar & R. Ramayanti
Department of Child Health and Psychiatry, Sumatera Utara, Medan, North Sumatera, Indonesia

ABSTRACT: Obstructive sleep disorder breathing is assumed to be associated with primary enuresis in children. Prolonged enuresis may cause developmental disorders, poor school performance and emotional disorders. A cross-sectional study was conducted in the Muara Batang Gadis district, North Sumatera in April 2016. The samples of the study were children aged from 5 to 14 years old. The Sleep Disturbance Scale for Children (SDSC) questionnaire was used for measuring the symptoms of sleep disorder breathing and the International Relationship Child and Adolescent Psychiatry and Allied Professions (IACAPAP) questionnaire for the presence of primary enuresis. Data were analysed using a chi-square test and logistic regression. The p-value of <0.05 was considered significant. Out of the 110 children, 27 (24.5%) snored more than three nights per week (habitual snorers), and 18 (16.4%) had primary enuresis. The habitual snorers with a history of primary enuresis outnumbered non-habitual snorers (9.1% versus 15.4%) with a p-value <0.05. There is a significant relationship between habitual snoring and primary enuresis.

Keywords: enuresis, habitual snoring, children

1 INTRODUCTION

Enuresis is strongly related to sleep disorder breathing (snoring), which frequently occurs in children (Von Gontard, 2012; Baird et al., 2014). Enuresis has long-term effects if it is not managed seriously (Heba et al., 2013; Kalorin et al., 2010) and may cause an impact on children's development (Khaleghipour et al., 2013). Children may experience internal or external behavioural disorders. Children will develop low esteem, get low grades in school and even develop emotional disturbances (Maternik et al., 2015; Prasetyo, 2015).

Habitual snoring is associated with enuresis. Snoring is the most common clinical manifestation occurring in children with Obstructive Sleep Apnoea (OSA) (Jeyakumar et al., 2012). Children with OSA do not have a good quality of sleep, resulting in decreased Antidiuretic Hormone (ADH).

ADH secretion will cause micturition at night (nocturnal enuresis) (Yousefichaijan et al., 2015).

Sex, age, poorly educated parents, low socioeconomic status, and a history of enuresis in the family are the variables that are associated with enuresis and habitual snoring in children (Alexopoulos et al., 2014). The relationship between enuresis and habitual snoring is becoming a problem in developing countries, including Indonesia, especially in the Muara Batang Gadis district.

2 METHODS

This is a cross-sectional analytic study to determine the relationship between enuresis and habitual snoring in children. This study was conducted in the Muara Batang Gadis district,

Mandailing Natal regency. This study was conducted in April 2016. The target population in this study was children aged between 5 and 14 years. The eligible population was children aged between 5 and 14 years in the Muara Batang Gadis district, Mandailing Natal regency. The sample was obtained using a simple random sampling method. The inclusion criteria was children aged between 5 and 14 years, and the exclusion criteria were spina bifida, cerebral palsy, and diabetes mellitus. Informed consent was obtained from each parent or person who was responsible for the sample. This study was approved by the Health Research Ethical Committee, Medical School, Universitas Sumatera Utara.

3 RESULTS

A total of 110 samples were enrolled in this study. The mean age of the samples was 9.23 years (SD 2.16). Based on sex, the number of male and female samples were equal. From a physical examination it was seen that 57.3% of the samples had normal tonsils. Urinalysis using a rapid urine test was conducted to exclude urinary tract infections. Blood glucose level was measured using a rapid bedside test (GlucoDr) to exclude hyperglycaemia in this study. There was no sample with neurological, urinary tract or metabolic disorders. There was also no history of medication usage, which may affect diuresis.

The sample distribution based on sex in the snoring group was equal. In the snoring group, there was a predominance of females (13.6%), while in the non-snoring group we found a male predominance (39.1%). Tonsillar examination showed that 15 (13.6%) samples in the snoring group had enlarged tonsils (T3-T3). In the non-snoring group, most samples (54.5%) had normal tonsils. There was a variation in sample distribution based on the history of enuresis in siblings, father and mother. In the snoring group, a history of enuresis in siblings and father is more frequent, whereas a history of enuresis in a mother is smaller. The non-enuresis group showed a different pattern. Most samples had no enuresis history in siblings, father or mother. There were two samples in this study who had obesity and they were in the snoring group and non-enuresis group.

In the enuresis group, 10 (9.1%) of the samples were male, while the non-enuresis group was dominated by females (42.7%). In both groups, physical examination revealed normal tonsils (T1-T1) in the samples in different proportions (6.4% and 50.9%, respectively). A history of enuresis in the father and mother of those in the non-enuresis group was higher compared to the enuresis group (40.0% vs 9.1% and 25.5% vs 9.1%) and a history of enuresis in siblings of the enuresis group was higher than in the non-enuresis group (11.8% vs 4.5%). Based on obesity status, sample characteristic distribution did not differ significantly in both groups.

Logistic regression was conducted to determine the risk factors of enuresis and snoring in this study. Age, sex, obesity, number of siblings, history of enuresis in siblings, fathers and mothers, number of house dwellers, and tonsils were the risk factors analysed in this study.

Table 1. Risk factors for enuresis in habitual snoring samples.

	Constant	Wald	P-value*
Age	0.973	0.012	0.912
Sex	6.037	2.456	0.117
Number of siblings	1.751	0.510	0.475
History of enuresis in siblings	2.721	1.060	0.303
History of enuresis in fathers	0.117	2.879	0.900
History of enuresis in mothers	18.132	5.420	0.020
Number of house dwellers	0.459	0.833	0.361
Obesity	0.000	0.000	1.000
Tonsil size	0.140	8.488	0.004

*Regression logistic test.

Table 2. Relationship of habitual snoring and enuresis.

	Enuresis		No enuresis		
	n	%	n	%	P-value*
Snoring	10	9.1	17	15.4	
No snoring	8	7.3	75	68.2	0.001
Total	18	16.4	92	83.6	

*Chi-squared test.

The results showed that a history of enuresis in mothers and tonsil size were related to enuresis in the samples with snoring (p-values of 0.020 and 0.004, respectively). Of the two factors, one of them was a protective factor. The protective factor was tonsil size. Based on statistical analysis, we found that the incidence of enuresis in the samples with snoring was decreased 0.14 times along with increasing tonsil size. On the other hand, the risk factor for enuresis in the samples with snoring in this study was the history of enuresis in mothers. If the samples had mothers with a history of enuresis, the rate of enuresis would increase 18.132 times compared to samples without that risk factor.

A chi-squared test was done to determine the relationship between snoring and enuresis. The result showed that there was a statistically significant relationship between snoring and enuresis in children with a p-value of 0.001.

4 DISCUSSION

Enuresis is a frequently neglected problem, mainly in children and adolescents. Several recent studies have shown that the prevalence of enuresis in children and adolescents is high enough. Penbegül et al. (2013) conducted a study involving 4,203 children and reported a prevalence of enuresis of 25.9%. Another study reported a lower prevalence rate. Solanki et al. (2013) found that the prevalence of enuresis in children in rural areas in India was 11.13%. Karnicnik et al. (2012) conducted a study in Slovenia and reported a prevalence of 12.8%. A similar result was reported by Makrani et al. (2015) in Iran with a prevalence rate of 11.01%. The prevalence of enuresis in Indonesia from several studies was about 10.9% (Windiani & Soetjiningsih, 2010).

The risk factors of enuresis are socioeconomic, psychological and genetic. Von Gontard (2012) stated that 70–80% of children with enuresis had genetic disorders. In their study, Solanki and Desai (2014) had a different opinion. They found that the risk factors of enuresis were socioeconomic status and the presence of a urinary tract infection. The latter result was similar to a report from Makrani et al. (2015), who found that psychological factors, socio-economic levels and urinary tract infections were the risk factors of enuresis.

In this study, we found 18 out of 110 children with enuresis based on the International Relationship for Child and Adolescent Psychiatry and Allied Professions questionnaire. The prevalence of enuresis was 16.4%, with 10 (9.1%) male and 8 (7.3%) female.

Snoring is an important sign that leads to airway problems. Habitual snoring needs to be managed further because it can develop into Obstructive Sleep Apnoea Syndrome (OSAS) and causes serious problems in children. The incidence of OSAS is approximately 0.1%–5.7% and increases along with age, obesity, tonsil enlargement, and the other risk factors (Brock-mann et al., 2012).

Nafiu et al., in their study in the United States that enrolled children aged 6–18 years, reported a prevalence rate of 27.3% for snoring. A similar result was reported by this study. The prevalence rate for snoring in children aged 5–14 years in this study was 24.5% (Nafiu et al., 2011).

The relationship between habitual snoring and enuresis in children is still debatable. Sakel-laropoulou et al. (2012) conducted a study with 42 children aged from 3.5 to 14.5 years who had sleep disturbances. In their study they used polysomnography as the gold standard in measuring sleep quality to identify habitual snoring, and reported that seven children (16.7%) had enuresis. This concluded that there was a relationship between habitual snoring and enuresis in children.

Alexopoulos et al. (2006) did a study to determine the relationship between habitual snoring and enuresis in children. The samples in this study were 1,821 children aged 5–14 years. The study reported that 135 (7.3%) children had habitual snoring and 7.4% of them had nocturnal enuresis. The study found that habitual snoring was related to enuresis.

Satti et al. (2015) examined 290 children with tonsillar hypertrophy in Saudi Arabia. The study aimed to determine the relationship between tonsillar hypertrophy accompanied by snoring with enuresis. From the study, they reported that 114 (39.3%) children with tonsillar hypertrophy had enuresis. They concluded that children with enuresis must be examined for tonsillar enlargement.

Ahmadi et al. (2013) conducted a study in Iran to determine the prevalence of enuresis in children who had undergone a tonsillectomy. A total of 420 children were enrolled, and 92 of them had a history of enuresis. After a tonsillectomy was done, each sample was discharged and was followed for three months. Enuresis was not found in 51 (60.7%) children who had a tonsillectomy and 22 (26.2%) children had improved enuresis symptoms (p <0.001). The study concluded that the prevalence of enuresis would decrease after a tonsillectomy.

In our study, we found a relationship between habitual snoring and enuresis in children. In this study, 18 (16.4%) children who had habitual snoring also had enuresis. It was proven that there was a relationship between habitual snoring and enuresis in this study.

Snoring may cause a non-deep state sleep. This will cause a decrease in ADH secretion. The decreased ADH disrupts water retention so that urine production will be increased. That is the pathophysiology on how habitual snoring in children can cause enuresis. This was observed in our study where habitual snoring caused enuresis in children (Alexopoulos et al., 2006; Kaditis et al., 2015).

Despite all of these results, this study still has weaknesses. The sample in this study is not large enough and this makes the results different from the previous studies.

5 CONCLUSION

There is a relationship between habitual snoring and enuresis in children in this study. A history of enuresis in mothers and tonsil size are risk factors of enuresis in this study. In contrast, a history of enuresis in fathers and siblings and tonsillar hypertrophy are not risk factors of enuresis.

REFERENCES

Ahmadi, M.S., Amirhassani, S. & Poorolajal, J. (2013). The effect of adenotonsillectomy on pediatric nocturnal enuresis: A prospective cohort study. *Iranian Journal of Otorhinolaryngology*, 25, 37–40.

Alexopoulos, E.I., Kostadima, E., Pagonari, I., Zintzaras, E., Gourgoulianis, K.G. & Kaditis, A. (2006). Relationship between primary nocturnal enuresis and habitual snoring in children. *Pediatric Urology*, 68, 406–409.

Alexopoulos, E.I., Malakasioti, G., Varlami, V., Miligkos, M., Gourgoulianis, K. & Kaditis, A.G. (2014). Nocturnal enuresis is associated with moderate-to-severe obstructive sleep apnea in children with snoring. *International Pediatric Research Foundation*, 76(6), 555–559.

Baird, D.C., Seehusen, D.A. & Bode, D.V. (2014). Enuresis in children: A case-based approach. *American Family Physician*, 90(8), 560–568.

Brockmann, P.E., Urschitz, M.S., Schlaud, M. & Poets, C.F. (2012). Primary snoring in school children: Prevalence and neurocognitive impairments. *Sleep & Breathing*, 16, 23–29.

Heba, H.A., Lobna, M.E., Ahmed, E.M.B., Wael, S. & Ashraf, K.A. (2013). Effect of adenotonsillectomy on nocturnal enuresis in children with OSA. *Egyptian Journal of Chest Diseases and Tuberculosis*, 62, 275–280.

Jeyakumar, A., Rahman, S.I., Armbrecht, E.S. & Mitchell, R. (2012). The relationship between sleep-disordered breathing and enuresis in children. *Laryngoscope*, *122*(8), 1873–1877.

Kaditis, G.A., Alonso Alvarez, M.L., Boudewyns, A., Alexopoulos, E.I., Ersu, R., Joosten, K., ... Verhulst, S. (2015). Obstructive sleep-disordered breathing in 2–18-year-old children: Diagnosis and management. *European Respiratory Journal*, *25*, 1–18.

Kalorin, C.M., Mouzakes, J., Gavin, J.P., Davis, T.D., Feustel, P. & Kogan, B.A. (2010). Tonsillectomy does not improve bedwetting: Results of a prospective controlled trial. *The Journal of Urology*, *184*, 2527–2532.

Karnicnik, K., Koren, A., Kos, N. & Varda, N.M. (2012). Prevalence and quality of life of Slovenian children with primary nocturnal enuresis. *International Journal of Nephrology*, *2*, 1–6.

Khaleghipour, S., Masjedi, M. & Kelishadi, R. (2013). The effect of breathing exercises on the nocturnal enuresis in the children with the sleep-disordered breathing. *Iranian Red Crescent Medical Journal*, *15*(11), e8986.

Makrani, A.H., Moosazadeh, M., Nasehi, M.N., Abedi, G., Afshari, G., Farshidi, G. & Aghaei, S. (2015). Prevalence of enuresis and its related factors among children in Iran: A systematic review and meta-analysis. *International Journal of Pediatrics*, *2*, 1–6.

Maternik, M., Krzeminska, K. & Zurowska, A. (2015). The management of childhood urinary incontinence. *Pediatric Nephrology*, *30*, 41–50.

Nafiu, O.O., Burke, C.C., Chimbira, W.T., Ackwerh, R., Reynolds, P.I. & Malviya, S. (2011). Prevalence of habitual snoring in children and occurrence of peri-operative adverse events. *European Journal of Anaesthesiology*, *28*, 340–345.

Penbegül, N., Çelik, H., Palancı, Y., Yıldırım, K., Atar, M., Kemal, N. & Nuri, M. (2013). Prevalence of enuresis nocturnal among a group of primary school children living in Diyarbakır. *Turkish Journal of Urology*, *39*, 101–105.

Prasetyo, R.V. (2015). Tatalaksana inkonteinensia urine pada Anak. In N.A. Soemyarso, W. Suryaningtyas, R.V. Prasetyo (Eds.), *Gangguan berkemih pada Anak* (pp. 27–45). Surabaya, Indonesia: Airalangga University Press.

Sakellaropoulou, A.V., Hatzistilianou, M.A., Emporiadou, M.N., Aivazis, V.T., Goudakos, J., Markou, K. & Athanasiadou-Piperopoulou, F. (2012). Relationship between primary nocturnal enuresis and habitual snoring in children with obstructive sleep apnoea-hypopnoea syndrome. *Archives of Medical Science*, *8*(3), 521–527.

Satti, S.A., Medani, S.A. & Elabyad, M. (2015). Primary nocturnal enuresis in children presenting to the outpatient Department of Khartoum ENT Teaching Hospital with adenotonsillar hypertrophy, Khartoum, Sudan. *Basic Research Journal of Medicine and Clinical Sciences*, *4*(1), 15–19.

Solanki, A.N. & Desai, S.G. (2014). Prevalence and risk factors of nocturnal enuresis among school-age children in rural areas. *International Journal of Research in Medical Sciences*, *2*, 202–205.

Von Gontard, A. (2012). Enuresis. In J.M. Rey (Ed.), *IACAPAP e-textbook of child and adolescent mental health*. Geneva, Switzerland: International Relationship for Child and Adolescent Psychiatry and Allied Professions.

Windiani, I.G.A.T. & Soetjiningsih. (2010). Prevalensi dan faktor risiko enuresis pada anak taman kanak-kanak di kotamadya Denpasar. *Sari Pediatri*, *10*, 151–157.

Yousefichaijan, P., Khosrobeigi, A., Zargar, S. & Salehi, B. (2015). Sleep disorder in children with overactive bladder. *International Journal of Clinical Pediatrics*, *4*(2–3), 145–148.

Stem Cell Oncology – Adella (Ed.)
© 2018 Taylor & Francis Group, London, ISBN 978-0-8153-9272-9

Association between hypertension and health-related quality of life in adolescents

N. Rosari, O.R. Ramayani, E. Effendy, R. Siregar & B. Siregar
Department of Child Health and Psychiatry, Faculty of Medicine, Universitas Sumatera Utara, Medan, North Sumatera, Indonesia

ABSTRACT: The prevalence of hypertension in children, particularly those of school age, is increasing and is related to a change in the quality of life. To assess the relationship between hypertension and the quality of life in adolescence, a cross-sectional study was conducted in 13–18 year old adolescents in Singkuang, North Sumatra. Anthropometry and blood pressure measurements were done. The quality of life was assessed using the PedsQL questionnaire. From a total of 79 samples, 19 (24.1%) children were hypertensive and 60 (75.9%) were not. There were 67 (84.8%) children with good and 12 (15.2%) with poor quality of life. There were 14 (17.7%) hypertensive children with good and 5 (6.3%) with poor quality of life. A chi-squared test was done with a value of $p = 0.121$ ($PR = 2.256$ and $CI\,95\% = 0.809–6.287$). There is no relationship between hypertension and quality of life in adolescents.

Keywords: adolescent hypertension, health-related quality of life

1 INTRODUCTION

Hypertension is one of the most common chronic diseases and is a major cause of morbidity and mortality worldwide (Berendes et al., 2013). Hypertension can occur in children. Often hypertension that occurs in adults started in childhood (Sekarwana et al., 2011).

The prevalence of hypertension amounts to more than one billion people worldwide and hypertension in children, especially those of school age, has increased (NHBP, 2004). In children and adolescents aged from 3 to 18 years, the prevalence of hypertension is 3.6% and of prehypertension is 3.4%. From a cross-sectional study of adolescents, there was a prevalence of hypertension of 3.2% and a prevalence of prehypertension of 15.7% (Falkner, 2010).

Primary hypertension is more often diagnosed in adolescence than in childhood. Data from the National Childhood Blood Pressure found that in adolescents with 2- and 4-year interval blood pressure measurements showed 14% prehypertensive adolescents, which progressed to hypertension in 2 years: about 7% per year (Falkner, 2010). In Indonesia, according to basic health research (*Riskesdas*), in 2007 the prevalence of hypertension at age 15–17 years is 8.3%.[5] A study in RSU Zainal Abidin Banda Aceh found a hypertension prevalence of 23.4% in children aged 4–16 years (Infodatin Pusat, 2016).

Childhood hypertension should receive serious attention, because the disease can carry on into adulthood, so early detection is required every year after a three-year-old child (Lurbe et al., 2016). Childhood hypertension is asymptomatic hypertension, which is associated with changes in Health-Related Quality of Life (HRQoL) and which remains controversial (Erickson et al. 2001). Therefore, this study aims to investigate the HRQoL in children with hypertension, including aspects such as their physical condition, emotions and social aspects related to health, and research will be conducted in Singkuang Village, Muara Batang Gadis sub-district, Mandailing Natal, North Sumatra Province (village assisted by the Department of Health Sciences Faculty of Medicine, University of North Sumatra).

2 METHOD

The design of this study is a cross-sectional comparative study to determine the relationship between hypertension with the quality of life of adolescents. This study was conducted at Al-Fath Integrated Islamic Boarding Junior High School, Singkuang Village, Muara Batang Gadis Sub-district, Mandailing Natal Regency from 18 June 2016 until 31 September 2016.

The population that met the inclusion criteria were given a PedsQL questionnaire regarding the quality of life of the child. Anthropometric measurements and blood pressure measurements were performed. The collected data were analysed statistically to obtain sample characteristics and the relationship of the quality of life with hypertension in adolescents. Bivariate analysis was conducted on this research data. Data analysis of each of the nominal dichotomous variables was undertaken using a chi-square test to determine the relationship of hypertension with the quality of life of adolescents. Data processing was done with SPSS software, where p <0.05 was considered significant.

3 RESULTS

The number of samples collected in this study were 103 people from three classes in the school. Of the total of 103 students, there were 24 children who did not meet the inclusion criteria for being under 13 years old, so that the number of samples aged 13–18 years was 79 children.

Table 1 shows that the mean age of the adolescents who became respondents in the study was 13.86 (SB 0.91). The most respondents were male (42.42%) and female (37.8%). There were 22 (27.8%) grade 7 adolescents, 23 people (29.1%) were grade 8 and 34 people (43.0%) were grade 9. The mean body weight was 38.34 (SB 8.17) kg. The mean height was 143.34 (SB 7.16) cm with a mean systolic pressure of 110.58 (SB 9.74) mmHg and a diastolic pressure of 72.23 (SB 6.59) mmHg. The number of hypertensive adolescent children was 27 persons (34.2%) and there were 52 people (65.8%) without hypertension. Using PedsQL, the quality of life of adolescents report assessment that was done covered physical aspects, emotional, social, and school aspects, with the result showing that 64 people (81.0%) had a good quality of life and 15 people (19.0%) had a poor quality of life, with a mean score of 80.04 (SB 12.11).

Table 2 shows the results of a chi-squared test used to assess the relationship between hypertension and the quality of life in adolescents. Hypertension is divided into two groups: hypertensive and not hypertensive. Quality Of Life (QoL) is divided into two groups: good

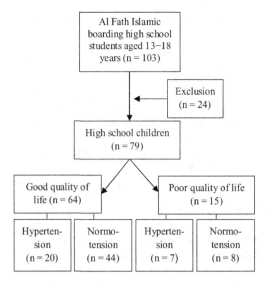

Figure 1. Study profile.

34

Table 1. Characteristics distribution.

Characteristic	Sample N = 79
Sex, n (%)	
Boys	42 (53.2)
Girls	37 (46.8)
Grade, n (%)	
Grade 7	22 (27.8)
Grade 8	23 (29.1)
Grade 9	34 (43.0)
Parents earning, n (%)	
500.000	18 (22.8)
500.000–1.000.000	46 (58.2)
1.000.000–3.000.000	15 (19.0)
Blood pressure, n (%)	
Hypertension	19 (24.1)
Normotension	60 (75.9)
PedsQL, n (%)	
Good	67 (84.8)
Poor	12 (15.2)
Mean age, years (SD)	13.86 (0.91)
Mean weight, kg (SD)	38.34 (8.17)
Mean height, cm (SB)	143.34 (7.16)
Mean blood pressure, mmHg (SB)	
Systolic	109.05 (8.82)
Dyastolic	71.32 (6.41)
Mean QoL score, (SB)	80.03 (11.34)

Table 2. Association between hypertension and quality of life.

	Quality of life			P	PR	CI 95%
	Poor	Good	Total			
Hyper tension				0.121	2.256	0.809–6.287
Yes	5	14	19			
No	7	53	60			
Total	12	67	79			

and poor. Based on the results of the chi-squared test, there is no relationship between hypertension and quality of life, with $P = 0.257$ (RP = 1.685 and CI 95% = 0.684–4.151).

4 DISCUSSION

Primary hypertension can be detected in childhood and adolescence if there are family factors of hypertension, obesity and lifestyle. The death and disability of children due to hypertension does not occur, but organs can be damaged from childhood onwards, such as left ventricular hypertrophy, thickening of the carotid blood vessel walls, changes in retinal vessels and cognitive changes. Asymptomatic hypertension occurs in more than 3% of children and less than 3% of children are prehypertensive, so hypertension in childhood is a long-term health problem (Falkner, 2010).

The prevalence of hypertension in the world varies by region. The lowest prevalence is 0.9%. The prevalence of obese children with hypertension has reached 7.1% (Trevisol et al., 2012). The prevalence of hypertension and prehypertension is 3.6% and 3.4% in children aged 3–18 years (Falkner, 2010).

A cross-sectional study in Aligarth in 2007, which examined 5–17 year old children, found a higher prevalence of females with hypertension (9.4%) than males (9.36%).

Another study in Germany showed a prevalence of boys with hypertension of 6% and girls of 1.4% at age 14–17 years, whereas by the age of 16.5–19 years, the prevalence of boys with hypertension was 5.5% and girls was 1.9%.[11] In Indonesia, according to basic health research (*Riskesdas*) in 2007, childhood hypertension in 15–17 year olds had a prevalence of 8.3%.[5] Research in Zainal Abidin Hospital Banda Aceh found a prevalence of hypertension of 23.4% in children aged 4–16 years. The prevalence of hypertension with quality of life and psychological disorders at the age of 11–17 years was around 10.7% (Berendes et al., 2013).

The prevalence of hypertension is influenced by weight, increased physical activity and diet or nutritional modification (Lurbe et al., 2016). Body mass index affects physical and emotional health and blood pressure (Neuhauser et al., 2009). In adults, a 4 mmHg increase in blood pressure causes a 20% risk of death due to stroke (Neuhauser et al., 2011).

There are four aspects related to the phenomenon of quality of life in children with hypertension among other factors 1) belief in the effect of hypertension on the concerns of serious illness, 2) a feeling of condition that tends to worsen, 3) the relationship between pain and social role, and 4) an illustration that the disease will cripple (Bardage & Isacson, 2001)

In this study, which was conducted in children aged 13–18 years, it was found that the average adolescent weight was 38.34 kg and height was 143.34 cm with a mean of 109.05 mmHg systolic pressure and diastolic pressure of 71.32 mmHg. Fourteen people (17.7%) with a good quality of life were affected by hypertension and five people (6.3%) with a poor quality of life were affected by hypertension.

Each hypertensive patient has an impact and influence on the quality of life (Korhonen et al., 2011). The quality of life of individuals with hypertension is slightly worse than that of those with normotension (Trevisol et al., 2011). The quality of life of individuals who are treated for hypertension is better because this will decrease the symptoms over time. Optimal drug therapy is an important goal in everyday clinical practice (Kjellgren et al., 1998). But other studies have shown that hypertensive patients with antihypertensive use will have fewer symptoms and quality of life. This is caused by a disturbance of the physical symptoms that may be associated with hypertension. Hypertension lowers quality of life in physical and social areas but does not decrease the emotional aspects (Erickson et al., 2001).

The quality of life of hypertensive patients in terms of physical roles, such as body pain, social function and emotional roles, is higher than for normotensive individuals (Trevisol et al., 2011). A study that assessed the physical activity of a child with hypertension found that the child had no activity disorders and had few behavioural dimension problems (Wang et al., 2009). Another study found the physical capacity of children with lower hypertension (Kjellgren et al., 1998). In addition, psychological and psychophysiological aspects are associated with baroreceptors, which play a role in the response to pain (Rau & Elbert, 2001) However, most studies show that hypertension can interfere with vitality, social function, mental health, mood and psychological function. Hypertension is also associated with symptoms such as headache, dizziness, depression, anxiety and fatigue (Wang et al., 2009).

One study showed an association of quality of life with hypertension where the results showed no difference in the symptoms of hypertension and not hypertension. Symptoms associated with hypertension may not be diagnosed by the same conditions as the symptoms of normotension. These symptoms emerged after more than 16 years (Korhonen et al., 2011).

In this study, assessing the quality of life of adolescents based on PedsQL reports covering the physical, emotional, social, and school aspects, found that hypertensive children had the same quality of life as children with normotension.

This study still has many limitations because it does not examine other aspects related to hypertension. Many aspects that can affect hypertension with quality of life include socio-demography, personal and environmental characteristics, physical omission or weight stabilisation symptoms associated with hypertension, continued comorbidities and other related diseases. This study also has a high prevalence of hypertension rates in the study sites so that further research is needed on the causes of these figures.

5 CONCLUSION

The results of this study indicate that there is no relationship between quality of life with hypertension in adolescents.

REFERENCES

Bardage, C. & Isacson, D.G. (2001). Hypertension and health-related quality of life an epidemiological study in Sweden. *Journal of Clinical Epidemiology*, *54*, 172–178.

Berendes, A., Meyer, T., Wette, M.H. & Lingen, C.H. (2013). Association of elevated blood pressure with low distress and good quality of life. *Psychosomatic Medicine*, *75*, 422–428.

Durrani, A.M. & Wasseem, F. (2011). Blood pressure distribution and its relation to anthropometric measurements among school children in Aligarh. *Indian Journal of Public Health*, *55*, 121–124.

Erickson, S.R., Williams, B.C. & Gruppen, L.D. (2001). Perceived symptoms and health related quality of life reported by uncomplicated hypertensive patients compared to normal controls. *Journal of Human Hypertension*, *15*, 539–548.

Falkner, B. (2010). Hypertension in children and adolescents epidemiology and natural history. *Pediatric Nephrology*, *25*, 1219–1224.

Haris, S., Dimiati, H. & Anwar, M.S. (2013). Profil Hipertensi pada Anak di RSUD Dr. Zainoel Abidin Banda Aceh. *Sari Pediatri*, *15*(2), 105–110.

Infodatin Pusat data dan Informasi Kementeriaan Kesehatan RI. (2007). Diunduh dari. Retrieved from http//www.riskesdas.litbang.depkes.go.id.

Kjellgren, K.I., Ahlner, J., Dahlo, F.B., Gill, H., Hedner, T. & Saljo, R. (1998). Perceived symptoms amongst hypertensive patients in routine clinical practice. A population based study. *Journal of Internal Medicine*, *244*, 325–332.

Korhonen, P.E., Kivela, S.L., Kautiainen, H., Jarvenpa, A.S. & Kantola, I. (2011). Health-related quality of life and awareness of hypertension. *Journal of Hypertension*, *29*, 2070–2074.

Lurbe, E., Alcon, J.J., Redon, J. & Lande, M.B. (2016). Systemic hypertension. In R.M. Kliegman, B.F. Stanton, J.W. St Geme III, N.F. Schor, & R.E. Behrman (Eds.), *Nelson textbook of pediatrics* (20th ed., pp. 2294–2303). Philadelphia, PA: Elsevier.

Mohr, P., Rodriguez, M., Slavikova, A. & Hanka, J. (2011). The application of vagus nerve stimulation and deep brain stimulation in depression. *Neuropsychobiology*, *64*, 170–181.

National High Blood Pressure (NHBP) Education Program Working Group on High Blood Pressure in Children and Adolescents. (2004). The fourth report on the diagnosis, evaluation, and treatment of high blood pressure in children and adolescents. *Pediatrics*, *114*, 555–576.

Neuhauser, H.K., Schaffrath, R.S., Thamm, M. & Ellert, U. (2009). Prevalence of children with blood pressure measurements exceeding adult cut offs for optimal blood pressure in Germany. *European Journal of Cardiovascular Prevention and Rehabilitation*, *16*, 195–200.

Neuhauser, H.K., Thamm, M., Ellert, U., Hense, H.W. & Schaffrath, R.A. (2011). Blood pressure percentiles by age and height from non-overweight children and adolescents in Germany. *Pediatrics*, *127*, 978–988.

Rau, H. & Elbert, T. (2001). Psychophysiology of arterial baroreceptors and the etiology of hypertension. *Biological Psychology*, *57*, 179–201.

Sekarwana, N., Rachmadi, D. & Hilmanto, D. (2011). Penyunting [Editorial]. In *Konsensus tata laksana hipertensi pada anak* (pp. 7–13). Jakarta, Indonesia: Unit Kerja Nefrologi Ikatan Dokter Anak Indonesia.

Trevisol, D.J., Moreira, L.B., Kerkhoff, A., Fuchs, S.C. & Fuchs, F.D. (2011). Health related quality of life and hypertension: A systematic review and meta-analysis of observational studies. *Journal of Hypertension*, *29*, 179–188.

Trevisol, D.J., Moreira, L.B., Fuchs, F.D. & Fuchs, S.C. (2012). Health-related quality of life is worse in individuals with hypertension under drug treatment result of population based study. *Journal of Human Hypertension*, *26*, 374–380.

Wang, R., Zhao, Y., He, X., Ma, X., Yan, X., Sun, Y., ... He, J. (2009). Impact of hypertension on health related quality of life in a population based study in Shanghai China. *Public Health*, *123*, 534–539.

Ware, J.E. & Dewey, J.E. (2000). Health status and outcomes assessment tools. *The International Electronic Journal of Health Education*, *3*, 138–148.

Stem Cell Oncology – Adella (Ed.)
© 2018 Taylor & Francis Group, London, ISBN 978-0-8153-9272-9

Effect of smoking on superoxide dismutase levels in DM with pulmonary TB patients

M.I. Sari & S.S. Widjaja
Department of Biochemistry, Faculty of Medicine, Universitas Sumatera Utara, Medan, North Sumatera, Indonesia

Z. Amir
Department of Pulmonology, Faculty of Medicine, Universitas Sumatera Utara, Medan, North Sumatera, Indonesia

D.M. Darlan
Department of Parasitology, Faculty of Medicine, Universitas Sumatera Utara, Medan, North Sumatera, Indonesia

D.D. Wijaya
Department of Anaesthesiology and Intensive Care, Faculty of Medicine, Universitas Sumatera Utara, Medan, North Sumatera, Indonesia

ABSTRACT: Cigarette smoke contains free radicals. This condition can lead to the decrease of antioxidants. This study aims to determine the effect of cigarette smoking on Superoxide Dismutase Antioxidant (SOD) levels in Diabetes Mellitus (DM) with pulmonary Tuberculosis (TB) patients. The study was conducted on 30 male patients with DM with pulmonary TB. Smoking data was obtained by questionnaire. The SOD level was determined according to the ELISA technique. The mean values of SOD were analysed using SPSS software. There was no significant difference ($p = 0.56$) in the SOD levels of DM with pulmonary TB patients in non-smoker groups compared to those in smoker groups. The level of SOD had significant differences ($p = 0.000$) in smoker subjects by Brinkman index classification. Cigarette smoking can affect the SOD level in DM with pulmonary TB patients depending on the length of time a person has been smoking and the number of cigarettes per day that are smoked.

Keywords: smoking, SOD, DM, TB

1 INTRODUCTION

Smoking has become a community lifestyle; a habitual thing in Indonesian society. Smoking behaviour can cause a negative impact on health. The estimation of the number of deaths that will be caused by smoking in 2030 could reach 10,000,000 people every year and 80% of deaths happen in the developing countries (WHO, 2008). The data shows that Indonesia is in third position of the ten countries with the most smokers in the world. Various serious effects of smoking can happen in the early days. The damage to organs can happen from the time that the first cigarette is consumed (Barber et al., 2008).

Cigarette smoke is one of the exogenous sources of free radicals (oxidants). This is a factor in the occurrence of systemic disease and organ damage, including the pancreas. It happens via the pathway of the phosphatidylinositol-3-kinase enzyme. Inhibition of this enzyme causes a decrease of adiponectin secretion. This process can decrease the insulin sensitivity, which directly disrupts the process of glucose metabolism (Hilawe et al., 2015). Oxidative stress also increases the levels of the hormones epinephrine and norepinephrine. These hormones affect the sympathetic nervous system and increase the rate of gluconeogenesis and glycogenolysis that causes hyperglycaemia (Vu et al., 2014). Both of these pathways will cause metabolic disorders such as Diabetes Mellitus (DM) (Hilawe et al., 2015; Vu et al., 2014). The condition of hyperglycaemia in people with DM will lead to auto oxidative glucose reactions, protein glycation and the activation of polyol metabolism pathways that will accelerate the formation of free radicals, and this can cause damage to the organs.

Since the beginning of the 20th century, researchers have found a risk of TB in patients with DM. The data of WHO shows that DM will increase the risk of pulmonary TB infection to three times larger than that of the normal population (WHO, 2011). This condition triggers the formation of free radicals.

Naturally, there are antioxidant defence systems of enzymes against free radicals, such as Superoxide Dismutase (SOD), catalase and glutathione peroxidase enzymes, in the body. Based on previous studies, it was reported that SOD is the leading line of defence against free radical compounds (Alvarez, 1987).

In normal circumstances there is an appropriate balance between free radicals and antioxidants. However, this balance can shift when the production of free radicals is increased. The decreasing of antioxidants in the SOD of smokers has been found in a previous study (Pasupathi et al., 2009). In other research, the decrease of SOD antioxidant activity was also found in the conditions of DM and pulmonary TB (Moses et al., 2008; Mohod et al., 2011; Taheri et al., 2012). Therefore, the aim of this study was to evaluate the effect of cigarette smoking on SOD levels in DM in pulmonary TB patients. Previous research regarding the effect of cigarettes on the level of SOD of healthy subjects has been done. But there was no research regarding the effect of cigarettes on the level of SOD in DM in pulmonary TB patients.

2 METHODS

This study was conducted after getting permission from the ethical committee of the Faculty of Medicine of the University of Sumatera Utara (North Sumatra) No.327/KEPK FK USU-RSUP HAM/2017. This research was conducted on 30 male DM with pulmonary TB patients from the clinic, in Medan, who were aged over 20 years. Patients were excluded as study participants if they were: 1) using enzymatic antioxidant supplements (superoxide dismutase, catalase, glutathione peroxidase) as well as non-enzymatic antioxidants (vitamin A, vitamin C, carotenoids, flavonoids, curcumin); 2) suffering from HIV infection.

Patients that agreed to participate in the study were required to fill out and sign the informed consent after being given an explanation about the purposes and benefits of the research. The status of smoking and the level of smoking were determined by using questionnaires. The participants were grouped by smoking category: non-smoker and smoker groups. The level of smoking was determined by using the Brinkman Index (BI). BI values were calculated as the number of cigarettes smoked per day multiplied by the number of years of smoking. The categories of smoking of the smokers were mild if the BI value was <200, moderate if the BI value was 200–600 and severe if the BI value was >600 (Brinkman & Coates, 1963).

The blood samples were collected (5 mL) through peripheral venipuncture after at least 12 hours of fasting. The serum over the blood was separated in a plain vacuum tube, aliquoted and stored at -20 °C and used for the following assays of blood glucose and SOD. The blood glucose and SOD levels of the subjects in this research were conducted at the Integrated Laboratory of the Faculty of Medicine, University of North Sumatra. The blood glucose level was determined by using a spectrophotometer with a wavelength of 546 nm using the GOD-PAP method. SOD activity was determined according to the Enzyme-Linked Immunosorbent Assay (ELISA) technique using a human ELISA kit manufactured by the bioassay technology laboratory.

The mean and standard deviation values of SOD that were obtained from the subjects were calculated. The mean value of SOD was compared between the non-smoker group and the smoker group using a Mann–Whitney U-test by SPSS statistical software. The mean of SOD on the smoker BI group was compared using a Kruskall–Wallis test in SPSS software.

3 RESULTS AND DISCUSSION

In the present study, Table 1 presents the information regarding the characteristics of the subjects.

Thirty subjects who met the inclusion and exclusion criteria were obtained. The average age of the subjects was 53.26 years old, and these consisted of 20 smoker subjects and ten non-smoker subjects. The mean value of blood glucose of the subjects was 291.20 mg%. The mean value of the blood glucose of the subjects of this study is above the normal value. In healthy people, normal blood glucose levels are below 120 mg%. Blood glucose levels above 120 mg% are referred to as hyperglycaemia. This condition occurs in patients with DM (Murray et al., 2012).

Persistent hyperglycaemia in patients with DM is a risk factor of increasing free radicals. The increase of free radical production will affect the level and function of endogenous enzymatic antioxidants. Endogenous enzymatic antioxidants work as the first line antioxidant defence of SOD. Excessive free radical production affects the production of SOD. The decrease of SOD production means that the scavenger function does not work optimally (Alvarez, 1987; Dembinska-Kiec et al., 2008). In this research, the mean value of SOD was 136.71 U/L. The value of SOD in the subjects in this study were classified at low ranges because they were based on the kit used in this study, where normal SOD levels were in the range of 3–900 U/L. This was possible because the subjects in this study were DM patients with pulmonary TB, the group who were at risk of getting decreasing SOD levels.

DM is one of the most important risk factors for pulmonary TB. The mechanisms underlying the association of DM with TB are still not understood today, although there have been a number of hypotheses about the role of proinflammatory cytokines in DM patients as an important molecule in the human defence mechanisms against pulmonary TB. This condition will increase the production of free radicals (Podell, 2014).

Smoking will worsen the condition of DM with pulmonary TB patients. Blood glucose levels will increase and the free radicals formed cannot be offset by the production of antioxidants such as SOD. The effects of cigarettes on the SOD levels of patients with DM who are also infected with pulmonary TB can be seen in Table 2.

The normality of the distribution of SOD data was analysed by the Shapiro–Wilk test. The Shapiro–Wilk test results get $p < 0.05$, which means that the data was considered to be an abnormal distribution. There was a differentiation in the SOD levels of DM with pulmonary

Table 1. Characteristics of study population.

Variable	Mean, SD	Min; Max
Age (year)	53.26 ± 1.74	36.00; 77.00
Smoker (N)	20	
Non-smoker (N)	10	
Blood-glucose (mg%)	291.20 ± 11.29	20.00; 460.00
SOD (U/L)	136.71 ± 20.97	70.34; 532.20

Table 2. The mean difference test between superoxide dismutase in non-smoker and smoker subjects.

	Non-smoker	Smoker	p*
SOD (U/L)	148.57 ± 44.08	30.79 ± 23.26	0.56

*Mann–Whitney U.

41

TB patients in non-smoker groups (the mean value of SOD is 148.57 U/L) compared to smoker groups (the mean value of SOD is 130.79 U/L), but the Mann–Whitney U-test of the groups shows no significance ($p = 0.56$).

The results of this study are different from the results of the research in India that showed that the SOD levels of saliva and blood from non-smokers were higher than those of the smokers, with a significance of $p < 0.05$ (Gavali et al., 2013). In addition, research was also done in Saudi Arabia, Iraq and Taiwan, which stated that the level of SOD in smokers was lower than that in non-smokers (Ahmed, 2013; Abdul-Rasheed et al., 2013; Jenifer et al., 2015).

The main ingredient in cigarettes is tobacco. Tobacco contains approximately 4,000 elements and at least 200 of them are harmful to health. The main toxins of tobacco that are capable of adverse health effects are nicotine, tar, carbon monoxide gas and various heavy metals. Cigarette smoke generated from tobacco burning can increase the production of free radicals in body cells. Free radicals are molecules containing unpaired electrons in their outermost orbits. This unpaired electron makes it very reactive, because free radicals can attack important molecules, such as DNA, enzyme proteins and lipids, causing cell damage such as to the pancreatic cells and other cells (Britton & Edwards, 2007).

Free radicals from cigarette smoke can be suppressed by antioxidant activity. The difference in the results of this research compared with the previous research can be analysed if levels of other antioxidant endogenous enzymes in the body are known. There are endogenous antioxidants in addition to SOD in the body, such as catalase and glutathione peroxidase (Murray et al., 2012). Antioxidant catalase and peroxydase glutathione also play a role in tackling the free radicals in the body. The amount of antioxidant activity against the free radicals can decrease the SOD levels in the smokers that were not significant than non-smokers.

The characteristics of the smoker groups in this study, based on BI category, can be seen in Table 3.

Table 3 shows that the mean value of the smoking period on smoker subjects was 16.30 years and the mean value of the number of cigarettes smoked/day were 15.80 cigarettes. Based on BI, 10 subjects in this group of smokers are categorised as heavy smokers. Nicotine in cigarettes is addictive, although the concentration in cigarettes is only about 1–1.3 mg. Nicotine will increase levels of dopamine in the brain and if nicotine levels drop in the smoker's brain, there will be induced anxiety and stress on the smokers. To handle these things, the tendency of people to keep enjoying cigarettes is very large. With the recurrent exposure to nicotine in the smoker, the ability of the brain to adapt to nicotine begins to increase (Benowitz, 2010). This could be the cause of the high number of heavy smokers in this study. The longer the period that a person is a smoker, the greater the increase in the number of cigarettes per day.

The effect of cigarettes based on the length of years of smoking and the number of cigarettes smoked on SOD levels can be seen in Table 4.

There was a difference in the SOD levels in the smoker DM with pulmonary TB patients based on BI group. The mean value of SOD in mild smokers (274.9 U/L) was higher compared to moderate smokers (116.94 U/L). The mean value of SOD in mild and moderate smokers was higher compared to severe smokers (81.72 U/L). Based on the Kruskal-Wallis test, the mean values of SOD were compared between mild, moderate and severe smokers and the result was significant differences ($p = 0.000$).

Table 3. Characteristics of smoker subjects.

Variable	Mean, SD	Min; Max
Smoking period (yr)	16.30 ± 8.14	3.00; 3.00
No of cigarettes smoked/day	15.80 ± 6.67	4.00; 24.00
Brinkman index (N)		
Mild	4	
Moderate	6	
Severe	10	

Table 4.　SOD in Brinkman index of smoker subjects on DM with pulmonary TB patients.

Brinkman index	SOD U/L	p*
Mild	274.92 ± 85.50	0.000
Moderate	116.94 ± 17.52	
Severe	81.72 ± 6.10	

*Kruskal–Wallis test.

Determined by using the BI, a severe smoker was a smoker whose BI value was >600. This means that the subjects in the severe smoker groups were smoking for long periods and had taken a lot of cigarette smoke per day (Brinkman & Coates, 1963). The consequences of this condition create more free radical production due to the effects of tobacco burning. A higher production of free radicals will correlate negatively to the amount of antioxidants. The length of time that a person has been smoking and the number of cigarettes per day that are taken by a person affect the levels of SOD (Pasupathi et al., 2009).

4　CONCLUSIONS

In this research on DM with pulmonary TB patients, it was found that the SOD levels of smokers were lower than those of non-smokers. The SOD levels were the lowest in severe smokers compared to mild smokers and moderate smokers. Nevertheless, statistical analysis showed that there was no effect of cigarettes on the level of SOD in DM with pulmonary TB patients compared to normal subjects. Cigarette smoking can affect SOD levels in DM with pulmonary TB patients depending on the length of time a person has smoked and the number of cigarettes per day that are taken by a person.

ACKNOWLEDGEMENTS

The authors gratefully acknowledge that this research is supported by the Institute of Research, Universitas Sumatera Utara (USU), as Talenta Research USU of 2017 with contract no. 5338/UN5.1.R/RPM/2017, 22 May 2017.

REFERENCES

Abdul-Rasheed, M.O.F. & Al-Rubayee, W.T. (2013). Effects of cigarette smoking on lipid peroxidation and antioxidant status in Iraqi men at Baghdad city. *International Journal of Basic and Applied Sciences*, 2(1), 47–50.
Ahmed, A.M. (2013). Salivary antioxidants superoxide dismutase and glutathione peroxidase in smokers comparing to non-smokers. *Journal of Biosciences Research*, 4(1), 4–9.
Alvarez, J.G. (1987). Spontaneous lipid peroxidation and production of hydrogen peroxide and superoxide in human spermatozoa: Superoxide as major enzyme protectant against oxygen toxicity. *Journal of Andrology*, 8, 338–348.
Barber, S., Ahsan, A., Adioetoomo, S.M. & Setyonaluri, D. (2008). *Tobacco economics in Indonesia*. Paris, France: International Union Against Tuberculosis and Lung Disease.
Benowitz, N.L. (2010). Nicotine addiction. *The New England Journal of Medicine*, 362(24), 2295–2303.
Brinkman, G.L. & Coates, E.O.J. (1963). The effect of bronchitis, smoking, and occupation on ventilation. *American Review of Respiratory Disease*, 87, 684–693.
Britton, J. & Edwards. F. (2007). Tobacco smoking, harm reduction, and nicotine product regulation. *Lancet*, 317(9610), 441–445.
Dembinska-Kiec, A., Mykkanen, D., Kiec-Wilk, B. & Mykkanen, H. (2008). Antioxidant phytochemicals against type-2 diabetes. *British Journal of Nutrition*, 99(1), 109–117.

Gavali, Y., Deore, D., Surwase, S.P. & Zingade, U. (2013). Study of the serum superoxide dismutase levels in smoking and non-smoking patients with COPD. *International Journal of Recent Trends in Science and Technology*, *5*(3), 121–126.

Hilawe, E.H., Yatsuya, H., Li, Y., Uemura, M., Wang, C., Chiang, C., … Aoyama, A. (2015). Smoking and diabetes: Is the association mediated by adiponectin, leptin, or C-reactive protein? *Journal of Epidemiology / Japan Epidemiological Association*, *25*(2), 99–109. doi:10.2188/jea.JE20140055.

Jenifer, H.D., Bhola, S., Kalburgi, V., Warad, S. & Kokatnur, V.M. (2015). The influence of cigarette smoking on blood and salivary superoxide dismutase enzyme levels among smokers and nonsmokers-A cross sectional study. *Journal of Traditional and Complementary Medicine*, *5*(2), 100–105.

Mohod, K., Dhok, A. & Kumar, S. (2011). Status of oxidants and antioxidants in pulmonary tuberculosis with varying bacillary load. *Journal of Experimental Sciences*, *2*, 35–37.

Moses, A.O., Emmanuel, O.O., Ganiyu, A.O., Fidelis, A.A. & Dickson, A.O. (2008). Assessment of antioxidants and nutritional status of pulmonary tuberculosis patients in Nigeria. *European Journal of General Medicine*, *5*(4), 208–211.

Murray, R.K., Granne, D.K. & Rodwell, V.W. (2012). *Harper's illustrated biochemistry* (29th ed.). New York, NY: McGraw-Hill.

Pasupathi, P., Saravanan, G. & Farook, J. (2009). Oxidative stress bio markers and antioxidant status in cigarette smokers compared to nonsmokers. *Journal of Pharmaceutical Sciences & Research*, *1*(2), 55–62.

Podell, B.K. (2014). *The pathogenesis of diabetes-tuberculosis comorbidity* (Doctoral dissertation, Colorado State University, Fort Collins, CO).

Taheri, E., Mahmoud, D., Ahmad, S., Ali, M.M., Abolghase, D. & Mostafa, Q. (2012). The relationship between the activates of antioxidant enzymes in red blood cells and body mass index in Iranian type 2 diabetes and healthy subjects. *Journal of Diabetes & Metabolic Disorders*, *11*, 3.

Vu, C.U., Siddiqui, J.A., Wadensweiler, P., Gayen, J.R., Avolio, E., Bandyopadhyay, G.K., … Mahata, S.K. (2014). Nicotinic acetylcholine receptors in glucose homeostasis: The acute hyperglycemic and chronic insulin-sensitive effects of nicotine suggest dual opposing roles of the receptors in male mice. *Endocrinology*, *155*(10), 3793–3805. doi:10.1210/en.2014–1320.

World Health Organization. (2008). *WHO report on the global tobacco epidemic*. Retrieved from http://whqlibdoc.who.int/publications/2008/mpower_report_full_2017/_eng_full.pdf.

World Health Organization. (2011). *Non communicable disease report*. Retrieved from http://www.who.int/nmh/publications/ncd_report_chapter1.pdf.

Stem Cell Oncology – Adella (Ed.)
© 2018 Taylor & Francis Group, London, ISBN 978-0-8153-9272-9

Family support, coping strategies and anxiety in cancer patients

D.K. Sari
Faculty of Medicine, Universitas Sumatera Utara, Medan, North Sumatera, Indonesia

W. Daulay
Faculty of Nursing, Universitas Sumatera Utara, Medan, North Sumatera, Indonesia

R. Dewi
Master Nursing Programme, Faculty of Nursing, Universitas Sumatera Utara, Medan, North Sumatera, Indonesia

ABSTRACT: This study aims to test the association between family support, coping strategies and anxiety at Dr. Pirngadi General Hospital, Medan. The samples are 102 cancer patients undergoing chemotherapy who were assessed, and the results of the bivariate analysis showed a significant positive association ($p = 0.001 < 0.05$) and strong correlation ($r = 0.612$) between family support and the Problem-Focused Coping (PFC) strategy, while there was a significant negative association ($p = 0.001$) and moderate correlation ($r = -0.462$) with the Emotion-Focused Coping (EFC) strategy. A significant negative association ($p = 0.001$) and strong correlation ($r = -0.646$) was found between family support and anxiety. The multivariate analysis showed a dominant association ($p = 0.001$) between family support and the PFC strategy (Odds Ratio = 12.2), EFC (OR = 0.142) and anxiety (OR = 0.039). The conclusion was that there is an association between good family support and effective coping strategies and lower anxiety levels in cancer patients undergoing chemotherapy.

Keywords: Family support, Cancer, Coping strategies, Chemotherapy

1 INTRODUCTION

Over half of cancer patients are treated with chemotherapy (Prawirohardjo, 2010). Chemotherapy leads to various physiological and psychological side effects. The psychological side effects that may occur include stress, anxiety and depression. This stress leads to individuals using coping strategies to prevent further psychological disorders (Karabulutlu et al., 2010).

A study by Muhamad et al. (2011) stated that support from all family members, especially the spouse, plays an important role in decision-making and survival strategy.

The objective of this study is to test the association between family support, coping strategies and anxiety in cancer patients undergoing chemotherapy at Dr. Pirngadi General Hospital, Medan.

2 METHODS

This is a quantitative study using a correlational descriptive design with a cross-sectional approach. The study population is cancer patients undergoing chemotherapy in Dr. Pirngadi Hospital, Medan, Indonesia, with a purposive sampling technique resulting in 102 individuals. Data collection was performed directly from the respondents by using questionnaires about family support, coping strategies and anxiety.

3 RESULTS

3.1 *Characteristics of subjects*

Table 1, which shows the characeristics of cancer patients, shows that most of the patients were women, which is related to the highest prevalence being of breast cancer.

Table 2 shows that, of the 102 cancer patients undergoing chemotherapy, as many as 70 subjects (68.6%) had good family support, while poor family support was observed in 32 subjects (31.4%).

Table 3 shows that, of the 102 cancer patients undergoing chemotherapy, as many as 67 subjects (65.7%) were highly likely to use the Problem-Focused Coping (PFC) strategy, while the remaining 35 subjects (34.3%) were less likely to use the PFC strategy.

Table 4 shows that, of the 102 cancer patients undergoing chemotherapy, as many as 71 subjects (69.6%) were less likely to use the Emotion-Focused Coping (EFC) strategy, while the remaining 31 subjects (30.4%) were highly likely to use the EFC strategy.

Table 1. Characteristics of cancer patients undergoing chemotherapy (n = 102).

No	Characteristics	Freq.	(%)
1	Age (Years)		
	26–45 (Adult)	32	31.3
	46–65(Pre-elderly)	58	56.9
	>65 (Elderly)	12	11.8
2	Sex		
	Male	39	38.2
	Female	63	61.8
3	History of chemotherapy		
	1–3	65	63.7
	>3–6	37	36.3
4	Cancer type		
	Breast cancer	45	44.1
	Colorectal cancer	27	26.5
	Ovarian cancer	15	14.7
	Nasopharyngeal cancer (NPC)	13	12.7
	Prostate cancer	2	2.0
	Total	102	100

Table 2. Frequency distribution of family support (n = 102).

Family support	Freq.	(%)
Good	70	68.6
Poor	32	31.4
Total	102	100

Table 3. Frequency distribution of the Problem-Focused Coping (PFC) strategy (n = 102).

PFC strategy	Freq.	(%)
High	67	65.7
Low	35	34.3
Total	102	100

Table 4. Frequency distribution of the Emotion-Focused Coping (EFC) strategy (n = 102).

EFC strategy	Freq.	(%)
High	31	30.4
Low	71	69.6
Total	102	100

Table 5. Frequency distribution of anxiety at Dr. Pirngadi General Hospital, Medan, in 2017 (n = 102).

Anxiety	Freq.	(%)
Severe	2	2.0
Moderate	53	52.0
Mild	47	46.0
Total	102	100

Table 5 shows that, of the 102 cancer patients undergoing chemotherapy, as many as 53 subjects (52.0%) experienced moderate anxiety, and only 2 subjects (2.0%) experienced severe anxiety.

This study showed that there was a significant association with PFC strategy ($p < 0.05$). The value of 0.612 for the correlation coefficient (r) indicated a strong positive correlation, which means that subjects receiving better family support were more likely to use the PFC strategy. Similarly, a significant association was observed with the EFC strategy ($p < 0.05$).

There was a significant association with anxiety ($p < 0.05$). The value of –0.646 for the correlation coefficient (r) indicated a strong negative correlation, which means that subjects receiving better family support experienced milder anxiety.

This study showed that family support is a dominant variable that is significantly associated with the use of the PFC strategy, with an Odds Ratio (OR) of 12.2, indicating that cancer patients undergoing chemotherapy with good family support are 12.2 times more likely to use the PFC strategy.

Family support is a dominant variable that is significantly associated with the use of the EFC strategy, with an OR of 0.142 (OR < 1 = negative association), indicating that cancer patients undergoing chemotherapy with good family support are 0.142 times more likely to not use the PFC strategy.

Family support is a dominant variable that is significantly associated with anxiety, with an OR of 0.039 (OR < 1 = negative association), indicating that cancer patients undergoing chemotherapy with good family support were 0.039 times more likely to experience mild anxiety.

4 DISCUSSION

4.1 *Association between family support and coping strategies in cancer patients undergoing chemotherapy*

A significant association between family support and the PFC strategy indicated a strong positive correlation, which meant that subjects receiving better family support were more likely to use the PFC strategy. A significant association between family support and the EFC strategy at Dr. Pirngadi General Hospital, Medan, indicated a moderate negative correlation, which meant that subjects receiving better family support were less likely to use the EFC strategy.

These findings are similar to a study by Tan (2007), which stated that there is an association between social support and coping strategies in cancer patients, with a positive correlation between social support and the PFC strategy and a negative correlation between social support and the EFC strategy. The support from all family members, particularly the spouse, greatly affected decision-making and survival strategies in managing emotions (emotional support), providing information on health, lifestyle and diet, as well as supporting the provision of facilities (instrumental support), which are very helpful for breast cancer patients undergoing therapy and help to increase the survival of cancer patients (Muhamad et al., 2011).

Potter and Perry (2009) stated that individual coping strategies are determined by the type of stress experienced by the individual, the individual's life goals, beliefs about oneself and the world, and personal individual resources. An individual tends to use the PFC strategy when he/she believes that the demands from a situation or stressor can be changed, and to use the EFC strategy when he/she believes that only little or no changes can be conducted with regards to the pressure of the situation. However, in a stressful situation, an individual generally combines the PFC and the EFC strategies (Sarafino & Smith, 2011).

Effective coping strategies when facing a chronic disease such as cancer, particularly for those undergoing treatment such as chemotherapy, will greatly affect the compliance of the patient in routinely attending chemotherapy sessions and the presence of physical and psychological symptoms. From the results of this study, it can be concluded that good family support is one of the personal resources that contribute to the effectively high use of the PFC strategy and the effectively low use of the EFC strategy, thereby increasing the compliance of cancer patients in undergoing chemotherapy.

4.2 *Association between family support and anxiety in cancer patients undergoing chemotherapy*

Subjects with better family support were more likely to experience lower anxiety levels. These findings are similar to a study by Lekka et al. (2014), which stated that there was a moderate negative correlation between family support and anxiety, which meant that better family support was associated with lower anxiety levels in lung cancer patients. Meanwhile, the study by Sadeghi et al. (2015) found that there was a moderate negative correlation between social support (emotional support, instrumental support and information support) and anxiety in patients undergoing haemodialysis. A study by Ng et al. (2015) stated that social support is an important factor for cancer patients undergoing treatment in order to decrease their anxiety levels and to increase their quality of life.

From the study results, it can be concluded that good family support for cancer patients undergoing intense, cyclic and long chemotherapy requiring repeated admissions, along with the physiological and psychological side effects that may appear, such as moderate anxiety, will help to decrease the anxiety levels and increase the quality of life and survivability of cancer patients.

4.3 *Variables dominantly associated with coping strategies in cancer patients undergoing chemotherapy*

These results are similar to the findings by Kim et al. (2010), which stated that social support for breast cancer patients is associated with the use of coping strategies. Nasir and Muhith (2011) stated that an effective coping strategy is one that helps an individual to tolerate and accept a psychologically stressful situation and ignore the stressors that cannot be managed.

From these results, it can be concluded that in a cancer patient undergoing intense, cyclic and long chemotherapy requiring repeated admissions, good family support will increase the compliance of the cancer patient in undergoing chemotherapy to increase the quality of life.

4.4 *Variables dominantly associated with anxiety in cancer patients undergoing chemotherapy*

This result showed that only family support had a significant negative association with anxiety, indicating that cancer patients undergoing chemotherapy with a lack of family support experienced severe anxiety.

The results are similar to that from a study by Aberha et al. (2016), which stated that the lack of social support in patients with hypertension was the factor most associated with anxiety. Social interaction plays a role in the adaptation of a patient towards a chronic disease. An individual with anxiety will show poor physical, cognitive and emotional responses and is at risk of maladaptive behaviour that will prevent the individual from learning various methods to alleviate anxiety, and therefore social support, particularly from the family, may influence the individual to form new adaptive behaviours to help him/her adapt and learn (Videbeck, 2008).

From the results, it can be concluded that in a cancer patient undergoing intense, cyclic and long chemotherapy requiring repeated admissions, good family support will help the patient to adapt and decrease their anxiety towards chemotherapy, in order to increase their quality of life.

5 CONCLUSIONS

From the study results, it can be concluded that family support is significantly associated with coping strategies (PFC and EFC) as well as with anxiety in cancer patients undergoing chemotherapy. It is hoped that the results of this study are used as an input for providing health education for the family members of patients on the importance of family support, which would increase the quality of life of the patients.

REFERENCES

Aberha, M., Gebeyehu, A. & Ayano, G. (2016). Prevalence and factors associated with anxiety among patients with hypertension on follow up at Menelik-II Referral Hospital, Addis Ababa Ethiopia. *Journal of Psychiatry, 19*(4), 378. doi:10.4172/2378–5756.1000378.

Karabulutlu, E.Y., Bilici, M., Cayir, K., Tekin, B.S. & Kantarci, R. (2010). Coping, anxiety and depression in Turkish patients with cancer. *European Journal of General Medicine, 7*(3), 296–302.

Kim, J., Han, Y.J., Shaw, B., McTavish, F. & Gustafson, D. (2010). The role of social support and coping strategies in predicting breast cancer patients' emotional well-being. *Journal of Health Psychology, 15*(4), 543–552. doi:10.1177/1359105309355338.

Lekka, D., Pachi, A., Tselebis, A., Zafeiropoulos, G., Bratis, D., Evmolpidi, A., … Syrigos, K.N. (2014). Pain and anxiety versus sense of family support in lung cancer patients. *Pain Research and Treatment, 2014*, Article ID 312941. doi:10.1155/2014/312941.

Muhamad, M., Afshari, M. & Kazilan, F. (2011). Family support in cancer survivorship. *Asian Pacific Journal of Cancer Prevention, 12*, 1389–1397.

Nasir, A. & Muhith, A. (2011). *Dasar-Dasar Keperawatan Jiwa; Pengantar dan Teori*. Jakarta, Indonesia: Salemba Medika.

Ng, G., Mohamed, S., See, H.M., Harun, F., Dahlu, M., Sulaiman, H.A. & Zainal, Z.N. (2015). Anxiety, depression, perceived social support and quality of life in Malaysian breast cancer patients: A 1-year prospective study. *Health and Quality of Life Outcomes, 13*, 205. doi:10.1186/s12955-015-040 1–7.

Potter, P.A. & Perry, A.G. (2009). *Fundamental Keperawatan [Fundamentals of nursing]* (Book 2, 7th ed.). Jakarta, Indonesia: Salemba Medika.

Prawirohardjo, S. (2010). *Buku Acuan Nasional Onkologi Ginekologi*. Jakarta, Indonesia: YBP-SP.

Sadeghi, H., Saeedi, M., Rahzani, K. & Esfandiary, A. (2015). The relationship between social support and death anxiety in hemodialysis patients. *Iranian Journal of Psychiatric Nursing, 2*(8).

Sarafino, P.E. & Smith, W.T. (2011). *Health psychology: Biopsychosocial interaction* (7th ed.). Hoboken, NJ: John Wiley & Sons.

Sastroasmoro, S. (2011). *Dasar-dasar metodologi penelitian klinis*. Jakarta, Indonesia: CV Sagung Seto.

Tan, M. (2007). Social support and coping in Turkish patients with cancer. *Cancer Nursing, 30*(6), 498–504. doi:10.1097/01.NCC. 0000300158.60273.ba

Videbeck, S.L. (2008). *Buku Ajar Keperawatan Jiwa*. Jakarta, Indonesia: EGC.

Stem Cell Oncology – Adella (Ed.)
© *2018 Taylor & Francis Group, London, ISBN 978-0-8153-9272-9*

Vitamin D supplementation in tuberculosis patients: A cross-sectional study

D.K. Sari & N.K. Arrasyid
Faculty of Medicine, Universitas Sumatera Utara, North Sumatera, Indonesia

R.L. Kusumawati
Epidemiology Graduate Programme, Faculty of Medicine, Prince of Songkla University, Hat Yai, Thailand

Y.S. Harahap
Teladan Community Health Service, North Sumatera, Indonesia

ABSTRACT: Previous studies have not been able to show with certainty the effect of vitamin D supplementation in tuberculosis patients. The objective of this study is to determine whether vitamin D supplementation to patients with tuberculosis could influence 25-hydroxyvitamin D (25(OH)D) and calcium serum levels. Results: after 28 days, the vitamin D supplementation showed significant increase of 25(OH)D serum level at the end point ($p = 0.001$), but not for the calcium serum level ($p = 0.3$). Conclusions: supplementation with 1,000 IU vitamin D per day increased the 25(OH)D serum level but there was no association with the calcium serum level. These results suggest a.

Keywords: Calcium, Tuberculosis, Vitamin D

1   INTRODUCTION

Vitamin D supports the induction of pleiotropic antimicrobial responses in tuberculosis patient, resulting from an immunomodulatory effect (Coussens et al., 2012). Vitamin D supplementation accelerates sputum smear conversion and enhanced tuberculosis treatment (Martineau et al., 2011; Siempos et al., 2008).

Vitamin D is also known to be essential to *Mycobacterium tuberculosis* containment and killing through the activation of 25-hydroxyvitamin D (25(OH)D) receptors, present in all immune cells (Liu et al., 2006).

Deficiency in vitamin D is found in healthy people, especially women in tropical countries (Sari et al., 2017a, 2017b). Low sunlight exposure, vitamin D intake, physical activity, and vitamin D receptor gene polymorphism are risk factors for vitamin D deficiency (Sari et al., 2017c). However, low 25(OH)D serum level does not affect calcium serum level (Sari et al., 2017d).

Calcium signalling in tuberculosis infection plays a significant role in the pathogenesis of tuberculosis (Sharma, 2017). Calcium is also known to be a ubiquitous second messenger, which can control multiple processes and is included in cellular activities like division, motility, stress response, and signalling. However, Ca is thought to be a regulative molecule regarding tuberculosis infection but its binding relation with proteins which are influenced by Ca concentrations in host pathogen (Chan, 2017).

We therefore conducted a clinical trial to determine the effect of 1,000 IU vitamin D for 28 days on the 25(OH)D and calcium serum levels.

2 METHODS

The objective of this study is to determine the effect of 1,000 IU per day vitamin D supplementation for 28 days on the 25(OH)D and calcium serum levels in tuberculosis patients who lived in three community health centre areas in Medan City, North Sumatera, Indonesia between June and September 2017. This is a randomised control trial involving 48 patients: 24 tuberculosis patients for vitamin D supplementation, and a placebo group.

The subjects of this study consisted of tuberculosis patients from community health centres with a higher tuberculosis prevalence, in Medan, North Sumatera, Indonesia. The 32 men and women studied had various occupations, and were sampled purposively. The inclusion criteria were tuberculosis patients in the age range of 18–60 years. Exclusion criteria were subjects with a history of diabetes mellitus, myocardial infarction, and renal or liver dysfunction. In addition to those exclusion criteria, subjects who were pregnant and lactating were also excluded.

We measured 25(OH)D serum concentration by Chemiluminescent Immunoassay (CLIA) technology (Diasorin, Stillwater, MN). Measures were between 4.0 and 150 ng/mL. The lowest value was 4.0 ng/mL, which is based on an inter-assay precision of 3.90% CV. Reference ranges were <20 ng/mL, categorised as deficiency, 20–30 ng/mL (insufficiency), and 30–100 ng/mL (sufficiency) (Holick, 2007). To convert ng/mL to nmol/L, multiply by 2.496. Calcium serum was measured by ADVIA Bayer Assayed Chemistry Controls, with principal procedure: calcium ions form a violet complex with o-cresolphthalein complexone in an alkaline medium. The reaction is measured at 545/658 nm, and normal concentration of calcium was 8.3–10.6 mg/dL.

Continuous variables were expressed as continuous variables as means ± standard deviations (SDs). Categorical variables were expressed as percentage proportions, using chi-squared to express significant differences between two groups, and the Fischer test if the data did not meet the criteria. Values of $p < 0.05$ were considered statistically significant. We used the SPSS program (version 11.5; SPSS Inc., Chicago, IL) to perform the analysis.

This study was carried out after ethical approval was obtained from the Health Research Ethics Committee of Sumatera Utara University Medical School (No. 264/TGL/KEPK FK USU-RSUP HAM/2017) and all participants gave written informed consent to the study procedures.

3 RESULTS

3.1 *Characteristics of subjects*

Table 1 shows the characteristics of the two groups, one receiving vitamin D supplementation and the other a placebo; there were no significant differences between the two groups.

Table 2 shows the difference before and after intervention in the intervention group. After supplementation, there was a significant increase in vitamin D intake, while there was no significant difference in any of the nutrient intakes in the control group.

Table 1. Demographic and lifestyle characteristics of subjects before intervention.

Characteristic	Intervention (D) group (n = 24)	Control (C) group (n = 24)	p-value
Age (years)	37 ± 2.5	33.8 ± 9.1	0.4
Body mass index (kg/m^2)	19.8 ± 3.9	20.3 ± 3.1	0.2
Serum 25(OH)D (ng/mL)	19.7 ± 6.6	19.3 ± 4.6	0.1
Serum calcium (mg/dL)	9.0 ± 0.5	9.1 ± 0.5	0.3

Table 2. Energy and nutrient intake of subjects before and after intervention in the D group.

Nutrient intake	Intervention (D) group (n = 24)		
	Before	After	p-value
Energy (kcal)	710.3	760.9	0.25
Protein (g)	25.4	28.3	0.10
Calcium (mg)	219.1	198.4	0.47
Vitamin D (μg)	**3.6**	**31.1**	**0.01**

Table 3. Mean serum 25(OH)D and calcium levels before and after intervention.

Variable	Baseline	Endpoint	p-value
Serum 25(OH)D (ng/mL)			
Intervention (D) group	19.7 ± 6.6	27.3 ± 3.1	**0.04**
Control (C) group	19.3 ± 4.6	21.9 ± 2.4	0.01
p-value		**0.01**	
Serum calcium (mg/dL)			
Intervention (D) group	9.0 ± 0.5	8.9 ± 0.3	0.34
Control (C) group	9.1 ± 0.5	8.9 ± 0.4	0.1
p-value		0.5	

Table 3 shows the difference before and after intervention in both groups. After supplementation, there was a significant increase in vitamin D intake, while there was no significant difference in any of the nutrient intakes in the control group.

4 DISCUSSION

Vitamin D helps the body to effectively absorb calcium; there is an interaction between vitamin and mineral. Calcium is known to be a ubiquitous second messenger that can control multiple processes, has a role in tuberculosis infection, and a significant role in pathogenesis.

Calcitriol, the active metabolite of vitamin D, induces innate antimicrobial responses and suppresses proinflammatory cytokine responses in vitro (Martineau, 2007). This microbial activity is mediated via induction of reactive nitrogen intermediates, reactive oxygen intermediates, antimicrobial peptides, and autophagy (Hewison, 2011). These studies report similar findings to previous studies of tuberculosis patients that found vitamin D deficiency (Martineau et al., 2011; Salahuddin et al., 2013). However, after vitamin D supplementation, baseline patients categorised in deficiency, resulting in greater weight gain and a more rapid radiographic clearing of disease, as compared to the placebo (Salahuddin et al., 2013; Sari et al., 2017d). The previous study showed that high dose of vitamin D (which in that study was 600.000 IU vitamin D intramuscular) accelerated clinical, radiographic improvement in all tuberculosis patients and increased host immune activation, but the study lasted 12 weeks (Salahuddin et al., 2013). In this study, the length was 28 days (4 weeks), and the tuberculosis patients received 1,000 IU oral vitamin D supplementation per day. However, this study also showed an increase of 25(OH)D serum level at the end point.

Hypercalcaemia found in tuberculosis patient; the previous study confirmed that serum calcium is raised in tuberculosis, but the effect may be reduced by a low calcium intake and a low parathyroid hormone level. Although the calcium and vitamin D metabolism appeared to be altered in tuberculosis, no direct relationship between serum calcium and 1,25(OH)2D, was found (Chan, 2017). Our study reported normal calcium serum levels and no significant difference before and after vitamin D supplementation. But we found that serum

Our study had limitations. We did not assess parathyroid hormone, nor other clinical tuberculosis parameters such as chest X-ray or blood examination (C-reactive protein).

5 CONCLUSION

From the study results, it can be concluded that in tuberculosis patients there were vitamin D deficiency and insufficiency, but the calcium serum level was normal. No association was found between 25(OH)D and calcium serum level.

ACKNOWLEDGEMENTS

The authors gratefully acknowledge that the present research is supported by the Ministry of Research and Technology and the Higher Education Republic of Indonesia, Research and Community Service, Universitas Sumatera Utara. The support is under the research grant TALENTA of the year 2017 Contract Number 212/UN5.2.3.1/PPM/KP-TALENTA USU/2017.

REFERENCES

Coussens, A.K., Wilkinson, R.J., Hanifa, Y., Nikolayevsky, V., Elkington, P.T., Islam, K., … Martineau, A.R. (2012). Vitamin D accelerates resolution of inflammatory responses during tuberculosis treatment. *Proceedings of the National Academy of Sciences*, *109*(38), 15449–15454.

Hewison, M. (2011). Antibacterial effects of vitamin D. *Nature Reviews Endocrinology*, *7*(6), 337–345.

Holick, M.F. (2007). Vitamin D deficiency. *The New England Journal of Medicine*, *2007*(357), 266–281.

Liu, P.T., Stenger, S., Li, H., Wenzel, L., Tan, B.H., Krutzik, S.R., … Modlin, R.L. (2006). Toll-like receptor triggering of a vitamin D-mediated human antimicrobial response. *Science*, *311*(5768), 1770–1773.

Martineau, A.R., Timms, P.M., Bothamley, G.H., Hanifa, Y., Islam, K., Claxton, A.P., … Griffiths, C.J. (2011). High-dose vitamin D3 during intensive phase treatment of pulmonary tuberculosis: A double-blind randomised controlled trial. *The Lancet*, *15*, 242–250.

Salahuddin, N., Ali, F., Hasan, Z., Rao, N., Aqeel, M. & Mahmood, F., (2013). Vitamin D accelerates clinical recovery from tuberculosis: Results of the SUCCINCT Study [Supplementary Cholecalciferol in recovery from tuberculosis]. A randomized, placebo-controlled, clinical trial of vitamin D supplementation in patients with pulmonary tuberculosis. *BMC Infectious Diseases*, *13*(1), 22.

Sari, D.K., Tala, Z.Z., Lestari, S., Hutagalung, S. & Ganie, R.A. (2017a). Vitamin D receptor gene polymorphism among Indonesian women in North Sumatera. *Asian Journal of Clinical Nutrition*, *9*(1), 44–50.

Sari, D.K., Tala, Z.Z., Lestari, S., Hutagalung, S. & Ganie, R.A. (2017b). Lifestyle differences in rural and urban areas affected the level of vitamin D in women with single nucleotide polymorphism in North Sumatera. *Asian Journal of Clinical Nutrition*, *9*(2), 57–63.

Sari, D.K., Tala, Z.Z., Lestari, S., Hutagalung, S. & Ganie, R.A. (2017c). Body mass index but not 25(OH)D serum is associated with bone mineral density among Indonesian women in North Sumatera: A cross-sectional study. *Asian Journal of Clinical Nutrition*, *9*(2), 37–43.

Sari, D.K., Tala, Z.Z., Lestari, S., Hutagalung, S. & Ganie, R.A. (2017d). Vitamin D supplementation in women with vitamin D receptor gene polymorphisms: A randomized controlled trial. *Asian Journal of Clinical Nutrition*, *9*(2), 89–96.

Sharma, S. & Meena, L.S. (2017). Potential of Ca in Mycobacterium tuberculosis HRv pathogenesis and survival. *Applied Biochemistry and Biotechnology*, *181*(2), 762–771.

Siempos, I.I., Vardakas, K.Z., Kopterides, P. & Falagas, M.E. (2008). Adjunctive therapies for community-acquired pneumonia: A systematic review. *Journal of Antimicrobial Chemotherapy*, *62*(4), 661–668.

Stem Cell Oncology – Adella (Ed.)
© *2018 Taylor & Francis Group, London, ISBN 978-0-8153-9272-9*

Effect of different media on Adipose-Derived Stem Cell (ADSC) proliferation

A. Rilianawati, Arifah Zahra, Sarah Imanissa & Subintoro
Centre of Pharmaceutical and Medical Technology, Agency for the Assessment and Application of Technology, Indonesia

B. Ago Halim
JMB Clinic, Jakarta, Indonesia

ABSTRACT: Currently, adult stem cells can be obtained not only from the spinal cord and peripheral vessels, but also from fat tissues of the human body, where they can be isolated as adherent stem cells: Mesenchymal Stem Cells (MSCs). Fat tissue is considered as the source of MSCs for autologous tissue engineering because it is readily available in abundant quantities through minimally invasive procedures, as well as being easily cultured and propagated. Further, the fat tissue is a type of Adult Stem Cell (ASC) that is capable of metamorphosis/ trans differentiation into various strains, because of its nature of high plasticity. Therefore, it is possible to proliferate in the desired direction of the network. The purpose of this research was to investigate the effect of different media on Adipose-Derived Stem Cell (ADSC) proliferation from human subcutaneous adipose tissue.

Keywords: Different Media, Adipose-Derived Stem Cells (ADSCs), Proliferation

1   INTRODUCTION

Mesenchymal Stem Cells (MSCs) are a prospective object for use in cell therapy and are intensely studied by many research groups. MSCs are characterised primarily by the expression of surface markers and differentiation potential. MSCs express a series of specific markers (e.g. CD44, CD90, CD105, and CD13) and should differentiate into cells of mesodermal origin, such as adipocytes, osteoblasts, and chondrocytes. Due to the prospective clinical application, MSCs from different sources are actively studied. For example, MSCs are isolated from the bone marrow and fat tissue (Musina et al., 2006). Because of the easily accessible anatomical location and the abundant existence of subcutaneous adipose tissue, Adipose-Derived Stem Cells (ADSCs) hold the advantage of allowing a simple and, above all, less invasive harvesting technique.

Adipose is a complex tissue: its constituents are mostly adult adipose cells (90%) and the stromal vascular fraction, which are pra adipocytes, fibroblasts, smooth muscle, endothelial cells, monocytes/macrophages, implicit, and ADSCs (Mizuno, 2012). ADSCs can be isolated from adipose tissue using the 'lipectomy' method. Almost 1×10^7 to 6×10^8 stem cells with >90% survival potency can be isolated from 300 ml. Lipectomy has been known as being a safe procedure and a well-tolerated method, with very little chance of complication (<0.1%) (Locke, 2009). Adipose tissue produced by lipectomy will be treated as medical waste (Kang, 2003). It has been known that adipose tissue can produce more stem cells than the other part (Mizuno, 2012).

The composition of mesenchymal stem cell culture media is one of the key factors in the process of stem cell expansion. Chen et al. (2009) compared the growth of MSCs using Dulbecco's Modified Eagle's Medium (DMEM) and Minimum Essential Medium (MEM) culture media. Experimental results based on stem cell proliferation after culturing for 21 days, showed that proliferation cell on MEM culture media is bigger than on DMEM culture medium. Nakamura et al. (2008) measured the growth rate of MSCs in Mesenchymal Stem Cell Basal Medium (MSCBM) and DMEM culture medium. The experimental results showed that MSCs cultured in both media showed relatively similar growth rates.

2 METHOD

2.1 Isolation of adipose-derived stem cells

Human ADSCs were isolated from fat tissue, which was obtained from JMB Clinic in Jakarta, Indonesia. The contaminating layers were removed, and the remaining adipose tissue was washed using an autoclaved phosphate-buffered saline (PBS). The washed adipose was transferred into a sterile tube; then enzyme digestion was used. The mixture was incubated in 5% CO_2 and 37°C incubator for an hour. The layers formed at the end of incubation time: an upper adipose layer and an infranatant of the enzyme. The upper layer was aspirated off, and the remainder was transferred into a new sterile tube.

The filtered infranatant was then centrifuged at 1,200 rpm for 10 minutes. The supernatant was discarded, and the pellet was collected. The pellet was resuspended in lysis buffer and was centrifuged at 1,200 rpm for 10 minutes. The Stromal Vascular Fraction (SVF) pellet was resuspended in 1 ml of culture media. Stem cells in SVF were seeded in 75 cm^2 flasks containing 10 ml of culture media. The cells were incubated in 5% CO_2 and 37°C incubator, and allowed to grow confluently.

2.2 Cell counting using haemocytometer

Stem cells were trypsinised, then plated to 96 well-plates after confluently. This process was initiated by removing the culture media from the flask, and adding 2 ml of PBS. The flask was gently shaken, and then the liquid was discarded. Stem cells were trypsinised with trypsin-EDTA. Subsequently, stem cells were incubated in a 5% CO_2 and 37°C incubator for 5 minutes. The culture media served as a stop solution to cease the trypsin activity.

Following the addition of stop solution, stem cells were transferred into a new tube and centrifuged at 1,200 rpm for 10 minutes at 20°C. The resulting supernatant was discarded, and the pellet was resuspended in culture media. A 10 μl volume was taken from the resuspended pellet and mixed with 10 μl of trypan blue. The mixture was loaded into a haemocytometer, and then counted under a microscope. The desired concentration of cells was 10^5 cells per 100 μl, for MTT assay.

2.3 Plating and culture of ADSCs

The ADSCs were plated on 96 well-plates for MTT assay. Stem cells were plated on 96 well-plates at 1×10^5 cells/well. The 96 well-plates were incubated in a 5% CO_2 and 37°C incubator for 24 hours to allow the stem cells to the adherent.

2.4 Analysis of cell proliferation

The cells were incubated for 0, 1, 2, 3, 4, 5, 6, 7, 8, 9, 24, 48, 72, 96, 120, 144, and 168 hours. Hence, MTT reagent was added directly to the cells, and the cells incubated. The insoluble coloured formazan was dissolved in sodium dodecyl sulfate (SDS) and incubated overnight. The cells were processed on an enzyme-linked immunosorbent assay (ELISA) reader for absorption at 595 nm.

3 RESULTS

3.1 *Isolation of ADSCs*

Adipose tissue is considered to be a rich source of stem cells, especially with the increased incidence of obesity in modern populations (Kuhbier et al., 2010). For example, 1 g of adipose tissue has a greater number of MSCs than 1 g of bone marrow (Kitagawa et al., 2006; Fraser et al., 2006). Isolation of ADSCs involves centrifugation, digestion, and filtration,

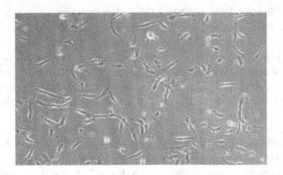

Figure 1.   ADSCs isolated using enzyme digestion.

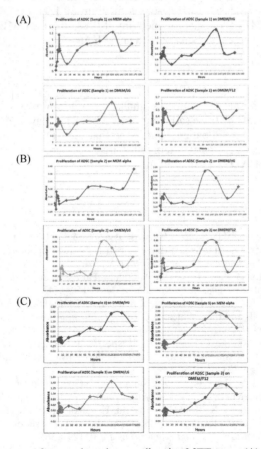

Figure 2.   Proliferation rates of mesenchymal stem cells using MTT assay: (A) Sample 1; (B) Sample 2; (C) Sample 3.

resulting in an adherent cell population containing MSCs. The digestion process involves collagenase enzyme, which has been known to act as a protease with specificity to degrade the triple-helical native collagen fibrils commonly found in connective tissue.

Figure 1 shows the ADSCs, which are isolated using enzyme digestion and incubated for four days, as observed under an inverted microscope. These cells were mostly detached, grew well, had normal spindle shape, and were fibroblastic.

3.2 *Effects of the different media on ADSC Proliferation*

The MTT results for Sample 1 shows that ADSC growth began to increase at 4 hours after incubation, with absorbance values: of 0.56 with MEM-alpha medium; 0.47 with DMEM/high-glucose medium; 0.47 with DMEM/low-glucose medium. However, the DMEM/F12 medium shows that the growth of ADSCs after 4 hours' incubation was 0.22, where ADSCs have not shown stable growth because ADSC growth is still increasing and decreasing. After 46 hours' incubation, ADSC growth shows a more stable growth rate. However, from the absorbance value it is found that ADSC growth with MEM-alpha medium is more stable compared to other culture media.

The MTT results for Sample 2 show that ADSC growth began to increase after 96 hours' incubation, with absorbance values: on MEM-alpha medium of 0.37; on DMEM/high-glucose medium of 0.64; on DMEM/low-glucose medium equal to 0.67; and on DMEM/F12 medium equal to 0.32. Measurement of proliferation in Sample 2 shows the growth of ADSCs has increased and decreased. It seems that ADSC proliferation is not stable and needs further study.

The MTT results for Sample 3 show that ADSC growth increased after 71 hours' incubation with absorbance values: on MEM-alpha medium of 1.30; on DMEM/high-glucose medium of 0.94; on DMEM/low-glucose medium of 0.88; and on DMEM/F12 medium of 0.65. Growth began to increase steadily over the next hour.

4 CONCLUSION

The absorbance value in Sample 2 appears smaller than in Samples 1 and 3. However, all three absorbance values of the three samples used varied. This may be due to the three samples being from different human/patient sources, so that the ADSC properties obtained also differ according to the character of the stem cell source. Further studies are required to investigate the metabolism of ADSC proliferation.

REFERENCES

Chen, H.H., Decot, V., Ouyang, J.P., Stoltz, J.F., Bensoussan, D. & De Isla, N.G. (2009). In vitro initial expansion of mesenchymal stem cells is influenced by the culture parameters used in the isolation process. *Bio-Medical Materials and Engineering*, *19*(4–5), 301–309.

Fraser, J.K., Wulur, I., Alfonso, Z. & Hedrick, M.H. (2006). Fat tissue: An underappreciated source of stem cells for biotechnology. *Trends in Biotechnology*, *24*(4), 150–154.

Kitagawa, Y., Korobi, M., Toriyama, K., Kamei, Y. & Torii, S. (2006). History of discovery of human adipose-derived stem cells and their clinical applications. *Japanese Journal of Plastic Reconstructive Surgery*, *49*(10), 1097–1104.

Kuhbier, J.W., Weyand, B., Radtke, C., Vogt, P.M., Kasper, C. & Reimers, K. (2010). Isolation, characterization, differentiation, and application of adipose-derived stem cells. *Advances in Biochemical Engineering/Biotechnology*, *123*, 55–105.

Musina, E.S., Bekchanova, E.S., Belyavskii, A.V. & Sukhikh, G.T. (2006). Differentiation potential of mesenchymal stem cells of different origin. *Bulletin of Experimental Biology and Medicine*, *141*(1), 147–151.

Nakamura, S., Yamada, Y., Baba, S., Kato, H., Kogami, H., Takao, M., ... Ueda, M. (2008). Culture medium study of human mesenchymal stem cells for practical use of tissue engineering and regenerative medicine. *Bio-Medical Materials and Engineering*, *18*(3), 129–136.

Thermo Fisher. (2013). Safety Data Sheets (SDS); Certificates of Analysis. Waltham, MA: Thermo Fisher Scientific. Retrieved from https://www.thermofisher.com/uk/en/home/technical-resources.html.

Stem Cell Oncology – Adella (Ed.)
© *2018 Taylor & Francis Group, London, ISBN 978-0-8153-9272-9*

Far lateral approach for removal of foramen magnum meningioma

R. Dharmajaya
*Department of Neurosurgery, Faculty of Medicine, Universitas Sumatera Utara, Medan,
North Sumatera, Indonesia*

ABSTRACT: Among the meningiomas of the posterior fossa, the Foramen Magnum (FM) meningioma deserves special consideration because of its characteristics in symptomatology, intriguing surgical anatomy, unique operative requirements, and outcome. When all meningiomas are considered, the FM meningioma has the worst outcome in terms of surgical results and operative morbidity. We report a 53-year-old female diagnosed as having FM meningioma, who had tumour removal surgery performed using a far lateral approach. Finally, a detailed technical operation and a classification system from various literature will also be explained.

Keywords: Foramen magnum meningioma, Far lateral approach

1   INTRODUCTION

Meningiomas represent 20% of all primary intracranial tumours and 75% of benign tumours of the Foramen Magnum (FM). However, FM meningiomas account for only 1.5 to 3.2% of all meningiomas (Bruneau & George, 2008; Bydon et al., 2014). FM meningiomas are categorised by their relative location to the medulla in the axial plane: anterolateral is the most common, posterolateral is the second most common, purely posterior lesions are the third, and the least common are entirely anterior (Bruneau & George, 2008; DeMonte et al., 2011). FM can be approached through transoral, suboccipital craniotomy, and far lateral approaches (Bruneau & George, 2008). For anterior midline, the FM meningioma transcondylar approach is preferred because it can give better visibility anterior to the brainstem, and also decreases the need for brainstem, cerebellar, and upper cervical retraction (Dobrowolski et al., 2016).

2   CASE REPORT

A 53-year-old female presented with chronic headache, numbness from the neck down, and weakness in both upper and lower extremities. Motor strength was 4 for all extremities and cape distribution of hypaesthesia was found. MRI showed a solid enhancing mass attached to the midline anterior FM, from the distal of clinoid to C1. The patient had undergone microsurgical resection (Simpson grade I) through a far lateral approach.

3   DISCUSSION

FM meningioma arises from the arachnoid at the craniospinal junction. The borders of this zone, as defined by George et al. (1997), range anteriorly from the lower third of the clivus, to the upper margin of the body of C2, laterally from the jugular tubercle to the upper margin of the C2 laminae, and posteriorly from the anterior edge of the squamous occipital bone to the C2 spinous process (George et al., 1997).

3.1   *Surgical anatomy*

When approximating FM meningioma, a precise affection of the normal anatomy is very important. Regional anatomy of the Vertebral Artery (VA) and the lower cranial nerves, and

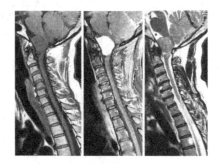

Figure 1.   MRI shows solitary mass, enhanced with contrast in cranio-cervical junction.

their displacement by space-occupying lesions, must be well recognised by the surgeon to ensure their protection.

The FM contains several critical neuroanatomical and vascular structures. The neural structures include the cerebellar tonsils, inferior vermis, fourth ventricle, caudal aspect of the medulla, lower cranial nerves (IX through XII), rostral aspect of the spinal cord, and upper cervical nerves (C1 and C2). (George & Lot, 1997; Kano et al., 2010).

Major arterial structures located within the FM include the VAs, Posterior Inferior Cerebellar Arteries (PICAs), anterior and posterior spinal arteries, and meningeal branches of the vertebral, external, and internal carotid arteries (George & Lot, 1997; Kano et al., 2010).

For an anatomic description, the VA is divided into four segments (Kano et al., 2010).

The first, 'pretransverse' (ostial, proximal) segment extends from its origin to the transverse process of the C6 vertebra (Kano et al., 2010).

The second 'transverse' segment runs inside the transverse processes of C6 through the axis (Kano et al., 2010).

Of special interest for surgery around the FM are the third and fourth segments. The V3 segment is also called the 'suboccipital segment' and extends from the transverse process of the axis to the dural penetration of the VA (Kano et al., 2010).

Anatomical relations of the VA are modified by head movements of rotation, as well as during surgical positioning. In neutral position, the vertical and horizontal portions of the V3 segment are perpendicular. On the contrary, after head rotation, as required during an anterolateral approach, both segments are stretched and run parallel, only separated by the posterior arch of the atlas, because the C1 transverse process is pushed anteriorly by this movement, away from the C2 transverse process. (Kano et al., 2010).

3.2   Classification system

The definitive objective of a classification system is to define preoperatively the surgical strategy, based on preoperative imaging characteristics of the lesion. The surgical strategy in cases of FM is the surgical approach, but also the anticipation of the modified vital structure position. In this classification system, FMs can be classified according to their compartment of development, their dural insertion, and to their relation to the VA (Komotar et al., 2010).

According to the compartment of development, FMs can be subdivided into: intradural, extradural, and intra-extra dural. According to the insertion on the dura, FM can be defined in the antero-posterior plane as: anterior, if insertion is on both sides of the anterior midline; lateral, if insertion is between the midline and the dentate ligament; and posterior, if insertion is posterior to the dentate ligament (Nader et al., 2014).

Surgical strategies vary according to the relation to the VA, FM having the possibility to develop: above the VA, below the VA, or on both sides of the VA (Nader et al., 2014).

3.3   Key steps of surgical procedure

The goal of this approach is to allow a tangential view of lesions located ventrally and ventrolaterally to the brainstem and upper cervical cord. This approach, along with control and

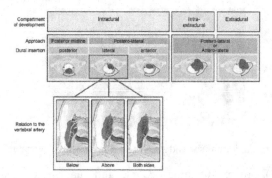

Figure 2. Classification of FM according to its location relative to the VA: below VA; above VA; on both sides of VA. Based on the compartment of development: intradural, extradural, or intra-extradural.

mobilisation of the VA, allows better visibility anterior to the brainstem, thus influencing favourably the safety and completeness of the operation. The advantages are: provides exposure of the lower third of the clivus, the FM, and the upper cervical spine; and decreases the need of brainstem, cerebellar, and upper cervical cord retraction, required to visualise the lower clivus and anterior FM (Pamir et al., 2010).

The patient is placed in the lateral recumbent position on the operating table, with the head positioned in the Mayfield holder. The head is laterally flexed −30 degrees, contralateral to the lesion, and flexed anteriorly so that the chin is 1 cm from the sternum.

The incision starts at the mastoid process, descending in a curve dorsal to the sternocleido-mastoid muscle and down to the level of C4. The dissection is carried through the subcutaneous tissues, the muscular fascia, and the fatty plane (Nader et al., 2014; Pamir et al., 2010).

Dissection through these anatomic layers, detaching each muscle from its lateral attachment, and displacing them medially and inferiorly, provides access to the transverse process of C1 and the lateral masses of the lower cervical vertebrae (Nader et al., 2014; Pamir et al., 2010).

By exposing the ipsilateral lamina of C2, and the posterior arch of C2, one can identify the VA with its venous plexus, located in the sulcus arteriosus lateral to the posterior arch of Cl, ventral to the C2 nerve root, and caudal to the inferior border of the inferior oblique muscle (Nader et al., 2014; Pamir et al., 2010).

A small craniotomy is performed with a high-speed drill, removing 1 cm of suboccipital bone from the FM. It is important to take this bony exposure far lateral to the junction with the occipital condyle. The posterior portion of the occipital condyle is drilled, while protecting the VA. The amount of resection of the condyle depends on the exact location (ventral or ventrolateral), size, nature of the lesion, the shape of the FM, and the relation of the VA to the lesion (Nader et al., 2014; Pamir et al., 2010).

A high-speed drill or rongeurs are used to remove the posterior arch of Cl. The foramen transversarium of Ct is unroofed with a drill. Using a subperiosteal dissection of the lamina and lateral mass, the VA is freed from the sulcus arteriosus of C1, and isolated to its entrance into the dura (Nader et al., 2014; Pamir et al., 2010).

Following isolation of the VA and appropriate bone removal, the dura is opened in a curvilinear fashion. The dural edges are retracted with sutures and the neurovascular structures are identified. The artery can be mobilised posteriorly and dissected from the lesion. After resection of the lesion, the dura can rarely be closed in a watertight fashion; therefore, a dural graft may be used (pericranium or fascia) and the defect covered with oxidised cellulose (Surgicel) and fibrin glue (Nader et al., 2014; Pamir et al., 2010).

3.4 *Outcomes and postoperative complications*

Yaşargil et al. (1980), in their review of the 114 operative cases reported in the literature between 1924 and 1976, found an operative mortality of approximately 13%, a good outcome in 69%, fair outcome in 8%, and a poor outcome in 10%. A low preoperative Karnofsky Per-

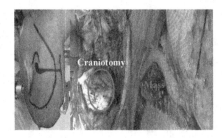

Figure 3. Plan of incision, craniotomy site and mass of the tumor with VA vertebral artery crossed over it.

formance Score (KPS), progressive clinical course, and quadriparesis were associated with increased operative risk and poor prognosis (Yaşargil et al., 1980). Recurrence is a major problem in skull base meningiomas (Yaşargil et al., 1980).

The most common complications are VA injuries, vertebral venous plexus bleeding (source of potential complication during surgery), neurologic disability from retraction of the neuraxis or arterial insult, delayed spinal cord and brainstem symptomatology from compromise of venous drainage, cerebral spinal fluid (CSF) leakage that leads to meningitis and pseudomeningocele, and C2 root neurapraxia from stretch injury (Pamir et al., 2010).

4 CONCLUSION

The far lateral approach has been used as the approach for the majority of the lesions located ventrolateral to the brainstem and in the upper cervical spinal cord. This approach pursues to remove the occipital bone, including the posterior aspect of the ipsilateral condyle and posterior arch of C1. Anatomical landmarks may be recognised for the neurosurgeon to avoid neurovascular injuries, especially to the VA and hypoglossal nerve.

REFERENCES

Bruneau, M. & George, B. (2008). Foramen magnum meningiomas: Detailed surgical approaches and technical aspects at Lariboisière Hospital and review of the literature. *Neurosurgical Review*, *31*(1), 19–33. doi:10.1007/sl 0143-007-0097-1.

Bydon, M., Ma, T.M., Xu, R., Weingart, J., Olivi, A., Gokaslan, Z.L., ... Bydon, A. (2014). Surgical outcomes of craniocervical junction meningiomas: A series of 22 consecutive patients. *Clinical Neurology and Neurosurgery*, *117*, 71–79.

DeMonte, F., McDermott, M.W. & Al-Mefty, O. (Eds.). (2011). *Al-Mefty's meningiomas* (2nd ed., pp. 297–307). New York, NY: Thieme.

Dobrowolski, S., Ebner, F., Lepski, G. & Tatagiba, M. (2016). Foramen magnum meningioma: The midline suboccipital subtonsillar approach. *Clinical Neurology and Neurosurgery*, *145*, 28–34.

George, B. & Lot, G. (1995). Foramen magnum meningiomas: A review from personal experience of 37 cases and from a cooperative study of 106 cases. *Neurosurgery Quarterly*, *5*(3), 149–167.

George, B., Lot, G. & Boissonnet, H. (1997). Meningioma of the foramen magnum: A series of 40 cases. *Surgical Neurology*, *47*(4), 371–379.

Kano, T., Kawase, T., Horiguchi, T. & Yoshida, K. (2010). Meningiomas of the ventral foramen magnum and lower clivus: Factors influencing surgical morbidity, the extent of tumour resection, and tumour recurrence. *Acta Neurochirurgica*, *152*(1), 79–86.

Komotar, R.J., Zacharia, B.E., McGovern, R.A., Sisti, M.B., Bruce, J.N. & D'Ambrosio, A.L. (2010). Approaches to anterior and anterolateral foramen magnum lesions: A critical review. *Journal of Craniovertebral Junction and Spine*, *1*(2), 86–99.

Nader, R., Gragnaniello, C., Berta, S.C., Sabbagh, A.J. & Levy, M.L. (2014). *Neurosurgery tricks of the trade. Cranial* (pp. 52–60). New York, NY: Thieme.

Pamir, M.N., Black, P.M. & Fahlbusch, R. (2010). *Meningiomas: A comprehensive text* (pp. 543–557). Philadelphia, PA: Saunders.

Yaşargil, M., Mortara, R.W. & Curcic, M. (1980). Meningiomas of basal posterior cranial fossa. In H. Krayenbühl (Ed.), *Advances and technical standards in neurosurgery* (pp. 3–115). Vienna, Austria: Springer-Verlag.

Stem Cell Oncology – Adella (Ed.)
© *2018 Taylor & Francis Group, London, ISBN 978-0-8153-9272-9*

The relationship between neck circumference and BMI with hypertension in children

S. Soraya & M. Lubis
Department of Paediatrics, Faculty of Medicine, Universitas Sumatera Utara, Medan, North Sumatera, Indonesia

I.I. Fujiati
Department of Public Health and Community, Faculty of Medicine, Universitas Sumatera Utara, Medan, North Sumatera, Indonesia

ABSTRACT: Hypertension is still becoming a global health problem. Body Mass Index (BMI) and Neck Circumference (NC) are anthropometric measurements to assess obesity, and are also reported to correlate with the risk of hypertension, to determine the relationship between NC, BMI, and hypertension in children. A cross-sectional study was conducted in North Sumatra, Indonesia. Samples were children aged 12–15 years old. The chi-square test was used to see the relationship between NC, BMI, and hypertension. Logistic regression was used to compare which one has a bigger influence on the increase in blood pressure. A p-value < 0.05 was significant. 264 children were included. Hypertension occurred in 9.8% of children with NC above the 90th percentile, and in 11.4% of children with overweight/obese BMI status. Children with overweight/obese BMI status showed a higher risk of hypertension. NC and BMI have been correlated with hypertension in children.

Keywords: Body Mass Index, Neck Circumference, Hypertension

1   INTRODUCTION

Obesity and being overweight are increasingly prevalent among children all over the world (WHO, 2015). Increased prevalence of obesity is also followed by an increase in comorbidity prevalence, such as hypertension, dyslipidaemia, and metabolic syndrome (IDAI, 2014; Mohammed, 2015; Haris & Tambunan, 2009).

The Body Mass Index (BMI) is an anthropometric index for assessing obesity in screening for regional body fat distribution (Androutsos et al., 2012), whereas the Neck Circumference (NC) is used to assess central obesity (Kuciene et al., 2015; Nafiu et al., 2014). The NC is also reported to have a positive correlation with the risk of hypertension and obesity (Nafiu et al., 2014; Hatipoglu et al., 2010; Guo et al., 2012).

2   METHODS

This study used cross-sectional design in Singkuang Village, North Sumatra. This research was conducted from March to May 2016. Inclusion criteria were all students of junior high school aged 12–15 years old, and parents signed the informed consent for research participation. The exclusion criterion was children with a deformity in the neck.

Body Weight (BW) was determined using the GEA body weight scale. Body Height (BH) was measured using a metal stadiometer. Next, BMI was assessed by using the BMI formula. NC was measured at the level of the thyroid cartilage, with the subject in the standing position and the head held erect. The measurements of the NC were projected on percentile for NC in Turkish children table for children aged six to 18 years. Then, a blood pressure measurement was performed using a mercury sphygmomanometer with cuff size adjusted to age. Blood pressure tables from *The Fourth Report from the NHBPEP Working Group on Children and Adolescents* (2004) were used.

Data processing used SPSS statistical software (version 19.0). Descriptive statistical analysis, mean and standard deviation (SD), was calculated for variables such as age, gender, weight, height, BMI, NC, and systolic and diastolic blood pressure. Univariate analysis was performed by using cross tabulation. Bivariate analysis was undertaken using chi-squared tests. Furthermore, multivariate analysis was analysed by using a logistic regression test.

3 RESULTS

There was a total of 278 students in both schools. The number of students in the junior high school was 170, and there were 108 students and in *pesantren*. There were 264 people eligible for the inclusion criteria, and 14 students were excluded from the study. The students who were excluded were made up of five students who were not present during the data collection, one student with a neck deformity, and eight students aged over 15 years.

Table 1 shows that the mean age of adolescents as subjects in the study was 13.8 years. Increased values of BMI, blood pressure, and NC were also found, but more in female subjects. Table 2 illustrates the relationship between risk factors such as age, gender, NC, and BMI, with blood pressure in subjects. There is a significant relationship between gender, NC, BMI, and increased blood pressure ($p < 0.05$). Table 3 shows the multivariate analysis. This suggests that BMI, gender, and NC variables jointly affected the increased blood pressure.

Table 1. Subject characteristics.

Characteristic	Boys $n = 123$	Girls $n = 141$	Total $n = 264$
Mean age, years (SD)	13.9 (0.95)	13.7 (1.04)	13.8 (1.00)
Mean weight, kg (SD)	39.8 (8.59)	42.2 (9.75)	41.1 (9.20)
Mean height, cm (SD)	149.0 (9.35)	144.6 (7.74)	146.4 (8.77)
NC, n (%)			
< P 90th	99 (37.6)	89 (33.8)	188 (71.2)
> P 90th	24 (8.7)	52 (19.8)	76 (28.8)
BMI, n (%)			
Underweight	27 (10.3)	22 (8.4)	49 (18.6)
Normal weight	83 (31.4)	62 (23.5)	145 (54.9)
Overweight	6 (2.3)	36 (13.7)	42 (15.9)
Obese	7 (2.7)	21 (8.0)	28 (10.6)
Blood pressure, n (%)			
Normal blood pressure	106 (40.3)	69 (26.2)	176 (66.70)
Pre-hypertension	12 (4.6)	38 (14.4)	50 (18.90)
Hypertension	4 (1.5)	34 (12.9)	38 (14.40)
Mean NC, cm (SD)	30.64 (2.44)	30.6 (2.33)	30.6 (2.37)
Mean BMI, kg/m^2 (SD)	17.8 (2.37)	20.5 (4.00)	19.1 (3.53)
Mean systolic, mmHg (SD)	102.1 (10.2)	109.7 (14.2)	106.1 (13.07)
Mean diastolic, mmHg (SD)	65.5 (7.46)	70.6 (9.97)	68.2 (9.21)

Table 2. The relationship between risk factors and hypertension.

Variable	Blood pressure		P	OR (95% CI)
	Normal blood pressure	Pre-Hypertension /Hypertension		
Age (years)				
12–13	74 (28.1)	36 (13.6)	0.860	1.05 (0.62–1.76)
14–15	102 (38.6)	52 (19.7)		
Gender				
Boys	107 (40.5)	16 (6.1)	0.001	6.97 (3.75–12.97)
Girls	69 (26.1)	72 (27.3)		
NC				
< P 90th	151 (57.2)	37 (14.0)	0.001	8.32 (4.57–15.14)
> P 90th	25 (9.5)	51 (19.3)		
BMI				
Under-/Normal weight	159 (60.2)	35 (13.3)	0.001	14.16 (7.33–27.33)
Overweight/Obese	17 (6.4)	53 (20.1)		

*Chi-squared.

Table 3. The effect of NC, BMI, and gender with risk of pre-hypertension and hypertension.

	P	OR	95% CI
NC (P > 90th)	0.001	4.436	2.14–9.21
Overweight/obese	0.001	5.871	2.79–12.32
Girls	0.001	4.964	2.41–10.22

*logistic regression.

4 DISCUSSION

The study found that the average increase in systolic and diastolic blood pressure was higher in female than in male subjects. Increased values in BMI, blood pressure, and NC were also experienced more by female subjects. Gender can indirectly affect blood pressure, although this is still under review (Azhim et al., 2007). The results of this study are in line with the research conducted by Ejike et al., which found that the BMI of girls was greater than that of boys, and that it increases as their age progresses, causing an increase in blood pressure, with the diastolic blood pressure of girls being higher than that of boys (Ejike, 2011).

Gender difference results in different body size. Body size affects arterial haemodynamic function, which is also influenced by blood flow velocity that indicates the vascular resistance and the elasticity of the blood vessels, which ultimately will affect blood pressure (Azhim et al., 2007).

It was found that there was a significant correlation between increased BMI and blood pressure. The results of this study are consistent with a study in Egypt involving adolescents aged 11 to 19, which found a significant correlation between increased BMI and the incidence of hypertension in children (Abolfotouh et al., 2011). Obesity and being overweight are two of the major global challenges, and are risk factors for cardiovascular disease (Hendy et al., 2013). Pathophysiology of hypertension in obesity is a highly complex matter. Some of the major mechanisms to consider include insulin resistance and hyperinsulinaemia, both of which are present in obesity (Flynn, 2013).

The results of this study are in line with a cross-sectional study conducted in the United States, showing that NC alone, or along with being obese/ overweight, is correlated with increased risk of high blood pressure in children and adolescents (Kuciene et al., 2015).

Some epidemiological studies have shown a relationship between increased NC and high blood pressure in children and adolescents (Ferreti et al., 2015).

The mechanism that can explain the relationship between NC and cardiometabolic risk is still under review. A size of NC above the 90th percentile leads to an increase in subcutaneous body fat. That is responsible for the release of most of the systemic fatty acids, especially in obese individuals. High concentrations of free fatty acids increase as a marker of oxidative stress. This provokes vascular endothelial injury and may play a role in the development of hypertension (Guo et al., 2012; Ferreti et al., 2015; Mazicioglu et al., 2010).

There are limitations in this study. There are a number of other factors that may effect an increase in blood pressure, such as lifestyle and unhealthy eating habits (e.g. high salt intake), lack of physical activity/having a sedentary life, history of parents suffering from hypertension, cholesterol, sleep disturbances, and stress conditions not analysed in adolescents who are overweight and obese with hypertension. In conclusion, this study found that there was a relationship between NC and BMI with hypertension in children.

REFERENCES

Abolfotouh, M.A., Sallam, S.A., Mohammed, M.S., Loutfy, A.A. & Hasab, A.A. (2011). Prevalence of elevated blood pressure and association with obesity in Egyptian school adolescents. *International Journal of Hypertension, 4061*, 1–8.

Androutsos, O., Grammatikaki, E., Moschonis, G., Roma-Giannikou, E.R., Chrousos, G.P., Manios, Y., … Gantenbein, C. (2012). Neck circumference: A useful screening tool of cardiovascular risk in children. *Pediatric Obesity, 7*(3), 187–195.

Azhim, A., Akioka, K., Akutagawa, M., Hirao, Y., Yoshizaki, K., Obara, S., … Kinouchi, Y. (2007). Effect of gender on blood flow velocities and blood pressure: Role of body weight and height. In *Conference Proceedings IEEE Engineering in Medicine and Biology Society* (pp. 967–970). New York, NY: Institute of Electrical and Electronics Engineers.

Ejike, C.E. (2011). Blood pressure to height ratios as simple, sensitive and specific diagnostic tools for adolescent (pre) hypertension in Nigeria. *Italian Journal of Pediatrics, 37*(1), 30.

Ferreti, R.L., Cintra, I.P., Passos, M.A.Z., Luis, G., Ferrari, G.L. & Fisberg, M. (2015). Elevated neck circumference and associated factors in adolescents. *BMC Public Health, 15*(1), 208.

Flynn, J. (2013). The changing face of pediatric hypertension in the era of the childhood obesity epidemic. *Pediatric Nephrology, 28*(7), 1059–1066.

Guo, X., Li, Y., Sun, G., Yang, Y., Zheng, L., Xingang, Z., … Li, J. (2012) Prehypertension in children and adolescents: Association with body weight and neck circumference. *Intern Med, 51*(1), 23–27.

Haris, S. & Tambunan, T. (2009). Hipertensi pada sindrom metabolik. *Sari Pediatri, 11*(4), 257–263.

Hatipoglu, N., Mazicioglu, M.M., Kurtoglu, S. & Kerdirci, M. (2010). Neck circumference: An additional tool of screening overweight and obesity in childhood. *European Journal of Pediatrics, 169*(6), 733–739.

Hendy, H., Sidiartha, I.G.L. & Nilawati, G.A.P. (2013). Obesity is associated with hypertension in adolescents. *Medicina, 44*(3), 150–156.

Ikatan Dokter Anak Indonesia (IDAI). (2014). Diagnosis, tatalaksana dan pencegahan obesitas pada remaja. UKK Nutrisi dan Penyakit Metabolik. Jakarta, Indonesia: Ikatan Dokter Anak Indonesia.

Juhász, M., Katona, E., Settakis, G., Paragh, G., Molnár, C., Fulesdi, B. & Páll, D. (2010). Gender-related differences in adolescent hypertension and in target organ effects. *Journal of Women's Health, 19*(4), 759–765.

Kuciene, R., Dulskiene, V. & Medzioniene, J. (2015). Association of neck circumference and high blood pressure in children and adolescents: A case-control study. *BMC Pediatrics, 15*, 1–10.

Mazicioglu, M.M., Kurtoglu, S., Ozturk, A., Hatipoglu, N., Cicek, B. & Ustunbas, H.B. (2010). Percentiles and mean values for neck circumference in Turkish children aged 6–18 years. *Acta Pediatrica, 99*(12), 1847–1853.

Mohammed, S.M. (2015). Childhood obesity: Epidemiology, determinants, and prevention. *Journal of Nutritional Disorders and Therapy, 5*(2), 1–4.

Nafiu, O.O., Zepeda, A., Curcio, C. & Prasad, Y. (2014). Association of neck circumference and obesity status with elevated blood pressure in children. *Journal of Human Hypertension, 28*(4), 263–268.

World Health Organization (WHO). (2015). *Interim report of the commission on ending childhood obesity*. Geneva, Switzerland: World Health Organization.

Stem Cell Oncology – Adella (Ed.)
© 2018 Taylor & Francis Group, London, ISBN 978-0-8153-9272-9

Trigeminal cardiac reflex in post-operative spheno-orbital meningioma

R. Dharmajaya
Faculty of Medicine, Universitas Sumatera Utara, Medan, North Sumatera, Indonesia

ABSTRACT: The Trigeminal Cardiac Reflex (TCR) is a phenomenon that is composed of bradycardia, arterial hypotension, apnoea, and gastric hypermobility. It mostly occurs during skull base surgery, at or around structures that are innervated by any sensory branch of the trigeminal nerve. We report a 48-year-old female who was diagnosed as having left spheno-orbital meningioma and had used a cranio-orbitozygomatic approach to remove the tumour. Six hours post-operatively, she had a sudden decrease in Heart Rate (HR), 31% decrease from baseline, and also a Mean Arterial Blood Pressure (MABP) decrease of 35% from baseline. Laboratory finding was normal, oxygen saturation was 100%, and no hyper-carbia occurred. She was suspected as having TCR. Intravenous administration of atropine abolished the reflex, and her HR and MABP slowly increased to normal.

Keywords: Spheno-orbital meningioma, Trigeminal cardiac reflex

1 INTRODUCTION

The Trigeminal Cardiac Reflex (TCR) happens in 10–18% of patients who have undergone skull base surgery (Gharabaghi et al., 2006). TCR leads to an immediate decrease in the Mean Arterial Blood Pressure (MABP) and Heart Rate (HR) of more than 20%, compared to the baseline levels with surgical-mechanical, electrical or chemical stimulation of the central part of any sensory branches of the trigeminal nerve, and to apnoea and gastric hypermobility coinciding with the surgical manipulation at or around any branch of the trigeminal nerve (Gharabaghi et al., 2006).

Since the 20th century, TCR has earned much clinical attention. The Oculocardiac Reflex (OCR) is the cardiac response (mainly bradycardia) associated with stimulation of the ophthalmic division of the trigeminal nerve during ocular surgeries (Schaller et al., 2009). Then, Schaller for the first time demonstrated that a similar reflex occurs with stimulation of the intracranial portion of the trigeminal nerve. Since then, much discussion has taken place about the reflex itself and treatment of TCR when it occurs during intracranial or extracranial procedures. Until now though, there has been no clear provision as to how to manage TCR.

2 CASE REPORT

A 48-year-old female presented with left proptosis bulbi as the chief complaint. This happened since six years. She could no longer see through her left eye, but its movement was still good. There was no history of headache, vomiting spit, convulsion, or one-sided paresis. She was diagnosed as having left spheno-orbital meningioma, and required a craniotomy tumour removal. A cranio-orbitozygomatic approach was used. She was transferred to intensive care for post-operative care with a stable haemodynamic profile. Six hours post-operatively, her HR suddenly decreased (baseline 80–88) to 55–60 beats per minute (31%

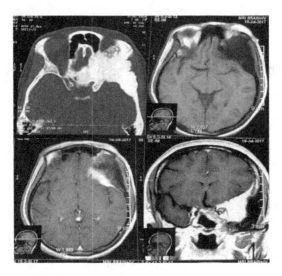

Figure 1.   Orbital CT, T1, T1 contrast, and T1 contrast coronal MRI scans of patient with spheno-orbital meningioma.

decrease). The ECG showed sinus rhythm. The MABP also decreased to 52 mmHg (baseline 80 mmHg; 35% decrease). Post-operative haemoglobin was 11 g/dL, central venous pressure was 12 mmHg, and other laboratory findings were normal. Her oxygen saturation was 100%, and no hypercarbia occurred. She was suspected of suffering TCR. Intravenous administration of atropine (2 mg) abolished the reflex, and HR and MABP slowly increased to normal.

3   DISCUSSION

The proposed mechanism for the development of TCR is that the sensory nerve endings of the trigeminal nerve send neuronal signals via the Gasserian ganglion to the sensory nucleus of the trigeminal nerve, forming the afferent pathway of the reflex arc (Schaller et al., 1999; Schaller, 2004). This afferent pathway continues along the short internuncial nerve fibres in the reticular formation to connect with the efferent pathway in the motor nucleus of the vagus nerve. Several lines of experimental evidence demonstrate that trigeminally induced cardiovascular reflexes could be mediated initially in the trigeminal nucleus caudalis and subsequently in the parabrachial nucleus, the rostral ventrolateral medulla oblongata, the dorsal medullary reticular field, and the paratrigeminal nucleus in animal models (Schaller et al., 2009).

TCR cases were defined as a drop in MABP and HR, both more than 20% from baseline levels, and had to fulfil at least two major criteria in plausibility and reversibility and two minor criteria in repetition and prevention, as described earlier by Schaller (Kumada et al., 1977). These points would help in clinical practice to assess whether the observed haemodynamic changes are related to a TCR phenomenon. In daily clinical practice, not all the criteria must or can always be required to confirm a TCR. However, the more of these criteria that are present, the more confirmed is a TCR.

3.1   *Type of TCR*

A central (proximal) TCR is triggered by the stimulation of the intracranial part of the trigeminal nerve, and thus upon the section which is located after the Gasserian ganglion. A peripheral (distal) TCR is therefore triggered by stimulation upon the extracranial course of the trigeminal nerve, distal to the Gasserian ganglion (Abdulazim et al., 2012). The peripheral

Table 1.   Major criteria (plausibility and reversibility) and minor criteria (repetition and prevention).

Evidence of TCR by Cause-Effect Relationship	
Plausibility	• The appearance of TCR must be explainable by an adequate stimulation of the trigeminal nerve. • TCR appears promptly after the stimulus is applied.
Reversibility	• Stimulus cessation abolishes the reflex, and cardiopulmonary parameters return to baseline.
Repetition	• Reapplication of the stimulus on cranial nerve V will result in similar haemodynamic changes.
Prevention	• A lighter stimulus of the same type does not result in the same severe TCR. • Trigeminal nerve block abolishes the TCR. • Application of anticholinergic drugs blocks the occurrence of the reflex.

Table 2.   The new classification of TCR.

Extended classification of TCR	Peripheral		Gasserian ganglion	Central
	Oculocardiac	Maxillo-mandibular		
Stimuli	Pressure on globe	V2 and V3 stimulation	Direct stimulation	Stimulation beyond ganglion
HR	Bradycardia	Bradycardia	Bradycardia/ tachycardia	Bradycardia
MABP	Hypotension/ normotension	Hypotension/ normotension	Hypotension/ hypertension	Hypotension
Respiration	Apnoea	Apnoea	Apnoea	Apnoea
Interventions	Strabismus surgery, intraocular injection, ocular trauma, acute glaucoma	Fracture reduction	Percutaneous ganglion ablation	CP angle, skull base tumours, trans sphenoidal cerebral aneurysm

TCR is further subdivided, based on the branch of the affected trigeminal nerve into the oculocardiac reflex (V1) and the maxillo-mandibular cardiac reflex (V2–V3). A TCR triggered at the Gasserian ganglion has, according to the latest studies (Abdulazim et al., 2012),.

3.2   Risk factor

As there is a lack of detailed knowledge of the physiology of TCR, the risk factors gain increased importance. The risk factors already known to increase the incidence of TCR include: (i) hypercapnia; (ii) hypoxaemia; (iii) light general anaesthesia; (iv) age (more pronounced in children); (v) the nature of the provoking stimulus (stimulus strength and duration); (vi) drugs (Schmeling et al., 1989; Blanc et al., 1983). Drugs known to increase TCR include: (i) potent narcotic agents (sufentanil and alfentanil) (Schmeling et al., 1989; Blanc et al., 1983); (ii) beta-blockers; (iii) calcium-channel blockers (Schmeling et al., 1989; Blanc et al., 1983).

3.3   Risk of TCR

Risk of TCR may range from mild bradycardia that responds to simple cessation of the stimulus to asystole and severe bradycardia requiring additional intervention with vagolytic drugs (Schmeling et al., 1989). In some rare but serious cases, it may lead to death if not detected early and appropriate measures taken. Also, hypotension that occurs during TCR may lead to myocardial and cerebral infarction in those who are at risk of these conditions (Schmeling et al., 1989).

3.4 *Management of TCR*

The best action in managing TCR is to prevent the risk factors above (Schaller, 2004). Intravenous anticholinergics, atropine and glycopyrrolate IV, may be used to treat and prevent TCR during operation (Hunsley et al., 1982). Hunsley et al. (1982) evaluated the efficacy of IV atropine and glycopyrrolate in the prevention of OCR in children operated on for strabismus. They tested different doses of the two drugs, glycopyrrolate 5 and 7.5 mg/kg and atropine 10 and 15 mg/kg. Overall, there was a reduction in the rate of bradycardia of between 23.8% and 33.3%. However, they noticed that even higher doses of the two drugs, atropine 15 mg/kg, and glycopyrrolate 7.5 mg/kg i.v., given five minutes before induction of anaesthesia, were not sufficient to protect completely against OCR in children (Hunsley et al., 1982).

4 CONCLUSION

TCR was defined as a drop in MABP and HR, both more than 20% from baseline levels, and had to fulfil at least two major criteria in plausibility and reversibility, and two minor criteria in repetition and prevention. The best management is prevention of the risk factor, and cholinergic agents are best to treat TCR during and post operation.

REFERENCES

Abdulazim, A., Stienen, M.N., Sadr-Eshkevari, P., Prochnow, N., Sandu, N., Bohluli, B. & Schaller, B. (2012). Trigeminocardiac reflex in neurosurgery – Current knowledge and prospects. In F. Signorelli (Ed.), *Explicative cases of controversial issues in neurosurgery* (pp. 3–18). Rijeka, Croatia: InTech. doi:10.5772/29607.

Arasho, B., et al. (2009). Management of the trigeminocardiac reflex: Facts and own experience. *Neurology India, 57*(4), 375–380.

Blanc, V.F., Hardy, J.F., Milot, J. & Jacob, J.L. (1983). The oculocardiac reflex: A graphic and statistical analysis in infants and children. *Canadian Anaesthetists' Society Journal, 30*(4), 360–369.

Gharabaghi, A., Koerbel, A., Samii, A., Kaminsky, J., Von Goesseln, H., Tatagiba, M. & Samii, M. (2006). The impact of hypotension due to the trigeminocardiac reflex on auditory function in vestibular schwannoma surgery. *Journal of Neurosurgery, 104*(3), 369–375.

Hunsley, J.E., Bush, G.H. & Jones, C.J. (1982). A study of glycopyrrolate and atropine in the suppression of the oculocardiac reflex during strabismus surgery in children. *British Journal of Anaesthesia, 54*(4), 459–464.

Kumada, M., Dampney, R.A. & Reis, D.J. (1977). The trigeminal depressor response: A novel vasodepressor response originating from the trigeminal system. *Brain Research, 119*(2), 305–326.

Schaller, B. (2004). Trigeminocardiac reflex. *Journal of Neurology, 251*(6), 658–665.

Schaller, B., Cornelius, J.F., Prabhakar, H., Koerbel, A., Gnanalingham, K., Sandu, N., ... Trigemino-Cardiac Reflex Examination Group (TCREG). (2009). The trigemino-cardiac reflex: An update of the current knowledge. *Journal of Neurosurgical Anesthesiology, 21*(3), 187–195.

Schaller, B., Probst, R., Strebel, S. & Gratzl, O. (1999). Trigeminocardiac reflex during surgery in the cerebellopontine angle. *Journal of Neurosurgery, 90*(2), 215–220.

Schmeling, W.T., Kampine, J.P. & Warltier, D.C. (1989). Negative chronotropic actions of sufentanil and vecuronium in chronically instrumented dogs pretreated with propranolol and/or diltiazem. *Anesthesia & Analgesia, 69*(1), 4–14.

Stem Cell Oncology – Adella (Ed.)
© 2018 Taylor & Francis Group, London, ISBN 978-0-8153-9272-9

Association between sedentary activities and parental obesity with childhood obesity

S.M. Lubis
Department of Child Health, Faculty of Medicine, Universitas Sumatera Utara,
H. Adam Malik General Hospital, Medan, North Sumatera, Indonesia

M. Fattah
Department of Molecular Biology, Prodia Widyahusada Laboratory, Jakarta, Indonesia

H.A. Damanik
Department of Internal Medicine, Faculty of Medicine, Universitas Sumatera Utara,
Medan, North Sumatera, Indonesia

Jose R.L. Batubara
Paediatric Endocrinology Division, Child Health Department, Faculty of Medicine,
University of Indonesia, Cipto Mangunkusumo Hospital, Jakarta, Indonesia

ABSTRACT: Across the world, the prevalence of overweight and obese children is high. The influences of several factors have been extensively described; this includes genetic, cultural, and environmental factors, such as sedentary activity in children. This study aims to determine the association between sedentary activities and parental obesity with obesity in children. A case-control study was carried out at ten elementary schools in Medan. The data about sedentary lifestyle and parental obesity was obtained by giving questionnaires to parents or guardians. Data was analysed by chi-squared tests, with $p < 0.05$ being considered as statistically significant. There were 212 children recruited, aged 6–12 years—105 children with obesity as the case group and 107 normal-weight children as a control group. This study found a significant association between parental obesity and sedentary activities with obesity in children ($p < 0.01$). It is important to make efforts to prevent obesity in children.

Keywords: Childhood obesity, sedentary behaviour, parental obesity

1   INTRODUCTION

In recent years, being overweight and obese have been increasing dramatically in many developing countries, particularly in urban settings and amongst high Socio-Economic Status (SES) groups. Overweight and obese children are likely to maintain their status into adulthood and are at higher risks of developing chronic diseases, such as hypertension, dyslipidaemia, type-2 diabetes, heart disease, stroke, gall bladder disease, osteoarthritis, sleep apnoea and respiratory problems, and certain cancers (Wang & Lim, 2012).

Obesity tends to run in families. Genetics plays a major role. A common explanation is that family members share a common attitude towards food, eating habits, and exercise. Children of heavier parents have been found to exhibit lower levels of physical activity, have a greater preference for high-fat foods, and a lower preference for healthier foods. The risk of obesity is low in children where neither parent is obese, greater when one parent is obese, and greatest when both parents are obese. An estimate says that heredity contributes about 5–25% of the risk of obesity (Kumar et al., 2010).

Obesity has been considered to result from lifestyle changes, especially in food consumption, physical activity, and sedentary tendencies, because the environment has grown more obesogenic in recent decades (Fuemmeler et al., 2013). The causes of children being over-weight and obese are complex. The decrease in physical activity and increased time spent in sedentary pursuits, such as television viewing and other electronic media use, are considered major contributors. With increasing levels of sedentary behaviour, there is reduced energy expenditure while energy intake remains unaltered. This will lead to a rising prevalence of overweight and obese children (Saliba, 2015). The objectives of this study were to determine the relationships between parental obesity and sedentary activities, with obesity in children.

2 METHODS

A case-control study was conducted in ten elementary schools in Medan, Sumatera Utara, Indonesia. Schools were selected from the school list, provided by the education department, by using simple random sampling. The case group was children with obesity and the control group was normal-weight children, aged 6–12 years. The study included a questionnaire for parents or guardians, and anthropometric measurements. The questionnaires requested information about the onset of obesity, date of birth, parental obesity, and sedentary behaviour.

Sedentary behaviour can be considered over multiple dimensions: time (amount of time spent in activity) and type (Must & Tybor, 2005). Respondents were asked to report the number of hours in a typical week over the past three months they spent watching television (including videos), and using a computer (including playing computer games and using the Internet). They were instructed to report leisure-time hours only and to exclude time spent on these activities at work or school. Respondents reported their weekly hours for sedentary activities in five categories: 5 or fewer, 6 to 10, 11 to 14, 15 to 20, or more than 20 hours (Shields & Tremblay, 2008). Children who were under steroid treatment, had chronic infection or disease, endocrine disorder, genetic disease, or short stature were excluded from this study. This study was approved by the Ethics Committee of the Medical School, University of Sumatera Utara, Medan, Indonesia. All children and parents gave written informed consent to the results of this study being used for scientific research purposes.

Anthropometric measurements included body weight (in kg), which was measured to the nearest 0.1 kg by a digital machine. Height (in cm) was measured to the nearest 0.1 cm by using a stadiometer. All instruments were validated following the manufacturer's protocol. Waist circumference (in cm) was determined at the midpoint between the iliac crest and lowermost margin of the ribs, by using a non-stretchable measuring tape while the child was in a standing position and after expiration. Body Mass Index (BMI) was calculated as weight (in kg) /height (in m) (Ogden & Flegal, 2010). Children who had a BMI of more than P95 based on age and gender-specific BMI (CDC Standards, 2000) were considered obese, and those who had a BMI of P3 to 85, by the same standards, were considered to have normal weight.

Data was analysed using SPSS software, version 24 (SPSS Inc., Chicago, IL, USA). Quantitative variables were expressed as mean ± Standard Deviation (SD). Descriptive statistics were used to analyse socio-demographic characteristics of the subjects. Anthropometric measurements between case and control groups were compared using student's t-test.

3 RESULTS AND DISCUSSION

There were 212 children recruited, aged 6–12 years, 105 children with obesity as the case group and 107 normal-weight children as the control group.

Characteristics of children in this study are shown in Table 1. Children in the case group had significantly higher levels of BMI and body weight. There was a significant association between age, body weight, height, waist circumference, and BMI, with nutritional status, $p < 0.05$. However, we did not find an association between sex and nutritional status.

Table 1. Characteristics of children in study.

	Case	Control	p
Age (years)	9.87 ± 1.49	9.17 ± 1.62	0.01
Sex: Male	67 (63.8)	64 (59.8)	0.55
Female	38 (36.2)	43 (40.2)	
Body weight (kg)	46.60 ± 10.44	27.90 ± 5.81	0.01
Body height (cm)	136.50 ± 9.90	130.68 ± 9.86	0.01
Waist circumference (cm)	76.39 ± 8.83	57.76 ± 6.96	0.01[†]
BMI (kg/m²)	24.73 ± 2.96	16.15 ± 1.48	0.01

BMI: Body mass index. Data are means ± SD, or percentages. Associations are considered significant when $p < 0.05$.

Table 2. Association between parental obesity and sedentary behaviour with BMI.

	Case	Control	p
Family history of obesity:			
Yes	72 (34.0)	26 (12.3)	0.01
No	33 (15.6)	81 (38.2)	
Sedentary lifestyles			
<5 hours	13 (6.1)	37 (17.5)	<0.001[†]
6–10 hours	11 (5.2)	45 (21.2)	
11–14 hours	10 (4.7)	14 (6.6)	
15–20 hours	34 (16.0)	6 (2.8)	
>20 hours	37 (17.5)	5 (2.4)	

[†]*Kolmogorov–Smirnov.*

There are many possible causes of obesity amongst children, and the scope to make causal inferences based solely on parental weight is limited. However, it seems reasonable to suggest that adult attitudes and behaviours that affect their weight are likely to influence their children's weight (McLoone & Morrison, 2012). Parental obesity has been identified as being a predominant risk factor for childhood obesity, probably owing to a combination of genetic, epigenetic, social, and environmental factors. Children with two obese parents have a higher risk of obesity than those with one or no obese parent (Svensson et al., 2011). Some recent studies have found a significant association between parental obesity with obesity in children (Bralić et al., 2005; Bahreynian et al., 2017; Devakumar et al., 2016). These results are consistent with our study; we reported the significant association between parental obesity and obesity in children ($p < 0.05$), and we found that the parental history of obesity was present for 72 (34%) of children with obesity and 33 (15.6%) of normal-weight children (Table 2).

Lifestyle changes in high-income countries have led to a decrease in the energy expenditure needed for daily life, and an increase in sedentary activities and weight gain. Sedentary behaviour is not simply a lack of physical activity but is also a cluster of individual behaviours, where sitting or lying is the dominant mode of posture and energy expenditure is very low; it is a multi-faceted behaviour that might take place at work, school, or home. Childhood and adolescence are crucial stages of development where lifestyle habits are formed and set (Al-Nakeeb et al., 2012).

Some studies reported a significant association between sedentary activities and obesity in children (Alqahtani et al., 2015; Shields & Tremblay, 2008). Other studies reported that normal-weight children spend less time in sedentary activities than children with obesity (Vilchis-Gil et al., 2015; Baruki et al., 2006; Kreuser et al., 2013). In our study, we also reported that most of the obese children had sedentary activities for more than 20 hours in a week; for normal-weight children, most of them had sedentary activities 6–10 hours a week. We found a significant association between sedentary activities and obesity in children (Table 2).

The American Academy of Pediatrics (2001) recommends some guidelines for parents regarding television use by children. These include a limitation of children's total media time to no more than one or two hours of quality programming per day, the removal of electronic media gadgets from children's bedrooms, discouraging television viewing for children younger than two years, monitoring of things children are doing with electronic gadgets, viewing programmes along with children and discussing the contents, and encouraging alternative entertainment for children, including reading, athletics, hobbies and creative play (Saliba, 2015).

Our study has several limitations. We use self-reported data for children's sedentary activities and parental obesity. However, the questionnaire has previously demonstrated satisfactory reliability and validity, and honest reporting was encouraged by ensuring confidentiality during data collection. The sedentary activities considered in this study were limited to screen-behaviours. Despite these limitations, our findings contribute to our understanding of the relationship between parental obesity, sedentary activities, and obesity amongst children.

Parents need to be involved in obesity prevention programmes. The health authorities need to launch public campaigns for the awareness of obesity amongst children and the importance of healthy nutrition and physical activity. Healthcare workers including family, doctors, and paediatricians, need to facilitate parental awareness of obesity. In addition, intervention studies are needed to establish the effectiveness of reducing obesity amongst children through increasing physical activity, in tandem with reducing sedentary behaviours, especially screen time.

4 CONCLUSION

This study shows a significant association between parental obesity and sedentary behaviour, with obesity in children. The reduction in childhood obesity is regarded as a public health priority, and our findings suggest that parental obesity and sedentary behaviour are responsible for childhood obesity. Family-based interventions are recommended to treat childhood obesity, aiming to change attitudes and behaviours towards food and physical activity within a family. Public health strategies to prevent childhood obesity by targeting overweight and obese parents are recommended to prevent childhood obesity.

ACKNOWLEDGEMENTS

We are grateful to the children who participated in our study, and to all fieldworkers and data personnel.

REFERENCES

Al-Nakeeb, Y., Lyons, M., Collins, P., Al-Nuaim, A., Al-Hazzaa, H., Duncan, M.J & Nevill, A. (2012). Obesity, physical activity, and sedentary behavior amongst British and Saudi youth: A cross-cultural study. *International Journal of Environmental Research and Public Health*, 9(4), 1490–1506.

Alqahtani, N., Scott, J. & Ullah, S. (2015). Physical activity and sedentary behaviors as risk factors of obesity among rural adolescents. *Journal of Child and Adolescent Behavior*, 3, 185.

Bahreynian, M., Qorbani, M., Khaniabadi, B.M., Motlagh, M.E., Safari, O., Asayesh, H. & Kelishadi, R. (2017). Association between obesity and parental weight status in children and adolescents. *Journal of Clinical Research in Pediatric Endocrinology*, 9(2), 111–117.

Baruki, S.B.S., Rosado, L.F.P.D., Rosado, G.P. & Ribeiro, R.D.C.L. (2006). Association between nutritional status and physical activity in Municipal Schools in Corumbá. *Revista Brasileira de Medicina do Esporte*, 12(2), 80e–84e.

Bralić, I., Vrdoljak, J. & Kovačić, V. (2005). Associations between parental and child overweight and obesity. *Collegium Antropologicum*, 29(2), 481–486.

Devakumar, D., Grijalva-Eternod, C., Cortina-Borja, M., Williams, J., Fewtrell, M. & Wells, J. (2016). Disentangling the associations between parental BMI and offspring body composition using the four-component model. *American Journal of Human Biology*, *28*(4), 524–533.

Fuemmeler, B.F., Lovelady, C.A., Zucker, N.L. & Østbye, T. (2013). Parental obesity moderates the relationship between childhood appetitive traits and weight. *Obesity*, *21*(4), 815–823.

Garver, W.S. (2011). Gene-diet interactions in childhood obesity. *Current Genomics*, *12*(3), 180–189.

Kreuser, F., Kromeyer-Hauschild, K., Gollhofer, A., Korsten-Reck, U. & Rottger, K. (2013). 'Obese equals lazy?' Analysis of the association between weight status and physical activity in children. *Journal of Obesity*, *2013*, 1–9.

Kumar, S., Raju, M. & Gowda, N. (2010). Influence of parental obesity on school children. *Indian Journal of Pediatrics*, *77*(3), 255–258.

McLoone, P. & Morrison, D.S. (2012). Risk of child obesity from parental obesity: Analysis of repeat national cross-sectional surveys. *The European Journal of Public Health*, *24*(2), 186–190.

Must, A. & Tybor, D.J. (2005). Physical activity and sedentary behavior: A review of longitudinal studies of weight and adiposity in youth. *International Journal of Obesity*, *29*, S84–S96.

Ogden, C.L. & Flegal, K.M. (2010). Changes in terminology for childhood overweight and obesity. *National Health Statistics Reports*, *25*, 1–5.

Saliba, M. (2015). Obesity and sedentary behaviour in children and their implications in adulthood. *The Journal of the Malta College of Family Doctors*, *4*, 11–15.

Shields, M. & Tremblay, M.S. (2008). Sedentary behaviour and obesity. *Health Reports*, *19(2)*, 19–29.

Svensson, V., Jacobsson, J.A., Fredriksson, R., Danielsson, P., Sobko, T., Schiöth, H.B. & Marcus, C. (2011). Associations between severity of obesity in childhood and adolescence, obesity onset, and parental BMI: A longitudinal cohort study. *International Journal of Obesity*, *35*(1), 46–52.

Vilchis-Gil, J., Galván-Portillo, M., Klünder-Klünder, M., Cruz, M. & Flores-Huerta, S. (2015). Food habits, physical activities, and sedentary lifestyles of eutrophic and obese school children: A case-control study. *BMC Public Health*, *15*(1), 1–8.

Wang, Y. & Lim, H. (2012). The global childhood obesity epidemic and the association between socio-economic status and childhood obesity. *International Review of Psychiatry*, *24*, 176–188.

Stem Cell Oncology – Adella (Ed.)
© *2018 Taylor & Francis Group, London, ISBN 978-0-8153-9272-9*

Use of C-Reactive Protein (CRP) and haematological score to predict positive blood cultures in sepsis

I.N.D. Lubis
Department of Immunology and Infection, London School of Hygiene and Tropical Medicine, UK

D.E.F. Liestiadi, E. Azlin & S. Nafianti
Department of Paediatrics, Faculty of Medicine, Universitas Sumatera Utara, Medan, North Sumatera, Indonesia

ABSTRACT: The diagnostic test C-Reactive Protein (CRP) and haematological scoring system provide results in a shorter time than cultures, and have been used to help to determine the diagnosis of neonatal sepsis. Objective: To evaluate the diagnostic value of CRP and haematological scoring systems in relation to positive blood culture results. The CRP test showed sensitivity and specificity of 92.8% and 62%, respectively. The haematological scoring system showed a sensitivity of 100% and specificity of 82.7%. Both the CRP and haematological scoring system were sensitive to prediction of positive blood culture. However, the haematological scoring system showed better specificity than CRP. Both tools can be used to assist in the diagnosis of neonatal sepsis in resource-limited settings.

Keywords: C-reactive protein, haematological scoring system, neonatal sepsis

1 INTRODUCTION

Sepsis is an infection (confirmed or suspected) evidenced by a systemic manifestation of the infection associated with haemodynamic changes and other clinical manifestations. Sepsis in neonates is classified into early-onset infection when it appears within the first 72 hours of life, and late-onset infection if infections occur after seven days of age (Gotoff, 2002; Shane et al., 2017). Premature infants are more vulnerable to infections, due to the impaired immune system, and sepsis becomes the second most common cause of neonatal death in preterm birth (Lawn et al., 2005; Shane & Stoll, 2014). The burden of neonatal sepsis varies between geographic region and income levels (Shane et al., 2017). In Indonesia, the incidence ranges between 20.7 and 38.7% (Zaidi et al., 2005).

The definitive diagnosis of neonatal sepsis is made by isolating the causative pathogens, commonly from blood cultures (Gotoff, 2002). Nevertheless, bacterial growth in culture requires time and it is not always possible to isolate the causative agents (Shane & Stoll, 2014). Other commonly used diagnostic tests include total and differential White Blood Cell (WBC) count, absolute and immature neutrophil counts, the ratio of Immature-to-Total neutrophils (IT ratio), Procalcitonin (PCT) and C-Reactive Protein (CRP) (Shane et al., 2017; Stocker et al., 2010; Canpolat et al., 2011). However, the availability of some of these tests is often limited to central hospitals. Another approach is to use a Haematological Scoring System (HSS), developed to facilitate the diagnosis of neonatal sepsis (Shane et al., 2017).

This scoring system incorporates different parameters, including leukocyte count, total neutrophil (polymorphonuclear cells, PMN) count, IT ratio, Immature-to-Mature neutrophil (IM ratio), total immature PMN, platelet count, and degenerative PMN. Each item is given an average weight of value 1 if it indicates an infection, and interpreted as having a sepsis when the score is ≥ 5, possible sepsis for a score of 3 to 4, and not having a sepsis for a score below 2 (Pal et al., 2014; Narasimha & Kumar, 2011).

The aim of this study is to evaluate the diagnostic value of CRP and HSS in relation to blood culture results for the diagnosis of neonatal sepsis.

2 METHOD

Patients were neonates admitted to the Neonatology Unit at Haji Adam Malik General Hospital, Medan, between April and August 2015. Neonates suspected of sepsis were examined, and had performed laboratory tests including complete blood count, IT ratio, IM ratio, PMN and degenerative PMN, CRP and blood culture. The laboratory results were then evaluated to calculate the score in the haematological scoring system. The score was then compared to the CRP value and against the blood culture results. Diagnosis of sepsis was made by physicians based on physical examination and laboratory results before blood culture results. Written informed consent was obtained from the parents or legal guardians. The study was approved by the Ethics Committee of the University of Sumatera Utara, Indonesia.

3 RESULTS

A total of 154 neonates were treated in the Neonatology Unit during the study period. Amongst them, 51 were suspected of sepsis and 43 were enrolled in the study. The incidence of suspected neonatal sepsis in the study was 33.1%.

CRP was positive in 24 (55.8%) out of 43 neonates, and blood cultures demonstrated bacterial growth in 13 neonates (Table 2). The sensitivity and specificity for CRP were 92.8% and 62%, respectively. The numbers of neonates with a haematological score above 4, suggesting a sepsis, were 19 (44.2%), with 14 neonates showing positive results in the blood cultures (Table 2). The sensitivity and specificity of the haematological scoring system were 100% and 82.7%, respectively.

Both positive results of CRP (OR 21.2; 95% CI 2.4–185.9; $P < 0.001$) and haematological scoring system (OR 3.8; 95% CI 1.8–8.1; $P < 0.001$) were highly associated with the positive results of the blood cultures.

Table 1. Patients' characteristics.

Characteristic	Confirmed sepsis* ($n = 14$)	Suspected sepsis ($n = 29$)
Female (%)	7 (50.0)	17 (58.6)
Gestational age (%)		
<37 weeks	6 (42.9)	20 (68.9)
≥ 37 weeks	8 (57.1)	9 (31.0)
Age on admission (%)		
<72 h	6 (42.9)	25 (86.2)
>72 h	8 (57.1)	4 (13.8)
Birth weight (%)		
<2500 g	2 (14.2)	20 (68.9)
2500–4000 g	12 (85.7)	9 (31.0)

*Confirmed sepsis is declared when blood culture is positive.

Table 2. Diagnostic value of CRP & HSS in relation to blood culture results.

	Blood culture		Sensitivity	Specificity	PPV*	NPV**
	Positive	Negative				
CRP						
Positive	13	11	92.8%	62%	54.1%	94.7%
Negative	1	18				
HSS						
Positive	14	5	100%	82.7%	73.6%	100%
Negative	0	24				

*PPV: Positive Predictive Value; **NPV: Negative Predictive Value.

4 CONCLUSIONS

The incidence of neonatal sepsis between April and August 2015 in Haji Adam Malik General Hospital was 33.1%. This study showed that the CRP and haematological scoring system were highly sensitive in predicting positive blood cultures, although the scoring system showed better specificity. With the lack of a more sensitive tool, such as PCT, to guide antibiotic use for patients with suspected sepsis in resource-limited settings, HSS has shown excellent sensitivity and specificity in predicting positive blood culture results.

REFERENCES

Canpolat, F.E., Yigit, S., Korkmaz, A., Yurdakök, M. & Tekinalp, G. (2011). Procalcitonin versus CRP as an early indicator of fetal infection in preterm premature rupture of membranes. *The Turkish Journal of Pediatrics*, *53*(2), 180–186.

Gotoff, S.P. (2002). Infections of the neonatal infant. In R.E. Behrman, R.M. Kliegman & H.B. Jenson (Eds.), *Nelson textbook of paediatrics* (16th ed., pp. 538–552). Philadelphia, PA: WB Saunders Company.

Lawn, J.E., Cousens, S., Zupan, J. & Neonatal Survival Steering Team. (2005). 4 million neonatal deaths: When? Where? Why? *The Lancet*, *365*(9462), 891–900.

Narasimha, A. & Kumar, M.H. (2011). Significance of hematological scoring system (HSS) in early diagnosis of neonatal sepsis. *Indian Journal of Hematology and Blood Transfusion*, *27*(1), 14–17.

Pal, K., Samanta, A.K. & Singh, R. (2014). A comparative study of early onset versus late onset neonatal sepsis with special reference to bacteriological, demographic and clinical profile. *International Journal of Current Research and Review*, *6*(3), 7–15.

Shane, A.L. & Stoll, B.J. (2014). Neonatal sepsis: Progress towards improved outcomes. *Journal of Infection*, *68*, S24–S32.

Shane, A.L., Sánchez, P.J. & Stoll, B.J. (2017). Neonatal sepsis. *The Lancet*, *390*(10104), 1770–1780.

Stocker, M., Fontana, M., El Helou, S., Wegscheider, K. & Berger, T.M. (2010). Use of procalcitonin-guided decision-making to shorten antibiotic therapy in suspected neonatal early-onset sepsis: Prospective randomized intervention trial. *Neonatology*, *97*(2), 165–174.

Zaidi, A.K.M., Huskins, W.C., Thaver, D., Bhutta, Z.A., Abbas, Z. & Goldmann, D.A. (2005). Hospital acquired neonatal infections in developing countries. *The Lancet*, *365*(9465), 1175–1188.

Stem Cell Oncology – Adella (Ed.)
© 2018 Taylor & Francis Group, London, ISBN 978-0-8153-9272-9

Differences in C-Reactive Protein (CRP) between depression levels in ischaemic stroke patients

S.N. Lubis
Department of Internal Medicine, Faculty of Medicine, Universitas Sumatera Utara, Medan, North Sumatera, Indonesia

W.H. Lubis
Department of Psychosomatics and Internal Medicine, Faculty of Medicine, Universitas Sumatera Utara, Medan, North Sumatera, Indonesia

I. Nasution
Department of Neurology, Faculty of Medicine, Universitas Sumatera Utara, Medan, North Sumatera, Indonesia

ABSTRACT: Post-Stroke Depression (PSD), characterised by mood abnormality, self-blame, and grief, is diagnosed in 40–72% of stroke patients. It can inhibit the healing of stroke patients and increase mortality rate. The aim is to investigate the difference in C-Reactive Protein (CRP) value between depression levels in ischaemic stroke patients. Forty-five consecutive ischaemic stroke patients at Adam Malik and affiliated hospitals had their CRP values assessed, and 15 days later, the Beck Depression Inventory (BDI) questionnaire was used to classify their depression levels. 51.1% of the PSD patients were men aged 60.71 ± 10.3 years old, and 64.4% were smokers and high school graduates. The mean CRP level in post-stroke patients with mild depression was 0.7 mg/dl, with moderate depression was 3 mg/dl, and with major depression was 9.4 mg/dl. There were significant differences in CRP value between depression levels in ischaemic stroke patients ($p = 0.001$). The highest CRP level occurred in cases of severe depression, followed by moderate depression, and then mild depression.

Keywords: BDI, CRP, Ischaemic Stroke, Post-Stroke Depression

1 INTRODUCTION

Depression is a mood disorder characterised by sadness, loss of interest or pleasure, guilt, trouble concentrating, disturbed sleep, change of appetite, and low energy. This problem can be chronic or recurrent (50–65%) and may disrupt a person's ability to perform daily activities. In severe cases, depression can cause a person to commit suicide (Canan et al., 2012).

Stroke is the second leading cause of death after coronary heart disease, and is a persistent source of disability worldwide. About 6.7 million people die from stroke every year, and it represents 12% of global deaths. As a disease associated with the ageing process, stroke prevalence has been rising significantly across the globe in recent years, especially in populations over 65 years of age (reaching approximately nine million people per year) (Van Eeden et al., 2015).

Post-Stroke Depression (PSD) is one of the most common stroke complications, characterised by mood abnormalities, self-blame, and sadness; it is diagnosed in 40–72% of stroke patients. PSD is a major factor that can inhibit the healing function of neurologic stroke patients and increase mortality. Depression will affect patient behaviours, such as medical rehabilitation, smoking, diet, medication adherence, and physical activity. Depression also affects physiological factors such as autonomic nervous system disorders and inflammation (Solnek & Seiter, 2002; Schuyler, 2000).

C-Reactive Protein (CRP) is an important biomarker in cardiovascular disease and ischaemic strokes. CRP concentrations increase rapidly in people with severe neurological deficits. Research by Wang et al. (2017) in China reported that CRP levels were positively correlated with the incidence of depression associated with dysfunction of the Hypothalamic-Pituitary-Adrenal (HPA) axis, the involvement of pro-inflammatory cytokines, such as TNF-α, IL-6, IL-1 and cortisol, which induce mood disorders that cause the symptoms of depression. The inflammatory cytokines circulating in the vessel may also decrease levels of serotonin and other neurotransmitters in the brain, and lead to depression (Winbeck et al., 2002; Kupfer et al., 2013; Craven et al., 1988; Valkanova et al., 2013). This study aims to determine the differences in CRP value between different levels of depression in patients with ischaemic stroke at Haji Adam Malik Hospital and affiliated hospitals (Universitas Sumatera Utara hospital and Pirngadi hospital).

2 METHODS

2.1 Data collection

This cross-sectional study of 45 consecutive PSD patients at Adam Malik Hospital and affiliated hospitals from April–July 2017 on ischaemic stroke patients, was based on history finding, neurological physical examination, and CT head scan. CRP levels were examined in patients with ischaemic stroke and then, on the 15th day, the Beck Depression Inventory (BDI) questionnaire was used to classify depression levels into mild, moderate and severe depression. The inclusion criteria were ischaemic stroke patients with depression, aged over 18 years old, and who had signed the informed consent. Ischaemic stroke patients were excluded from this study if they had a history of fever before onset, a history of blood disorders or malignancy, had used corticosteroids or anti-inflammatory drugs before, or had a previous history of depression.

2.2 Statistical methods

All data was analysed with SPSS statistical software (version 22). Demographic data was described as number and percentage. Data with normal distribution is reported as mean ± standard deviation, whereas with abnormal distribution is reported with the median value (minimum–maximum). Comparison of CRP levels between different levels of depression in ischaemic stroke patients is analysed using the Kruskal–Wallis test. When $p < 0.05$, it indicates a statistically significant value.

3 RESULTS

This study followed 45 patients who had met the inclusion criteria: 23 patients (51.1%) were male, and 22 patients (48.9%) were female; the mean age of all patients was 60.71 years. The majority ethnicity was Bataknese (71.1%). The majority of patients who became respondents in this study were entrepreneurs (37.8%), followed by retirees (17.8%), civil servants/soldiers (15.6%), and housewives (15.6%). The results of this study showed that 64.4% of patients were smokers and 35.6% were non-smoking patients. The mean Body Mass Index (BMI) of the respondents was 21.8 kg/m^2. The median value of serum CRP was 3.0 mg/dl, with a minimum value of 0.2 mg/dl and a maximum value of 21.6 mg/dl.

Based on the characteristics of research subjects in Table 1, it is known that there is no significant relationship between sex, age, ethnicity, occupation, education level, smoking status and BMI, with depression level in patients with ischaemic stroke, as indicated respectively by p-values of $p = 0.537$; $p = 0.909$; $p = 0.547$; $p = 0.850$; $p = 0.866$; $p = 0.066$; and $p = 0.271$.

Using the Kruskal–Wallis test, Table 2 shows that there was a significant difference of CRP value between different levels of depression in ischaemic stroke patients. CRP was highest in

Table 1. Characteristics of research subjects.

Characteristic	n = 45	p-value
Sex, n (%)		
Male	23 (51.1)	0.537
Female	22 (48.9)	
Age (mean ± SD)	60.71 ± 10.3	0.909
Ethnicity, n (%)		
Bataknese	32 (71.1)	0.547
Javanese	7 (15.6)	
Acehnese	6 (13.3)	
Occupation, n (%)		
Entrepreneur	17 (37.8)	0.850
Retiree	8 (17.8)	
Civil servant/Soldier	7 (15.6)	
Housewife	7 (15.6)	
Private employee	4 (8.9)	
Unemployed	2 (4.4)	
Education level, n (%)		
Senior High School	11 (24.4)	0.866
No School	10 (22.2)	
College	9 (20)	
Primary School	8 (17.8)	
Junior High School	7 (15.6)	
Smoking status, n (%)		
Yes	29 (64.4)	0.066
No	16 (35.6)	
BMI, median (min–max), kg/m^2	21.8 (17.7–27.2)	0.271
CRP, median (min–max), mg/dl	3.0 (0.2–21.6)	0.001

Table 2. Values of CRP for depression levels in ischaemic stroke patients.

Depression level	Median CRP (mg/dl)	Minimal CRP (mg/dl)	Maximal CRP (mg/dl)	P
Mild	0.7	0.2	3.0	0.001*
Moderate	3.0	0.8	19.3	
Severe	9.4	2.8	21.6	

*$p < 0.05$.

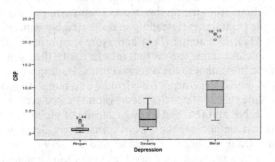

Figure 1. Boxplot comparison of CRP values between depression levels in ischaemic stroke patients.

patients with severe depression, followed by CRP with moderate depression, and then CRP with mild depression (p < 0.05).

4 DISCUSSION

PSD is a complication of stroke characterised by mood disorder, which will greatly affect the outcomes of the medical rehabilitation processes that patients will undergo. There will be an increased mortality, and a decrease in the quality of life associated with the inhibition of healing processes of neurology and daily activity in stroke patients (Wang et al., 2017; Zuidersma et al., 2011).

The results of this study showed that the median CRP levels in patients with post-stroke mild depression was 0.7 mg/dl, moderate depression was 3.0 mg/dl, and severe depression was 9.4 mg/dl. Using the Kruskal–Wallis test, there were significant differences of CRP value between different levels of depression in stroke ischaemic patients: CRP levels were significantly higher in severe depression, followed by moderate depression, and then mild depression, with p = 0.001.

The inflammatory process after the onset of ischaemic stroke has a complex role in the brain ischaemia. Induction of pro-inflammatory genes can occur very early after onset and may aggravate tissue damage. Acute phase response is an important mechanism of host reaction to tissue injury, which promotes the severity of organ involved through the mechanism of inflammation or thrombosis. This response is triggered by cytokines, and local defence cells such as microglia, which are activated and marked with the synthesis of acute phase proteins such as pro-coagulants and pro-inflammatories. CRP, globulin and fibrinogen are major acute phase proteins, which will trigger the collection/aggregation of erythrocytes. CRP will cause a decrease in the production of monoamine agents, affecting turnover of neurotransmitters (a decrease in serotonin, epinephrine, dopamine) and eventually resulting in behavioural changes, an impaired atmosphere, and the feeling and presentation of depressive symptoms (Miller et al., 2009; Shaikh et al., 2011; Ballantyne et al., 2015; Geng et al., 2016).

Wang et al. (2017) reported that CRP levels were positively correlated with the incidence of depression (r = 0.28 with p = 0.003) in 114 patients in China, associated with HPA dysfunction, involvement of pro-inflammatory cytokines, such as TNF-α, IL-6, IL-1 and cortisol, which cause a mood disorder resulting in the appearance of symptoms of depression. Increased inflammatory cytokines circulating in the circulation may also decrease levels of serotonin and other neurotransmitters in the brain, and trigger a depression condition (Valkanova et al., 2013; Wang et al., 2017).

A cross-sectional study by Brethour et al. (2011) in Alabama reported that high CRP levels at the time of ischaemic stroke were a significant predictive factor for the incidence of depression with p = 0.009, and decreased quality of life for patients with p = 0.002. Another study by McKechnie et al. (2010), involving 28 ischaemic stroke patients, showed that a median CRP of 16.04 mg/dl (7.12–36.14 mg/dl) was associated with PSD (p = 0.025) (Feng et al., 2014).

Emotional behaviour is governed by neurotransmitters such as monoamine, and monoamine dysfunction can cause various symptoms including depression. This hypothesis explains the location of the lesion being the pathogenesis of PSD. Cerebral lesions lead to disconnected ascending projections from the midbrain and brainstem, passing thalamus and basal ganglia, and reaching the frontal cortex, leading to decreased biogenic amine bioavailability, including serotonin (5-HT), Dopamine (DA) and Norepinephrine (NE), and resulting in depressive symptoms. The ischaemic lesions that interfere with the ascending axons contain biogenic amines from the brainstem to the cerebral cortex, leading to the decreased biogenic availability of amines in limbic structures of the frontal and temporal lobes, as well as in the basal ganglia. Monoamine theory states that depression is associated with low monoamine levels, in particular 5-HT, NE and DA, and the high density of global receptors for Monoamine Oxidase (MAO-A) that metabolises these neurotransmitters. Serotonergic and noradrenergic fibres, originating from the brainstem nuclei and conserving the limbic system, the prefrontal cortex, and other structures, are associated with mood regulation. The cholinergic system, through nicotinic acetylcholine receptors, is thought to be involved in the aetiology of major depression. Mesolimbic dopaminergic dysfunction can cause anhedonia. All of these pathways can be cut off by a stroke lesion, resulting in depression (Valkanova et al., 2013; Wang et al., 2017; Brethour et al., 2011).

5 CONCLUSION

There was a significant difference in CRP levels between different levels of depression in ischaemic stroke patients, in which cases, CRP levels were significantly higher in post-stroke severe depression, followed by moderate depression, and then mild depression.

REFERENCES

Ballantyne, C.M., Hoogeveen, R.C., Bang, H., Coresh, J., Folsom, A.R., Chambless, L.E., ... Boerwinkle, E. (2015). Lipoprotein-associated phospholipase A2, high-sensitivity C-reactive protein, and risk for incident ischemic stroke in middle-aged men and women in the Atherosclerosis Risk in Communities (ARIC) study. *Archives of Internal Medicine, 165*(21), 2479–2484.

Brethour, M., Albright, K.C., Vance, D.E., Alexandrov, A.V. & Alexandrov, A.W. (2011). The predictability of C-reactive protein, lipoprotein-associated phospholipase A2, and depression on later health outcomes in patients experiencing a first-time stroke. *Stroke, 43*(Suppl 1), A3253.

Canan, F., Dikici, S., Kutlucan, A., Celbek, G., Coskun, H., Gungor, A., ... Kocaman, G. (2012). Association of mean platelet volume with DSM-IV major depression in a large community-based population: The MELEN study. *Journal of Psychiatric Research, 46*(3), 298–302.

Craven, J.L., Rodin, G.M. & Littlefield, C. (1988). The Beck Depression Inventory as a screening device for major depression in renal dialysis patients. *The International Journal of Psychiatry in Medicine, 18*(4), 365–374.

Feng, C., Fang, M. & Liu, X.Y. (2014). The neurobiological pathogenesis of post-stroke depression. *The Scientific World Journal, 2014*, 521349. Retrieved from http://www.hindawi.com/journals/tswj/2014/521349/.

Geng, H.H., Wang, X.W., Fu, R.L., Jing, M.J., Huang, L.L., Zhang, Q., ... Wang, P.X. (2016). The relationship between C-reactive protein level and discharge outcome in patients with acute ischemic stroke. *International Journal of Environmental Research and Public Health, 13*(7), 636–640. doi:10.3390/ijerph13070636.

Kupfer, D.J., Regier, D.A. & Narrow, W.E. (Eds.) (2013). *Diagnostic and statistical manual of mental disorders* (5th ed.). Arlington, VA: American Psychiatric Association.

McKechnie, F., Lewis, S. & Mead, G. (2010). A pilot observational study of the association between fatigue after stroke and C-reactive protein. *The Journal of the Royal College of Physicians of Edinburgh, 40*(1), 9–12. doi:10.4997/JRCPE.2010.103.

Miller, A.H., Maletic, V. & Raison, C.L. (2009). Depression. *Biological Psychiatry, 65*(9), 732–741.

Schuyler, D. (2000). Depression comes in many disguises to the providers of primary care: Recognition and management. *Journal of the South Carolina Medical Association (1975), 96*(6), 267–275.

Shaikh, M.K., Makhija, P., Baloch, Z.A., Mughal, M.F., Devrajani, B.R., Shaikh, S. & Das, T. (2011). C-reactive protein in patients with ischemic stroke. *World Applied Sciences Journal, 15*(9), 1220–1224.

Solnek, B.L. & Seiter, T. (2002). How to diagnose and treat depression. *The Nurse Practitioner, 27*(10), 12–23.

Valkanova, V., Ebmeier, K.P. & Allan, C.L. (2013). CRP, IL-6 and depression: A systematic review and meta-analysis of longitudinal studies. *Journal of Affective Disorders, 150*(3), 736–744.

Van Eeden, M., Kootker, J.A., Evers, S.M.A.A., Heugten, C.M., Geurts, A.C.H. & Van Mastrigt, G.A.P.G. (2015). An economic evaluation of an augmented cognitive behavioural intervention vs computerized cognitive training for post-stroke depressive symptoms. *BMC Neurology, 15*(1), 266. doi:10.1186/s12883-015-0522.

Wang, Y., Zhen, Y.Z., Zhai, J.L., Wu, D., Liu, K.S., Zhao, Q.Z. & Liu, C. (2017). Depression is associated with increased C-reactive protein levels in patients with heart failure and hyperuricemia. *Journal of Geriatric Cardiology, 14*(4), 282–284. doi:10.11909/j.issn.1671-5411.2017.04.010.

Winbeck, K., Poppert, H., Ergen, T., Conrad, B. & Sander, D. (2002). Prognostic relevance of early serial C-reactive protein measurements after first ischemic stroke. *Stroke, 33*(10), 2459–2464.

Zuidersma, M., Thombs, B.D. & De Jonge, P. (2011). Onset and recurrence of depression as predictors of cardiovascular prognosis in depressed acute coronary syndrome patients: A systematic review. *Psychotherapy and Psychosomatics, 80*(4), 227–237.

Stem Cell Oncology – Adella (Ed.)
© 2018 Taylor & Francis Group, London, ISBN 978-0-8153-9272-9

Management of palpebral epidermoid cyst with Tenzel semicircular flap procedure

R.R. Lubis
Department of Ophthalmology, Faculty of Medicine, Universitas Sumatera Utara, Medan, North Sumatera, Indonesia

ABSTRACT: The epidermal cyst is a benign cyst that develops out of the ectodermal tissue. The epidermal cyst may have no symptoms. The definitive diagnosis is made after an excisional biopsy based on microscopic appearance. A 49-year-old woman presented with a painless left lower eyelid mass. Examination revealed a firm, globular mass that was fixed to the tarsal plate of the lower eyelid. An excisional biopsy was performed that revealed an epidermal cyst. As with epidermal cysts in other locations, surgical excision is the treatment of choice. The Tenzel semicircular flap procedure is selected for eyelid reconstruction in this case. Histopathologic sections demonstrated a cyst line by a squamous epithelium containing keratin, consistent with the diagnosis of an epidermal cyst. The moderately sized epidermal cyst of the lower eyelid was successfully managed by surgical excision using the Tenzel semicircular flap procedure, which gives the best outcome for palpebral epidermal cysts, especially those of moderate size.

1 INTRODUCTION

Epidermoid cysts represent the most common cutaneous cysts. While they may occur anywhere on the body, they occur most frequently on the face, scalp, neck, and trunk (Handa et al., 2002).

The term epidermal inclusion cyst refers specifically to an epidermoid cyst that is the result of the implantation of epidermal elements in the dermis (Aloi et al., 1993; Barr et al., 1986). Studies have suggested that Human Papillomavirus (HPV) and exposure to ultraviolet (UV) light may play a role in the formation of some epidermoid cysts (Egawa et al., 1998). Epidermal cysts are benign slow-growing tumours, resulting from the proliferation of epidermal cells. A cyst of the eyelid typically presents during adolescence and late adulthood, as a solitary, elevated, round, freely mobile subcutaneous mass with smooth overlying skin (Swygert et al., 2007).

Epidermoid cysts are usually asymptomatic; however, they may become inflamed or secondarily infected, resulting in swelling and tenderness (Braun-Falco, 2000). Here we are reporting a case of an epidermal cyst of the upper eyelid.

A reconstructed lid requires three main elements: an outer layer of skin, an inner layer of the mucosa, and a semirigid skeleton between the two. The lid should be well-opposed to the globe, with neither entropion nor ectropion. The tumours of the lid necessitate careful judgement and planning to provide the therapy. The choice of treatment depends on several factors. Among these are the type, size and location of the lesion, with particular emphasis on the possible involvement of any adnexal structures (Stewart, 1994).

2 CASE

A 49-year-old female patient visited H. Adam Malik Hospital with a left lower eyelid mass. The patient gave the history of this swelling for last two months, for which she had been treated elsewhere. There was no associated pain or redness. There was no history of any ocular trauma. On examination, the right upper eyelid showed a large round swelling of around 1.6 cm in diameter. On palpation, the swelling was well-defined, cystic but firm in consistency, and was free from skin and bony margins. There was no sign of inflammation, and the overlying skin was normal. The posterior segment was normal. Examination of the right eye was normal. We planned for the surgery, keeping in mind that the cyst was an epidermal cyst. Repair of lower eyelid defects involving the eyelid margin, and extending from two thirds of the horizontal length of the eyelid margin, require advancement of adjacent tissue to effect the closure.

The author's choice to repair defects of moderate size (size defect 33%–75%) is the Tenzel semicircular rotation flap procedure, with minimal disturbance of the periorbital tissues and provision for adequate lid support.

A pentagonal-wide excision was required to remove the mass, including the margin of the left lower eyelid.

Reconstruction of the lower eyelid commenced with a semicircular incision, beginning at the lateral canthus, then curving superiorly and temporally. The diameter of the flap was about 3 cm, or twice the size of the defect. The flap was undermined subcutaneous widely to allow closure. A lateral canthotomy was performed, and the inferior limb of the lateral canthal tendon, the orbital septum, and the retractors were severed to allow maximal rotation movement. The tarsus, grey line, lid border was closed. Closure the lid margin, the tarsus was closed with 5–0 VICRYL, 5–0 PROLENE was passed at the grey line, and skin with 6–0 PROLENE.

The lateral canthal angle newly formed lid was splinted with a deep 5–0 VICRYL. Enough tension should be placed on the lower eyelid to prevent laxity. The skin flap was anchored to the periosteum of the lateral orbital rim. The tissue of the lateral canthal was then sutured

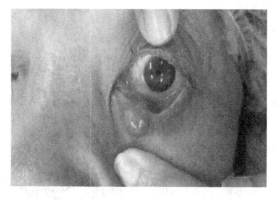

Figure 1.   A lower eyelid mass, 1.5 cm in diameter.

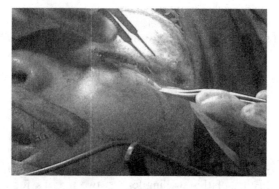

Figure 2.   Closure of the lateral canthal area.

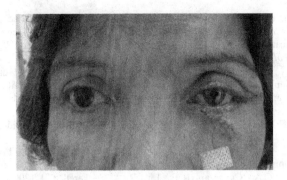

Figure 3. Five days after operation.

with 5–0 VICRYL and the skin closed at the lateral canthal area with 6–0 PROLENE. Antibiotic ointment was applied to the eye being operated upon. Two days after the operation, the patient was discharged from hospital.

Five days after the operation, the patient returned to H. Adam Malik Hospital. We evaluated the left eye. The sutures were good, there was no bleeding or pus, and the swelling of the inferior eyelid was reduced.

All sutures were removed after seven days, except for the lid margin sutures, which were left in place for 14 days. Histopathological examination revealed that the incised mass was an epidermal cyst.

3 DISCUSSION

Various mechanisms have been proposed for epidermoid cyst formation. It can be due to occlusion of the pilosebaceous follicles or surface epidermis, or can be due to implantation of epidermal elements that may be because of trauma or surgery. However, in recent studies human papillomavirus has been associated, but it is more commonly associated with epidermoid cysts of a plantar surface (Egawa et al., 2005).

The small asymptomatic epidermoid cyst can be managed with intralesional triamcinolone injection. Incision and drainage may be performed if a cyst wall is inflamed. Injection of triamcinolone into tissue surrounding the inflamed cyst results in faster improvement of the symptoms. However, it does not eradicate the cyst. The large symptomatic cyst should be excised in total, as in our case (Lucarelli et al., 2008).

4 CONCLUSION

A moderately sized epidermal cyst of the lower eyelid was successfully managed by surgical excision using the Tenzel semicircular flap procedure. The Tenzel semicircular flap procedure gives the best outcome for the palpebral epidermal cyst, especially for those of moderate size.

REFERENCES

Aloi, F., Tomasini, C. & Pippione, M. (1993). Mycosis fungoides and eruptive epidermoid cysts: A unique response of follicular and eccrine structures. *Dermatology, 187*(4), 273–277.
Barr, R.J., Headley, J.L., Jensen, J.L. & Howell, J.B. (1986). Cutaneous keratocysts of nevoid basal cell carcinoma syndrome. *Journal of the American Academy of Dermatology, 14*(4), 572–576.
Braun-Falco, O., Plewig, G., Wolff, H.H. & Burgdorf, W.H.C. (2000). Diseases of the sebaceous glands. In *Dermatology*. Berlin, Germany: Springer.

Egawa, K., Egawa, N. & Honda, Y. (2005). Human papillomavirus-associated plantar epidermoid cyst related to epidermoid metaplasia of the eccrine duct epithelium: A combined histological, immunohistochemical, DNA–DNA in situ hybridization and three-dimensional reconstruction analysis. *British Journal of Dermatology*, *152*(5), 961–967.

Egawa, K., Kitasato, H., Honda, Y., Kawai, S., Mizushima, Y. & Ono, T. (1998). Human papillomavirus 57 identified in a plantar epidermoid cyst. *British Journal of Dermatology*, *138*(3), 510–514.

Handa, U., Kumar, S. & Mohan, H. (2002). Aspiration cytology of epidermoid cyst of terminal phalanx. *Diagnostic Cytopathology*, *26*(4), 266–267.

Lucarelli, M.J., Ahn, H.B., Kulkarni, A.D. & Kahana, A. (2008). Intratarsal epidermal inclusion cyst. *Ophthalmic Plastic & Reconstructive Surgery*, *24*(5), 357–359.

Stewart, W.B. (1994). *Surgery of the eyelid, orbit, and lacrimal system* (Vol. 2). San Francisco, CA: American Academy of Ophthalmology.

Swygert, K.E., Parrish, C.A., Cashman, R.E., Lin, R. & Cockerell, C.J. (2007). Melanoma in situ involving an epidermal inclusion (infundibular) cyst. *The American Journal of Dermatopathology*, *29*(6), 564–565.

Stem Cell Oncology – Adella (Ed.)
© *2018 Taylor & Francis Group, London, ISBN 978-0-8153-9272-9*

The correlation between smoking and olfactory function using Sniffin' Sticks test

R. Lubis, D. Munir, S. Nursiah & H.R.Y. Herwanto
Department of Otolaryngology, Head and Neck Surgery, Faculty of Medicine,
Universitas Sumatera Utara, Medan, North Sumatera, Indonesia

ABSTRACT: This was an analytical observational study with a cross-sectional design, to determine the correlation between smoking and olfactory function. The population in this study is all employees, staff, residents, and family of patients present in the Ear, Nose and Throat Department, Haji Adam Malik Hospital in September 2016. Subjects had to be between 20–50 years old, currently smoking cigarettes, and not meet the following exclusion criteria: a medical history of recent viral infection, nasal/sinus surgery, nasal/brain tumours, head trauma, radiotherapy, chronic rhinitis in exacerbation, or tracheostomy. Out of 45 smokers, the proportion of olfactory dysfunction was 37.8%, while 62.2% did not suffer from olfactory dysfunction. The Threshold, Discrimination and Identification (TDI) score average was 30.80, with the lowest score average of 22.12 and the highest of 40. The results of this study indicate a significant correlation ($p < 0.05$) with olfactory dysfunction between the number of sticks per day and the number of years smoking.

Keywords: Smokers, Sniffin' Sticks

1 INTRODUCTION

The sense of smell is one of the several special senses that are essential for health (Shu et al., 2007). Olfactory disturbances can affect a person's safety (e.g. not being able to detect stale food, or smoke from a fire) and discomfort to the body itself, because the scent cannot be perceived, which sometimes affects the hygiene of a person (Hummel et al., 2010). Smoking is a risk factor for the smell dysfunction disorder. Many types of research suspected that there were side effects of smoking on the ability to sniff (Katotomichelakis et al., 2007).

The biological basis for decreased olfactory abilities associated with smoking is unclear. Inflammation and trigeminal stimulation due to exposure to cigarette smoke may inhibit the activation of the olfactory nerve and, in turn, odour perception. Long-term effects of smoking on the sense of smell may be caused by the influence of chemicals contained in cigarette smoke on the olfactory receptor cells in the olfactory mucosa. The role of apoptosis, the cellular mechanism responsible for the clearing of dead cells, can be triggered by a response to trauma. Some studies have shown an increase in apoptosis in olfactory nerve sinusitis and in ageing, but it is also found in animals exposed to tobacco smoke. Apoptosis is mediated by the caspase-3 enzymes, which show an increase in the epithelial activity of animals exposed to cigarette smoke, representing apoptotic cell death in the olfactory nerve. It has been mentioned as a cause of a loss of ability to smell (Katotomichelakis et al., 2007; Ishimaru & Fujii, 2007; Danielides et al., 2009).

The Sniffin' Sticks tools are an examination of nasal chemosensory function by using a pen-shaped tool that can emit odours. This examination consists of threshold scrubbing, discrimination of smell, and identification of smell. The result of these three subtests is the Threshold, Discrimination and Identification (TDI) score, which ranges from 0 to 48, with values ≤15 with anosmia, ≥ 30 for normosmia, and 16–29 for hyposmia (Orhan et al., 2011). This study aims to determine the correlation between smoking and olfactory function.

2   SUBJECTS AND METHOD

This research is an observational analytic research with the cross-sectional method to assess TDI for smokers at the Ear, Nose and Throat (ENT) polyclinic in Haji Adam Malik General Hospital, Medan, by using the Sniffin' Sticks extended test.

The research subjects chosen were smokers aged 20–50 years, performed history taking the procedure, routine examination of ENT, and who were willing to participate in the study by signing a letter of approval. The male and female inclusion criteria were: aged 20–50 years, having no sinonasal disease, no history of nasal trauma, no history of nasal surgery, no masses and polyps in the nasal cavity, and willing to participate in the study. The criteria for the exclusion of subjects was those who at the time of examination did not understand the instructions from the examiner.

3   RESULTS

Table 1 presents the results of the Sniffin' Sticks examination on all subjects. The mean of the subjects' threshold is 6.15 (SD = 3.48), with the smallest threshold value of 3.25, and the largest of 23.75. The mean discrimination value is 12.54 (SD = 2.32), with the smallest discrimination value of 3.8, and the largest of 16. The average identification value is 12.67 (SD = 1.72), with the smallest identification value of 7, and the largest of 15.5. The average value of TDI is 30.79 (SD = 3.54), with the smallest discrimination value of 22.12, and the largest of 40.

Table 2 presents the total mean number of sticks per day by subjects with olfactory dysfunction. There are as many as 11.06 sticks per day, with SD = 5.73 sticks per day. However, those subject groups who did not have any olfactory dysfunction had a mean total cigarette consumption of as many as seven sticks per day, with SD = 4.97 sticks per day. The mean score for number of years smoking in subjects with olfactory dysfunction is 10.41 years, with SD = 4.36 years. As for the group of subjects who did not have any olfactory dysfunction, the mean score for the number of years smoking is 7.21 years, with SD = 5.28 years. That is, the number of sticks per day p = 0.008 (p <0.05), and number of years smoking p = 0.007 (p < 0.05).

Table 1.   Olfactory function in relation to smoking.

	Mean	Median	SD	Min–Max
Threshold	6.15	5.25	3.48	3.25–23.75
Discrimination	12.54	13	2.32	3.8–16
Identification	12.67	13	1.72	7–15.5
Composite TDI score	30.79	31	3.54	22.12–40

Table 2.   Relationship between olfactory dysfunction and number of sticks per day and number of years smoking.

	Olfactory dysfunction		
	Yes	No	p*
Number of sticks per day, mean (SD)	11.06 (5.73)	7 (4.97)	0.008
Number of years smoking, mean (SD)	10.41 (4.36)	7.21 (5.28)	0.007

Based on the analytics using the Mann–Whitney test, it was found that there was a significant relationship between olfactory dysfunction and the number of sticks per day and the number of years smoking.

4 DISCUSSION

4.1 Olfactory function in relation to smoking

From this research, the average score of TDI is 30.80, with the lowest mean of 22.12 and the highest of 40. The same thing was also found in Katotomichelakis et al. (2007), where the numbers obtained were almost the same; that is, the average value of TDI in smokers is 36.3, the lowest 34.3, and the highest 38.3. Thus, in this study the scores of TDI subject smokers are still within the normal range.

4.2 Correlation between olfactory dysfunction and number of sticks per day and number of years smoking

The results of this study indicate that the average of the number of sticks per day is as much as 8.53 sticks, with the smallest consumption of two sticks, and the highest of 23 sticks. Katotomichelakis et al. (2007) found that the average number of sticks per day was 15 sticks, with a smallest number of five sticks, and a highest of 20 sticks.

The results of this study indicate that the average number of years smoking in the subjects is 8.42 years; the shortest consumption is two years and the longest is 23 years. In Japan, Katotomichelakis et al. (2007) found that the average number of years of smoking was ten, with a shortest time of one year, and a longest time of 45 years.

The results of this study indicate a significant correlation ($p < 0.05$) with olfactory dysfunction between the number of sticks per day and the number of years smoking. Frye et al. (1990) found that the correlation between olfactory dysfunction and number of sticks per day and number of years smoking, was statistically significant, with p-value of 0.03. The same was also reported by Da Silva and Panganiban (2006), who had a similar result in which the number of sticks per day and the number of years smoking had a significant correlation with olfactory dysfunction, with p-value of 0.019.

This is based on the fact that smoking has a dose–response relationship to the disturbance of smell (Vennemann et al., 2008). Long-term effects that can be caused by chemicals contained in cigarettes (acrolein, acetaldehyde, ammonia, and formaldehyde), can cause damage to receptors and mucous membranes, which occur in dose-related patterns (Frye et al., 1990).

5 CONCLUSION

This study proved that there was a statistically significant correlation ($p < 0.05$) with olfactory dysfunction between the number of sticks per day and the number of years smoking. A case-control comparison, the inclusion of older age groups, and a larger study population can further strengthen the understanding of the association between smoking and olfactory dysfunction.

REFERENCES

Da Silva, M.C.C. & Panganiban, W.D. (2006). A cross-sectional study on olfactory function among young adult smokers. *Philippine Journal of Otolaryngology Head and Neck Surgery*, *21*(1), 28–30.
Danielides, V., Katotomichelakis, M., Balatsouras, D., Riga, M., Tripsianis, G., Simopoulou, M. & Nikolettos, N. (2009). Improvement of olfaction after endoscopic sinus surgery in smokers and non-smokers. *Annals of Otology, Rhinology & Laryngology*, *118*(1), 13–20.
Frye, R.E., Schwartz, B.S. & Doty, R.L. (1990). Dose-related effects of cigarette smoking on olfactory function. *Journal of the American Medical Association*, *263*(9), 1233–1236.

Hummel, T., Pfetzing, U. & Lötsch, J. (2010). A short olfactory test based on the identification of three odors. *Journal of Neurology*, *257*(8), 1316–1321.

Ishimaru, T. & Fujii, M. (2007). Effects of smoking on odour identification in Japanese subjects. *Rhinology*, *45*(3), 224–228.

Katotomichelakis, M., Balatsouras, D., Tripsianis, G., Davris, S., Maroudias, N., Danielides, V. & Simopoulos, C. (2007). The effect of smoking on the olfactory function. *Rhinology*, *45*(4), 273–280.

Orhan, K.S., Karabulut, B., Keles, N. & Değer, K. (2011). Evaluation of factors concerning the olfaction using the Sniffin' Sticks test. *Otolaryngology—Head, and Neck Surgery*, *146*(2), 240–246.

Shu, C.H., Yuan, B.C., Lin, S.H. & Lin, C.Z. (2007). Cross-cultural application of the 'Sniffin' Sticks' odor identification test. *American Journal of Rhinology*, *21*(5), 570–573.

Vennemann, M.M., Hummel, T. & Berger, K. (2008). The association between smoking and smell and taste impairment. *Journal of Neurology*, *255*(8), 1121–1126.

Stem Cell Oncology – Adella (Ed.)
© 2018 Taylor & Francis Group, London, ISBN 978-0-8153-9272-9

The effect of andaliman fruit extract to blood glucose levels of mice with type 1 diabetes

M. Ridho
Faculty of Medicine, Universitas Sumatera Utara, Medan, North Sumatera, Indonesia

D. Lindarto
Department of Internal Medicine, Faculty of Medicine, Universitas Sumatera Utara, Medan, North Sumatera, Indonesia

ABSTRACT: Diabetes Mellitus (DM) is a disease for which treatment is expensive, therefore many researchers are looking for a cheap and effective treatment. The aim of this study is to evaluate the effect of andaliman fruit extract to blood glucose level of mice with type 1 diabetes. The study was conducted on 25 male mice. The mice were divided into five groups. Every group was injected with alloxan intraperitoneally and treated with aquades, andaliman extract and metformin for 15 consecutive days. The results showed that administration of andaliman extract with doses of 100, 200 and 300 mg/kg decreased the blood glucose levels significantly compared to the negative control group ($p \leq 0.05$). Andaliman extract of 100 and 200 mg/kg were not significantly different from the positive control group ($p \geq 0.05$). Blood glucose levels of mice with DM type 1 were decreased after andaliman extract was administered.

Keywords: andaliman fruit, type 1 diabetes mellitus, blood glucose level, alloxan

1   INTRODUCTION

Diabetes mellitus (DM) is a group of metabolic diseases characterised by hyperglycaemia which is caused by the disability of insulin secretion, insulin performance or both. Insulin is a hormone produced by beta cells in the pancreas which are needed to use glucose from digested food as a source of energy. Chronic hyperglycaemia in diabetes is associated with long-term damage, dysfunction or failure of several different organs, especially the eyes, kidneys, nerves, heart and blood vessels (American Diabetes Association, 2012).

The prevalence of DM is increasing rapidly worldwide and the World Health Organization has predicted that by 2030 the number of adults who suffer from diabetes will have increased twofold throughout the world, from 117 million people in 2000 to 370 million people. The experts observed that the incidence of diabetes will soar 65% by 2025, which means that 53.1 million people will be affected by this disease (Ozougwu et al., 2013).

The ability of developing countries to treat DM is doubtful because patent medicines for patients with DM are increasingly diverse. The cost for the treatment of diabetes is also more expensive and thus not affordable so funding and management that is cheap and effective are needed (Subroto, 2006, p. 16). The prevalence of the use of herbal medicines in conjunction with synthetic drugs is influenced by the relationship between demographic and socio-economic characteristics of the community. This is a powerful reason to examine the use of herbal medicines in health, including for people with DM (Adibe, 2009).

Andaliman fruit (Zanthoxylum acanthopodium DC) derived from the rutaceae family is a typical plant found in North Sumatra, Indonesia. The fruit is commonly used as a spice in traditional cooking of the Batak tribe (Siregar, 2002).

From the phytochemical test conducted by Tensiska (2001), it was found that andaliman fruit contains flavonoids and polyphenols that have antioxidant activity of through an antioxidant test with ransimat method. Flavonoids are also reported to have inhibitory activity against α-glucosidase enzymes. The activity of α-glucosidase inhibitors and antioxidants are the two things that affect DM (Suarsana et al., 2010). The seeds of most andaliman fruit are rich in oil that contains alkaloids in large quantities as well as unsaturated fatty acids which have antioxidant activity (Gupta and Mandi, 2013).

Therefore, andaliman fruit as a medicinal herb to treat DM will be examined.

2 METHOD

Twenty-five male mice weighing 20–35 g had fasted and weighed, fasting blood glucose level are measured, each mice induced by alloxan dose of 125 mg/kg bw intravenously. The mice were fed as usual, and their behaviour and body weight observed; they were considered diabetic when their fasting blood glucose levels ≥200 mg/dL (Ozougwu, 2013). The mice can be used for examination.

The rats were randomly divided into five groups. The negative control group was given aquades, the next group was given andaliman extract in quantities of 100, 200, 300 mg/kg bw and the positive control group was given 65 mg/kg bw of metformin. Each group consists of five rats. Every group was injected with alloxan intraperitoneally and treated for 15 consecutive days. The blood glucose level was observed with a glucometer on the 3rd, 6th, 9th, 12th and 15th days.

3 RESULTS AND DISCUSSION

The results of data analysis showed that there were significant differences between blood glucose level before and after induction of alloxan 125 mg/kg bw in all test groups ($p \leq 0,05$).

From the test results, the test group dose of 100, 200 mg/kg bw and positive controls show a decrease in blood glucose level from the third day and a decrease in the average blood glucose level to normal on day 15. The test group dose of 300 mg/kg bw and control negative did not show a decrease in blood glucose level on the third day; the blood glucose level in the test group dose of 300 mg/kg bw began to be seen on the 6th day and showed a decrease to the normal range on the 15th day. The negative control group showed an increase of blood glucose level on the 3rd, 6th and 9th days and a decline in blood glucose level on the 12th and 15th days.

The metformin dose of 65 mg/kg bw showed a decline of blood glucose level on the third day and a decrease in the average blood glucose level to normal on the 15th day. Provision of distilled water as a control group also decreased, but is still in the category of

Table 1.   Comparison of blood glucose level before and after induction of alloxan 125 mg/kg bw.

No	Test group	n	Blood glucose level before induction of alloxan Mean ± SD (mg/dL)	Blood glucose level after induction of alloxan Mean ± SD (mg/dL)	P Value
1	K(−)	5	112,6 ± 12,64	258 ± 44,74	0,001*
2	D1	5	69,6 ± 15,85	348,8 ± 115,28	0,003*
3	D2	5	67,4 ± 21,65	379,8 ± 132,59	0,006*
4	D3	5	94 ± 26,96	304,4 ± 67,60	0,003*
5	K(+)	5	114,6 ± 25,58	396,4 ± 121,88	0,009*
	Total	25			

*K(−) = Negative control group (aquades), D1 = andaliman fruit extract dose 100 mg/kg bw, D2 = andaliman fruit extract dose 200 mg/kg bw, D3 = andaliman fruit extract dose 300 mg/kg bb, K(+) = Positive control group (metformin dose 65 mg/kg bw).
*Significant ($p \leq 0,05$).

diabetes ($\geq$200 mg/dL). A decrease in blood glucose levels in the negative control group was supported by the regeneration of beta cells of Langerhans of the pancreas that are not broken down entirely so that they can secrete insulin (Diandra, 2011).

It is known that a dose of 100 mg/kg bw has the highest reduction percentage compared to the 200 and 300 mg/kg bw dose test group. Blood glucose level decreased at doses of 100 and 200 mg/kg bw and the positive control group did not differ much. On the 6th day, the dose of 300 mg/kg bw had the lowest reduction percentage compared to doses of 100 and 200 mg/kg bw.

Although blood glucose level reduction effects should strengthen with an increase in dose, the results of the analysis showed that increased doses of andaliman fruit extract were not followed by increased blood glucose level reduction effects in mice. This is presumably because it has saturated the receptors that it binds to in the interaction with bioactive chemical compounds contained in fruit andaliman. If the receptor has been saturated, the increased dose will not reach the maximum effect (Katzung, 2002).

Reduction of blood glucose level with andaliman fruit extracts can be caused by the presence of terpenoids, steroids and phenolic as well as their antioxidant activity. The result of identification with IR and UV-Vis showed that the main active compounds in the andaliman fruit are α-glucosidase inhibitors, antioxidants and flavonoids (class Auron) and flavanones (Gultom, 2011).

4 CONCLUSIONS

The results showed that andaliman fruit extract can lower blood glucose levels of mice models of DM type 1 induced by alloxan 125 mg/kg bw; and the andaliman fruit extracts dose of 100 mg/kg bw has the highest percentage reduction of blood glucose level.

Based on the results obtained from the studies that were conducted, further research is advised using larger samples and a variation of a larger dose and longer duration of administration to establish the optimal dose of andaliman fruit extracts that is antidiabetic. In addition, there should be further research to investigate the side effects of andaliman fruit extracts on the organs of mice in order to ascertain whether the andaliman fruit extract is safe for use as an herbal medicine.

REFERENCES

Adibe, M. O. (2009). Prevalence of concurrent use of herbal and synthetic medicines among outpatients in a mission hospital in Nigeria. *International Journal of Drug Development and Research, 1*(1), 66–60.

American Diabetes Association (ADA). (2012). Diagnosis and classification of diabetes mellitus. *Diabetes Care, 35*(1), 64–71.

Diandra. (2011). Pengaruh Pemberian Infusa Herba Sambiloto (*Andrographis paniculata Nees*) Terhadap Glibenklamid Dalam Menurunkan Kadar Glukosa Darah Tikus Putih Jantan Yang Dibuat Diabetes. *Skripsi*. Fakultas Matematika dan Ilmu Pengetahuan Alam UI. Depok.

Gultom, S. (2011). Flavonoid Buah Andaliman (Zanthoxylum acanthopodium DC) sebagai antioksidan dan inhibitor α-glucosidase. *Thesis*. Program Pascasarjana IPB. Bogor.

Gupta, D. D., & Mandi, S. S. (2013). Species specific AFLP markers for authentication of zanthoxylum acanthopodium & zanthoxylum oxyphyllum. *Journal of Medicinal Plants Studies, 1*(6), 1–9.

Hayati, F., Widyarini, S., & Helminawati. (2010). Efek antihiperglikemia infusa kangkung darat (*Ipomoea reptans* Poir) terhadap kadar glukosa darah mencit jantan yang diinduksi streptozotocin. *Jurnal Ilmiah Farmasi, 7*(1), 22–13.

Katzung, B. G. (2002). *Farmakologi dasar dan klinik*. Jakarta: Salemba Medika.

Kristanty, R. E., & Suriawati. J. (2014). Cytotoxic and antioxidant activity of petroleum extract of andaliman fruits (*Zanthoxylum acanthopodium* DC.). *International Journal of PharmTech Research, 6*(3), 1069–1064.

Ozougwu J. C., Obimba, K. C., Belonwu, C. D., & Unakalamba, C. B. (2013). The pathogenesis and pathophysiology of type 1 and type 2 diabetes mellitus. *Academic Journals, 4*(4), 57–46.

Piero, M. N., Nzaro, G. M., & Njagi, J. M. (2014). Diabetes mellitus—a devastating metabolic disorder. *Asian Journal of Biomedical and Pharmaceutical Sciences, 04*(40), 7–1.

Siregar, B. L. (2002). Andaliman (*Zanthoxylum acanthopodium* DC.) di Sumatera Utara: deskripsi dan perkecambahan. *Hayati, 10*(1), 40–38.

Suarsana, I. N., Priosoeryanto, B. P., Wresdiyati, T., & Bintang, M. (2010). Aktivitas Daya Hambat Enzim α-Glukosidase dan Efek Hipoglikemik Ekstrak Tempe pada Tikus Diabetes. *Jurnal Veteriner* 11(3), 195–190.

Subroto, M.A. (2006). *Ramuan herbal untuk diabetes mellitus*. Jakarta: Penebar Swadaya.

Tensiska. (2001). Aktivitas Antioksidan Ekstrak Buah Andaliman (Zanthoxylum acannhopodium DC) dalam Beberapa Sistem Pangan dan Kesetabilan Aktivitasnya Terhadap Kondisi Suhu dan pH. *Thesis*. Program Pascasarjana Universitas IPB. Bogor.

Yanling, W., Yanping, D., Yoshimasa, T., & Wen, Z. (2014). Risk factors contributing to type 2 diabetes and recent advances in the treatment and prevention. *Int. J. Med. Science, 11*(11), 1200–1185.

Stem Cell Oncology – Adella (Ed.)
© 2018 Taylor & Francis Group, London, ISBN 978-0-8153-9272-9

Association of birth weight and body mass index with cognitive function at Singkuang

M. Mardia, M. Lubis & I. Fudjiati
Department of Pediatric Medical School, Faculty of Medicine, Universitas Sumatera Utara, Medan, North Sumatera, Indonesia

ABSTRACT: Children with Low Birth Weight (LBW) have a generally increased incidence of neurological deficits or cognitive impairment during childhood compared with normal birth weight. Otherwise, that can affect cognitive function is a Body Mass Index (BMI). The purpose of this study was to determine the relationship between birth weight and BMI and cognitive function in children in primary school at Singkuang. A cross-sectional study was conducted in a primary school at Singkuang. The assessment of a child's cognitive function with the Mini Mental State Examination (MMSE). The results of this study indicate a significant association between birth weight and cognitive function ($P = 0.0001$). There is no relationship between BMI and cognitive function in children in primary school at Singkuang ($P = 0.356$).

There was a significant association between birth weight and cognitive function, and no association between BMI and cognitive function in children.

Keywords: body mass index, birth weight children, cognitive function

1   INTRODUCTION

Birth weight is considered to be one of the most important determinants of a child's health and survival and is seen as a good indicator of birth and lifelong health (Ayu, 2013). At present, one in ten infants in Indonesia are born with a low birth weight (LBW) of less than 2,500 grams. Previous research has shown that 35.6% of infants are born with a birth weight of less than 3,000 grams and 9.3% of infants with a birth weight of less than 2,500 grams (Karima, 2012).

Low birth weight babies (LBW) are still a problem in almost all countries. The World Health Organization (WHO) recorded that about 15% of live births in the world are LBW, with 6% of LBW incidence occurring in developed countries and 30% in developing countries (Simbolon, 2013). Based on the data of the number of babies born with LBW in 2007, LBW infants accounted for 295 out of 25,185 babies born. The incidence of LBW in hospitals in Indonesia is around 20%. In West Java regional referral centres each year record between 20–25% birth of LBW, while in rural areas the figure is 10.5%. In rural areas, most LBW die in the neonatal period (Risnah, 2009). Birth weight is considered to be one of the most important determinants of child health and survival and is seen as a good indicator of birth and lifelong health (Ayu, 2013). At present, one in ten infants in Indonesia is born under low birth weight (BBLR) is less than 2,500 grams. Previous research has shown that 35.6% of infants born with birth weight are less than 3,000 grams and 9.3% of infants born with birth weight less than 2,500 grams (Karima, 2012).

Low birth weight babies (LBW) are still a problem in almost all countries. WHO recorded about 15% of live births in the world are BBLR, 6% of LBW incidence in developed countries and 30% in developing countries (Simbolon, 2013). Based on the data of the number of babies born with BBLR in 2007, LBW infants accounted for 295 out of 25,185 babies born. The incidence of LBW in hospitals in Indonesia is around 20%. In West Java regional referral centres each year between 20–25% birth of **LBW**, while in rural areas 10.5%. In rural areas, most LBWs die in the neonatal period (Risnah, 2009).

According to **WHO**, **LBW** is closely related to neonatal mortality and morbidity, stunted growth and cognitive development, and chronic later disease (Setyo, 3013). Cognitive development consists of aspects of development including language and motor visual components (Dharmayanti, 2009). Cognitive function—often called cognition—is defined as a broad understanding of thinking and observing. In addition, cognitive function is also seen as a broad and inclusive concept that refers to the mental activities involved in the acquisition, processing, organisation and use of knowledge (Sayodi, 2016). Children with **LBW** exhibit lower academic scores than normal birth weight children, whose value is significant at the age of one year (Sherman, 2016).

Another factor which can affect cognitive function is body mass index (**BMI**). Measurements and assessments using **BMI** are associated with deficiency and excess of nutritional status (Adithya, 2016). Children with a low **BMI** for more than three years' experience an impairment of the development of cognitive function (Sherman, 2016). Referring from the results of the above research then conducted research on the relationship between birth weight and **BMI** with cognitive function in elementary schoolchildren in the Singkuang district.

2 MATERIALS AND METHOD

2.1 Population and sample

The study population is elementary schoolchildren in the village of Singkuang. The sample in this study is part of an affordable population that complies with the inclusion and exclusion criteria selected by consecutive sampling.

2.2 Data analysis

Data analysis was conducted by Chi-square to determine the relationship between categorical variables, with a significance level at $p < 0,05$. Data processing was through the use of a computer program.

3 RESULTS

The study was conducted in Singkuang village, Mandailing Natal Regency, North Sumatera. The total sample included in this study was 98 children who were in accordance with the inclusion and exclusion criteria. The female sex slightly dominated with a proportion of 33.3%.

The study also found that the majority of children have an underweight **BMI**. This study shows the association of birth weight with cognitive function in elementary schoolchildren in Singkuang village. The result of statistical test with a Chi-square test was a P value = 0.0001 which shows there is a significant correlation between birth weight with cognitive function in elementary schoolchildren in Singkuang village. In this study also showed relationship of

Table 1. Birth weight with cognitive function.

Birth weight	Cognitive function screening		Total	P Value
	Normal	Disturbance		
Normal	48	5	53	0,0001
Low	25	20	45	
Total	73	25	98	

Table 2. Body mass index with cognitive function.

Body mass index	Cognitive function screening		Total	P Value
	Normal	Disturbance		
Underweight	38	16	54	0,356
Normal	35	9	44	
Total	73	25	98	

BMI with cognitive function in elementary schoolchildren in Singkuang village. The result of statistical test with a Chi-square test was a P value = 0,356 where there is no correlation between BMI and cognitive function in elementary schoolchildren in Singkuang village.

4 DISCUSSION

This study showed that the percentage of LBW was higher than normal birth weight in elementary schoolchildren in Singkuang village. Previous research in Nepal has a relatively high prevalence of LBW, ranging from 14% to 32% (Maleqpour, 2004). The Ministry of Health of the Republic of Indonesia states that from 2005 to 2006 there was an increase in the prevalence of LBW by 24.3 per 1,000 live births to 25.9 per 1,000 live births. One of the main causes of high infant mortality is LBW (<2,500 grams). One of the efforts to try and tackle the problem of LBW is to assess the condition of the mother and various factors that affect her condition when pregnant. In general, level of education is a factor that affects birth weight, because the level of education can describe a person's level of knowledge about a matter related to health maintenance (Adi et al., 2015).

The study also found that the majority of children have an underweight BMI. In 2010, 3.7 million elementary schoolchildren had an underweight body mass. The majority of BMT underweight can be caused by risk factors from the development of body mass, one of which is that the problem of malnutrition is also higher in low income communities than people who have higher incomes. The nutritional deficiencies found in primary schoolchildren are lack of protein and less nutritional problems can not be overcome, especially in primary schools in poor and underdeveloped areas. A person's nutritional knowledge level affects attitudes and behaviours in choosing foods, which determine whether or not a person understands the nutritional benefits of the food consumed (Yudesti & Prayitno, 2013).

This study shows the association of birth weight with cognitive function in elementary schoolchildren in Singkuang village. The result of statistical test with Chi-square test was a P value = 0.0001 which shows there is a significant correlation between birth weight to cognitive function in elementary schoolchildren in Singkuang village. One of the effects of LBW is the slow growth of children seen in weight gain that does not reach normal levels when they are one year old. In addition, LBW is very susceptible to deficiencies and disturbances in the balance of various nutrients, making the child susceptible to permanent damage in physical and mental growth (Abadi et al., 2013). Many children who start life with a very LBW have problems when they start school. Other impacts of LBW include inability to focus on learning, visual-motor disturbance, answering skills of lower questions, and poor motor skills (Malekpour, 2004).

This study also showed the relationship of BMI to cognitive function in elementary schoolchildren in Singkuang village. The result of statistical test with Chi-square test was a P value = 0,356 where there is no correlation between BMI and cognitive function in elementary schoolchildren in Singkuang village. Lower BMI (underweight) and obesity tend to have lower cognitive scores (Julia et al., 2009). The results of this study may possibly be because the condition of cognitive function of children is influenced by environmental factors, including education in schools and community culture. This causes the child to be less motivated to learn new information and the potential of the child does not develop to the maximum, so not only the condition of cognitive function is influenced by the mass weight of the child.

101

5 CONCLUSION

From the results of this study it can be concluded that the initial screening of cognitive impairment with its relation to LBW and nutritional status is that there is a relationship between birth weight and cognitive function in elementary schoolchildren in Singkuang village with a P value 0.01; and no relationship between BMI and cognitive function in elementary school children in Singkuang village, with a P value 0.356.

REFERENCES

Abadi K, Wijayanti D, Ellen A, Erwina M, Sutrisna B. (2013). HipertensidanRisiko Mild cognitive impairment pada PasienUsiaLanjut. *Jurnal Kesehatan Masyarakat Nasional*, *8*, 119–124.

Adi S, Chundreyetti E, Yulistini. (2015). Faktorrisiko yang berpengaruhterhadapkejadianberatbadanlahirrendah di Rsupdr. M. Djamil Padang. *Jurnal Kesehatan Andalas*, *4* (3), 664–8.

Adithya A. Indeksmassatubuh (2016). http://eprints.undip.ac.id/44412/3/ADHITYA_PRADANA_22010110120064_BAB_2_KTI.pdf (Februari 6, 2016).

Ayu D, Trihandini I. Kehamilan yang. (2013). TidakDiinginkandanBeratBadanLahirBayi. *Jurnal Kesehatan Masyarakat Nasional*, *7*, 354–359.

Dharmayanti M, Herlina M. (2009). Skrininggangguankognitif fan bahasadenganmenggunakan *Capute Scales*. *Sari Pediatri J*, 11, 189–194.

Julia L, Mirnaw, Magda L. (2009). Cognitive and behavioral status of low birth weight preterm children raised in a developing country at preschool age. *Journal de Podiatrio*, 85.

Karima K, Endang L. (2012). Status gizidanberatbadanlahirbayi. *Jurnal Kesehatan Masyarakat Nasional*, *7*, 111–9.

Malekpour M. (2004). Low birth-weight infants and the importance of early intervention: Enhancing mother-infant interactions a literature review. *The British Journal of Developmental Disabilities*, *50*(2), 78–88.

Risnah. (2009). Hubungankadar hemoglobin plasma ibunifasdenganpanjangdanberatbadanbayilahir. *Jurnalkesehatan*, *2*, 35–42.

Setyo M, Paramita A. PolakejadiandandeterminanbayidenganBeratBadanLahirRendah (BBLR) di indonesiatahun 2013. BuletinPenelitianSistemKesehatan 2015, *18*, 1–10.

Shenlin S, Starr J, Rush M, Whalley L, Dewy I. (2016). *Birth weight and cognitive function at age 11 years: The Scottish mental survey*. Retrieved from http://adc.bmj.comlon.html (Februari 8, 2016).

Sherman T. (2016). *Low Birthweight and Developmental Delay: Research Issues in Communication Sciences and Disorder*. Retrieved from http://www.asha.org/uploadedFiles/asha/publications/cicsd/1997LowBirthweightandDevelopmentalDelays.pdf (Februari 6, 2016).

Simbolon D. (2013). Model prediksiindeksmassatubuhremajaberdasarkanriwayatlahirdan status gizianak. *Jurnal Kesehatan Masyarakat Nasional*, *8*, 19–27.

Simbolon D. (2013). Model prediksiindeksmassatubuhremajaberdasarkanriwayatlahirdan status gizianak. *Jurnal Kesehatan Masyarakat Nasional*, *8*(1), 19–28.

Yudesti I, Prayitno N. (2013). Perbedaan status gizianak SD kelas IV dan V di SD Unggulan Jakarta Timur 2012. *Jurnal Ilmiah Kesehatan*, *5*(1), 1.

Stem Cell Oncology – Adella (Ed.)
© 2018 Taylor & Francis Group, London, ISBN 978-0-8153-9272-9

Herbal medicine induces circulation and proliferation of Endothelial Progenitor Cell (EPC)

F. Sandra
Department of Biochemistry and Molecular Biology, Division of Oral Biology, Faculty of Dentistry, Trisakti University, Jakarta, Indonesia

D. Munir
PUI Stem Cell, Universitas Sumatera Utara, Medan, North Sumatera, Indonesia

ABSTRACT: Endothelial Progenitor Cells (EPC) can differentiate into mature endothelial cells as well as play a crucial role in the protection and improvement of vascular endothelium. Based on multivariate regression analysis, there was a strong correlation between the number of circulating EPC and the subjects' combined Framingham risk factor score. In hyperglycaemia, endothelial damage could occur over time, which may cause both micro- and macro-angiopathic complications. The number of EPC was reduced and was inversely related to levels of glycated haemoglobin (HbA1c) and type 2 diabetes mellitus. Additionally, hypercholesterolemic patients had lower EPC score compared to control subjects.

Keywords: endothelial progenitor cell, herbal medicine, proliferation

1 INTRODUCTION

Endothelial Progenitor Cell (EPC) is a type of stem cell with more limited ability in proliferation and differentiation. This cell is unipotent, which can differentiate into the mature endothelial cell. EPC has an important role in the formation of blood vessels and the remodelisation of endothelial cells on damaged blood vessels (Frisca, Sardjono & Sandra, 2008; Nababan et al., 2007). EPC is defined as a part of Mononuclear Cells that has molecule haematopoietic stem cell markers. The markers are: Cluster of Differentiation (CD)34, a glycoprotein mediating stem cell adhesion at bone marrow extracellular matrix; CD133, a molecule marker for more primitive stem cells; and Kinase Insert Domain Receptor (KDR), a protein that plays a crucial role in stimulating proliferation, formation of new blood vessels and angiogenesis (Frisca et al., 2008, 2010; Nababan et al., 2007; Sandra et al., 2010).

EPCs can be isolated from multiple sources, with the number of EPCs <1% in total in bone marrow and <0.01% in peripheral blood (PB) circulation (Frisca et al., 2008, Nababan et al., 2007). While the amount of EPC needed for use in human adult therapy is quite large in number, it is reported that it takes approximately 3–6 × 108 EPCs (Frisca et al., 2008). Therefore, it is necessary to increase the number of EPC. Expansion methods that have been developed are adherence assay using fibronectin, preplating or serial discarding with different induction of cytokines (Nababan et al., 2007).

Herbal medicine has been known to have potential in treating cardiovascular disease. For example, digoxin and digitoxin, derived from Digitalis lanata and Digitalis purpurea; reserpine, derived from Rauwolfia serpentina; and acetylsalicylic acid, derived from the willow bark (Liperoti et al., 2017). In cellular experiments, the herbal medicine was shown to have effects related to EPCs (Cai et al., 2013, Chen, Zhu & Zhang, 2013; Gao et al., 2010; Iijima et al., 2013; Lizandi et al., 2010; Lu et al., 2009; Tam et al., 2015; Widowati et al., 2012, 2014, 2016; Zhao, Li & Kong, 2014). In this article, various herbal medicines with their properties in EPC will be disclosed.

2   EPC IN CARDIOVASCULAR DISEASE (CVD)

Circulating EPC (CEPC) which is derived from bone marrow, can differentiate into mature endothelial cells as well as play a crucial role in the protection and improvement of vascular endothelium. The number of CPEC has been correlated with various factors. Based on multivariate regression analysis, there was a strong correlation between the number of CEPC and the subjects' combined Framingham risk factor score (Aragona et al., 2016; Hill et al., 2003). In smokers, the EPC count was correlated with a total number of risk factors and based on the individual risk factors analysis; smoking determined the numbers of CEPC (Aragona et al., 2016; Vasa et al., 2001). CEPC were significantly lower in smokers with coronary artery disease (CAD) compared to controls and non-smokers with CAD (Aragona et al., 2016; Yue et al., 2010).

Hyperglycaemia-induced endothelial damage over time may cause both micro- and macro-angiopathic complications (Aragona et al., 2016; Brownlee, 2005). The number of cultured EPC was reduced and was inversely related to levels of glycated haemoglobin (HbA1c) (Aragona et al., 2016; Loomans et al., 2004) and Type 2 Diabetes Mellitus (T2DM) (Aragona et al., 2016; Egan et al., 2008). EPC levels are low in diabetic populations both with/without vascular complications, therefore the EPC maturation/commitment process could be the cause, and not due to the EPC production/mobilisation failure from bone marrow (Aragona et al., 2016; Lombardo et al., 2012).

The EPC score was significantly lower in hypercholesterolemic patients when compared to control subjects (Aragona et al., 2016; Zhu et al., 2004). In an *in vitro* study, the exposure of cultured EPC to oxidised LDL induced a dose-dependent impairment of EPC activity. The impairment accelerated the rate of cell senescence and could be associated with a significant reduction in EPC numbers *in vivo* (Aragona et al., 2016; Imanishi et al., 2004).

3   HERBAL MEDICINE INCREASES NUMBER OF CEPC

There are experiments that show herbal medicine can increase the amount of CEPC and improve the function of CEPC which accelerates neovascularisation and re-endothelialsation in injured vessels. Among them, Xuezhikang, an extract of cholestin, was shown to increase CEPC. In a clinical study, after the treatment, CEPC in the Xuezhikang group (114.40 ± 6.55) was significantly higher than that in the antihypertensive drug treatment group (88.00 ± 6.32, $p < 0.01$) (Lu et al., 2009). Besides Xuezhikang, Tongguan capsule, a Chinese herbal preparation for supplementing qi and activating blood circulation showed an increase of CEPC as well. The number of EPC in the PB increased in the treatment group in comparison to the control group who were treated with placebos ($p < 0.05$). Also, the left Ventricular Ejection Fraction (LVEF) and Wall Motion Score Index (WMSI) was better in the Tongguan capsule-treated group than in the control group ($p < 0.05$) (Chen et al., 2013).

There are other herbal medicines that can induce the number of CEPC. Salvianic acid A, salvianolic acid B, and tanshinone IIA all increased the number of CEPC in the PB as well (Zhao et al., 2014). NF3, a Chinese 2-herb formula could significantly enhance the circulating CD34+/Vascular Endothelial Growth Factor (VEGFR)2+/CD45− EPC levels in diabetic foot ulcer rats by 60% ($p < 0.05$) through the partial elevation of Stromal Cell-Derived Factor 1 alpha (SDF-1α) (Tam et al., 2015).

4   HERBAL MEDICINE INCREASES PROLIFERATION OF EPC

Lycopene also significantly accelerates EPC proliferation in a time- and dose-dependent manner (Zhao et al., 2014). Regarding Xuezhikang, EPC proliferation capability in the Xuezhikang group (0.415 ± 0.018) was superior to those in the antihypertensive drug treatment group (0.333 ± 0.021, $p < 0.01$) (Lu et al., 2009). Studies on cultured EPC showed that ligustrazine, 3,4-dihydroxyacetophenone, breviscapine, and puerarin significantly stimulated the number of Clonal Formation Units (CFU) in a time- and dose-dependent manner (Zhao et al., 2014). Treatment with Saiko-Ka-Ryukotsu-Borei-To (SKRBT), a traditional herbal medicine that has been applied to treat stress-related neuropsychiatric disorders, increased EPC colony numbers significantly ($p < 0.05$) (Iijima et al., 2013).

A study in Curcuma longa L. and (-)-Epigallo Catechin-3-Gallate (EGCG) has shown that both these antioxidants, C. longa and EGCG, could enhance proliferation of Adipose-derived Mesenchymal Stem Cell (AD-MSC)-derived EPC. The highest proliferation rates were achieved by induction of C. longa in concentrations of 1 µg/mL, while induction of EGCG in a concentration of 0.25 µg/mL (Widowati et al., 2012). Meanwhile, β-carotene in the concentration of 20 µg/mL can also induce a proliferation of AD-MSC-derived EPC (Widowati et al., 2014). Another antioxidant, tea flavonoid, can induce proliferation of PB-derived EPC. Treatment of Epigallo Catechin Gallate (EGCG), Epicatechin Gallate (ECG), Epigallocatechin (EGC) and Catechin (C) of tea flavonoids increased the percentages of EPC marked by CD34, CD133, VEGFR-2 expressions (Widowati et al., 2016).

5 SIGNALLING TRANSDUCTION AND CELLULAR REPROGRAMMING OF EPC

Some signal transduction in mediating the proliferation of EPC has been reported. Among them, Phosphatidylinositol-4,5-bisphosphate3-Kinase (PI3K)/Akt signalling pathway has been widely reported. The PI3K/Akt signalling then led to some downstream signals such as Nuclear Factor (NF)κB/survivin (Li et al., 2012), Endothelial Nitric Oxide Synthases (eNOS) (Yu et al., 2014) or Forkhead Homeobox type O transcription factor (FOXO)3A (Huang et al., 2015). Besides PI3K/Akt, the Mitogen-Activated Protein Kinase (MAPK) signalling pathway has been shown as well (Xu et al., 2012; Oktaviono et al., 2014, 2016; Sandra et al., 2015). And among the MAPK family, p38 and p44/42 were shown to be correlated with the proliferation of EPC (Xu et al., 2012; Oktaviono et al., 2014, 2016; Sandra et al., 2015).

Cellular reprogramming as an approach has been proposed and shown in various cells, including EPC (Thal et al., 2012; Tendenan et al., 2017; Yoo et al., 2013). Intramyocard transplantation of reprogrammed EPC in acute myocardial infarction mouse models showed significant improvement in ventricular function, which is histologically supported by *de novo* cardiomyocyte differentiation and increased capillary density and fibrosis reduction (Thal et al., 2012). Interestingly, Human Dental Pulp Cells Induced Pluripotent Stem Cells (hDPC-iPSC) was shown capable of differentiating into the functional endothelial cell (Yoo et al., 2013).

6 SUMMARY

Herbal medicine can potentially increase the number of CEPC and induce proliferation of EPC so that optimal number of EPC for treatment can be achieved. The mechanism of EPC proliferation has been well disclosed, however, there is still a lack of information on how herbal medicine induces proliferation of EPC. EPC reprogramming to gain a more potent EPC in higher EPC number is a novel promising approach. There will be exciting further experiments in this research field.

REFERENCES

Aragona, C.O., Imbalzano, E., Mamone, F., Cairo, V., Lo Gullo, A., D'Ascola, A., Sardo, M.A., Scuruchi, M., Basile, G., Saitta, A. & Mandraffino, G. (2016). Endothelial Progenitor Cells for diagnosis and prognosis in cardiovascular disease. *Stem Cells International,* 2016, 8043792.
Brownlee, M. (2005). The pathobiology of diabetic complications: a unifying mechanism. *Diabetes,* 54(6), 1615–1625.

Cai, D.S., Zhou, H., Liu, W.W. & Pei, L. (2013). Protective effects of bone marrow-derived endothelial progenitor cells and Houttuyniacordata in lipopolysaccharide-induced acute lung injury in rats. *Cell Physiology and Biochemistry*, *32*(6), 1577–1586.

Chen, P., Zhu, C.L. & Zhang, M.Z. (2013). Effect of tongguan capsule on the number of endothelial progenitor cells in the peripheral blood of patients with coronary artery disease after PCI. *Zhongguo Zhong Xi Yi Jie He ZaZhi*, *33*(7), 873–877.

Egan, C.G., Lavery, R., Caporali, F., Fondelli, C., Laghi-Pasini, F., Dotta, F. & Sorrentino, V. (2008). Generalised reduction of putative endothelial progenitors and CXCR4-positive peripheral blood cells in type 2 diabetes. *Diabetologia, 51*(7), 1296–1305.

Frisca, Sardjono, C.T. & Sandra, F. (2008). Ekspansi endothelial progenitor cell. *Cermin Dunia Kedokteran*, *35*(161), 68–71.

Frisca, Sardjono, C.T. & Sandra, F. (2010). Berbagai paradigma pendefinisian endothelial progenitor cells. *Jurnal Kedokteran Maranatha*, *8*(1), 78–86.

Gao, D., Wu, L.Y., Jiao, Y.H., Chen, W.Y., Chen, Y., Kaptchuk, T.J., Lu, B., Song, J. & Chen, K.J. (2010). The effect of XuefuZhuyu decoction on in vitro endothelial progenitor cell tube formation. *Chinese Journal of Integrative Medicine*, *16*(1), 50–53.

Hill, J.M., Zalos, G., Halcox, J.P., Schenke, W.H., Waclawiw, M.A., Quyyumi, A.A. & Finkel, T. (2003). Circulating endothelial progenitor cells, vascular function, and cardiovascular risk. *The New England Journal of Medicine*, *348*(7), 593–600.

Huang, L., Wang, F., Wang, Y., Cao, Q., Sang, T., Liu F. & Chen, S. (2015). Acidic fibroblast growth factor promotes endothelial progenitor cells function via Akt/FOXO3a pathway. *PLoS One*, *10*(6), e0129665.

Iijima, H., Daikonya, A., Takamatsu, S., Kanno, A., Magariyama, K., Yoshikawa, K., Takamiya, T., Ueda, Y., Yakubo, S., Matsumoto, T., Ueno, T., Yamori, Y., Fukuda, N. & Kitanaka, S. (2013). Effects of the herbal medicine composition "Saiko-ka-ryukotsu-Borei-To" on the function of endothelial progenitor cells in hypertensive rats. *Phytomedicine, 20*(3–4), 196–201.

Imanishi, T., Hano, T., Sawamura, T. & Nishio, I. (2004). Oxidized low-density lipoprotein induces endothelial progenitor cell senescence, leading to cellular dysfunction. *Clinical and Experimental Pharmacology and Physiology*, *31*(7), 407–413.

Li, W., Wang, H., Kuang, C.Y., Zhu, J.K., Yu, Y., Qin, Z.X., Liu, J., Huang, L. (2012). An essential role for the Id1/PI3K/Akt/NFkB/survivinsignalling pathway in promoting the proliferation of endothelial progenitor cells in vitro. *Molecular and Cellular Biochemistry*, *363*(1–2), 135–145.

Liperoti, R., Vetrano, D.L., Bernabei, R. & Onder, G. (2017). Herbal medications in cardiovascular medicine. *Journal of the American College of Cardiology*, *69*(9), 1188–1199.

Lizandi, A.O., Sardjono, C.T., Frisca, Widowati, W., Gunanegara, R.F. & Sandra, F. (2010). GliSOD in meningkatkan potensi sel punca. *Cermin Dunia Kedokteran*, *37*(175), 107–110.

Lombardo, M.F., Iacopino, P., Cuzzola, M., Spiniello, E., Garreffa, C., Ferrelli, F., Coppola, A., Saccardi, R., Piaggesi, A., Piro, R., Mannino, D., Grossi, G., Lauro, D. & Irrera, G. (2012). Type 2 diabetes mellitus impairs the maturation of endothelial progenitor cells and increases the number of circulating endothelial cells in peripheral blood. *Cytometry Part A*, *81*(10), 856–864.

Loomans, C.J., de Koning, E.J., Staal, F.J., Rookmaaker, M.B., Verseyden, C., de Boer, H.C., Verhaar, M.C., Braam, B., Rabelink, T.J. & van Zonneveld, A.J. (2004). Endothelial progenitor cell dysfunction: a novel concept in the pathogenesis of vascular complications of type 1 diabetes. *Diabetes*, *53*(1), 195–199.

Lu, L., Zhou, J.Z., Wang, L. & Zhang, T.X. (2009). Effects of Xuezhikang and pravastatin on circulating endothelial progenitor cells in patients with essential hypertension. *Chinese Journal of Integrative Medicine*, *15*(4), 266–271.

Nababan, S.H.H., Purba, A.P., Frisca, Aini, N., Setiawan, B. & Sandra, F. (2007). Peranan endothelial progenitor cell dalam Neovaskularisasi. *Cermin Dunia Kedokteran, 34*(5), 257–259.

Oktaviono, Y.H., Sargowo, D., Widodo, M.A., Dirgantara, Y., Chouw, A. & Sandra, F. (2014). The proliferation of peripheral blood-derived endothelial progenitor cells from stable angina subjects. *The Indonesian Biomedical Journal*, *6*(2), 91–96.

Oktaviono, Y.H., Sargowo, D., Widodo, M.A., Dirgantara, Y., Chouw, A. & Sandra, F. (2016). Role of signal transduction Erk1/2 on the proliferation of endothelial progenitor cell (EPC) of patients with stable angina pectoris induced by growth factors. *Indonesian Journal of Clinical Pathology and Medical Laboratory*, *22*(3), 219–226.

Sandra, F., Murti, H., Aini, N., Sardjono, C. & Setiawan, B. (2010). Potensi terapi sel puncadalam dunia kedokterandan permasalahannya. *Jurnal Kedokteran Maranatha, 8*(1), 94–100.

Sandra, F., Oktaviono, Y.H., Widodo, M.A., Dirgantara, Y., Chouw, A. & Sargowo, D. (2015). Endothelial progenitor cells proliferated via MEK-dependent p42 MAPK signaling pathway. *Molecular and Cellular Biochemistry, 400*(1–2), 201–106.

Tam, J.C, Ko, C.H., Lau, K.M., To, M.H., Kwok, H.F., Siu, W.S., Lau, C.P., Chan, W.Y., Leung, P.C., Fung, K.P. & Lau, C.B. (2015). Enumeration and functional investigation of endothelial progenitor cells in neovascularization of diabetic foot ulcer rats with a Chinese 2-herb formula. *Journal of Diabetes, 7*(5), 718–728.

Tendean, M., Oktaviono, Y.H. & Sandra, F. (2017). Cardiomyocyte reprogramming: A potential strategy for cardiac regeneration. *Molecular and Cellular Biomedical Sciences, 1*(1), 1–5.

Thal, M.A., Krishnamurthy, P., Mackie, A.R., Hoxha, E., Lambers, E., Verma, S., Ramirez, V., Qin, G., Losordo, D.W. & Kishore, R. (2012). Enhanced angiogenic and cardiomyocyte differentiation capacity of epigenetically reprogrammed mouse and human endothelial progenitor cells augments their efficacy for ischemic myocardial repair. *Circulation Research, 111*(2), 180–190.

Vasa, M., Fichtlscherer, S., Aicher, A., Adler, K., Urbich, C., Martin H., Zeiher, A.M. & Dimmeler, S. (2001). The number and migratory activity of circulating endothelial progenitor cells inversely correlate with risk factors for coronary artery disease. *Circulation Research, 89*(1), E1–E7.

Widowati, W., Sardjono, C.T., Wijaya, L., Laksmitawati, D.R. & Sandra, F. (2012). Extract of Curcuma longa L. and (-)-Epigallo Catechin-3-Gallate Enhanced Proliferation of Adipose Tissue-derived Mesenchymal Stem Cells (AD-MSCs) and Differentiation of AD-MSCs into Endothelial Progenitor Cells. *Journal of US-China Medical Science, 9*(1), 22–29.

Widowati, W., Sardjono, C.T., Wijaya, L., Laksmitawati, D.R., Adiwinata, J. & Sandra, F. (2014). Effect of β-carotene on cell proliferation and differentiation of adipose-derived stem cells into endothelial progenitor cells. *Biotechnology: An Indian Journal, 9*(10), 407–412.

Widowati, W., Wijaya, L., Laksmitawati, D.R., Widyanto, R.M., Erawijantari, P.P., Fauziah, N., Bachtiar, I. & Sandra, F. (2016). Tea flavonoids induced differentiation of peripheral blood-derived mononuclear cells into peripheral blood-derived endothelial progenitor cells and suppressed intracellular reactive oxygen species level of peripheral blood-derived endothelial progenitor cells. *Natural Product Science, 22*(2), 87–92.

Xu, S., Wen, H. & Jiang, H. (2012). Urotensin II promotes the proliferation of endothelial progenitor cells through p38 and p44/42 MAPK activation. *Molecular Medicine Reports, 6*(1), 197–200.

Yoo, C.H., Na, H.J., Lee, D.S., Heo, S.C., An, Y., Cha, J., Choi, C., Kim, J.H., Park, J.C. & Cho, Y.S. (2013). Endothelial progenitor cells from human dental pulp-derived iPS cells as a therapeutic target for ischemic vascular diseases. *Biomaterials, 34*(33), 8149–8160.

Yu, J., Wang, Q., Wang, H., Lu, W., Li, W., Qin, Z. & Huang, L. (2014). Activation of liver X receptor enhances the proliferation and migration of endothelial progenitor cells and promotes vascular repair through PI3 K/Akt/eNOS signaling pathway activation. *Vascular Pharmacology, 62*(3), 150–161.

Yue, W.S., Wang, M., Yan, G.H., Yiu, K.H., Yin, L., Lee, S.W., Siu, C.W. & Tse, H.F. (2010). Smoking is associated with depletion of circulating endothelial progenitor cells and elevated pulmonary artery systolic pressure in patients with coronary artery disease. *The American Journal of Cardiology, 106*(9), 1248–1254.

Zhao, Q.T., Li, B.F. & Kong, H. (2014). Roles of Chinese medicine bioactive ingredients in the regulation of the cellular function of endothelial progenitor cells. *Chinese Journal of Natural Medicines, 12*(7), 481–487.

Zhu, J.H., Wang, X.X., Chen, J.Z., Tao, Q.M., Zhu, J.H. & Sun, J. (2004). Effects of hypercholesterolemia on the number and activity of endothelial progenitor cells in peripheral blood. *Zhonghua Nei Ke Za Zhi, 43*(4), 261–264.

Stem Cell Oncology – Adella (Ed.)
© *2018 Taylor & Francis Group, London, ISBN 978-0-8153-9272-9*

Relationship between Procalcitonin (PCT) and High-Density Lipoprotein (HDL) in bacterial sepsis

D. Tarigan, T. Kembaren & A. Rahimi
Department of Internal Medicine, Faculty of Medicine, Universitas Sumatera Utara, Medan, North Sumatera, Indonesia

ABSTRACT: Sepsis can decrease the anti-inflammatory and immunomodulator effects of High-Density Lipoprotein (HDL). Low HDL levels inversely correlate with the severity of sepsis and associate with an exaggerated systemic inflammatory response. Bacterial infection is a strong stimulus for PCT. To determine the correlation between PCT and HDL levels in bacterial sepsis an observational study with a case control design was conducted on 30 sepsis and 30 non-sepsis infection patients. Data was collected to fill out PCT and HDL level on the 1st, 3rd and 5th day and then analysed to assess their relationship. Statistically, a significant difference shows in the PCT and HDL levels between the sepsis and non-sepsis groups. There was a negative correlation between HDL and PCT, and a negative correlation between HDL level and the severity of sepsis, which show a medium strength correlation. Sepsis can be estimated when the HDL value less than 17,50 mg/dl. There was a significant relationship between PCT and HDL level in bacterial sepsis.

Keywords: sepsis, high-density lipoprotein, procalcitonin

1 INTRODUCTION

Sepsis is defined as an infection (whether a suspicion or evidence) accompanied by a systemic inflammatory response/SIRS (Systemic Inflammatory Response Syndrome). This condition originates from the interaction between pathogenic microorganisms and the immune system that triggers an excessive and irregular inflammatory response that is destructive. The new marker of sepsis, procalcitonin (PCT), has better accuracy values than previous markers (Wyllie et al., 2005), but is limited by relatively high prices and not all health facilities can afford it. Therefore it is necessary to find a marker that can predict sepsis and is also simple, cheap and easy to use in everyday practice without any additional cost (Wyllie et al., 2005; Christ dan Muller, 2005).

Low HDL levels are inversely related to the severity of sepsis and also associated with excessive systemic inflammatory responses. HDL can bind and neutralise lipopolysaccharide (LPS) of gram-negative bacteria and Lipoteichoic Acid (LTA) of gram-positive bacteria, thus supporting the clearance of this product (Badellino et al., 2008). This study was conducted to assess the association of HDL and PCT in patients with bacterial sepsis.

2 METHODS

The study design is case control. The study was conducted in the inpatient ward and Intensive Care Unit (ICU) of H. Adam Malik General Hospital from January to March 2017. Inclusion criteria were sepsis patients >17 years old. Exclusion criteria were sepsis patients with lipid-lowering drug use, sepsis patients with chronic kidney or liver disease, thyroid dysfunction, diabetes or malignancy; sepsis patients with chronic inflammatory diseases such as HIV, systemic lupus erythematosus or rheumatoid arthritis; and sepsis patients who died within 48 hours or were referred to another hospital.

There were 60 patients divided into two groups. The first group (30 people) were bacterial sepsis patients as the sample and the second group (30 people) were non-sepsis bacterial infection patients (30 people) as the control. Each patient was treated according to clinical conditions, and blood sampling was taken on the 1st, 3rd and 5th day for PCT and HDL checking, then the results processed and analysed using a computer program, with p < 0.05 significance. Ethical clearance was obtained from the Research Committee of the Medical Field Faculty of Medicine, North Sumatera University.

3 RESULTS

The study involved 30 subjects of sepsis and 30 non-sepsis patients, where no significant differences in baseline characteristics were found between the two groups (Table 1).

The results also explained that the PCT level in the sepsis group was higher than that in the non-sepsis group, whereas the HDL level in the sepsis group was lower than the HDL level in the non-sepsis group. Based on the Mann-Whitney test (because no normal distribution were data obtained), p < 0.05 for all HDL and PCT levels, meaning there was a significant difference between the sepsis and non-sepsis groups for both HDL and PCT levels (Table 2).

Spearman correlation test results obtained a significant negative correlation between HDL and the severity of sepsis with the correlation strength r = –0.586 showing moderate correlation. This indicates that the increase of the sepsis severity will decrease the value of HDL serum. The cut-off value of non-sepsis HDL was 17.50 mg/dl at baseline with a sensitivity of 80% and a specificity of 73%. So it can be estimated sepsis when the HDL levels lower than 17.50 mg/dl.

Table 1. The basic characteristics of research subjects.

Characteristics	Group Sepsis	Non-Sepsis	Total	P value
Age group (years)				
25–35	3 (10,0%)	3 (10,0%)	6 (10,0%)	0,987*
36–45	7 (23,3%)	6 (20,0%)	13 (21,7%)	
46–55	7 (23,3%)	9 (30,0%)	16 (26,7%)	
56–65	9 (30,0%)	8 (26,7%)	17 (28,3%)	
>65	4 (13,3%)	4 (13,3%)	8 (13,3%)	
Sex				
Male	14 (46,7%)	19 (63,3%)	33 (55%)	0,194**
Female	16 (53,3%)	11 (36,7%)	27 (45%)	
Total	30 (100%)	30 (100%)	60 (100%)	
Bacteria type				
Gram-positive	2 (6,7%)	3 (10%)	5 (8,3%)	0,146*
Gram-negative	15 (50%)	18 (60%)	33 (55%)	
Polymicrobial	5 (16,7)	0 (0%)	5 (8,3%)	
No microbes	8 (26,7%)	9 (30%)	15 (25%)	
Source of infection				
Lung	14 (46,7%)	16 (53,3%)	30 (50%)	0,791*
Abdomen	10 (33,3%)	7 (23,3%)	17 (28,3%)	
Urinary tract	5 (16,7%)	5 (16,7%)	10 (16,7%)	
Etc.	1 (3,3%)	2 (6,7%)	3 (5%)	

Fisher exact test*, Chi-square test**.

Table 2. The mean and median values of Procalcitonin (PCT) and HDL of the study subjects.

Laboratory characteristics	N	Mean	Std. Deviation	Median	P value*
1st day PCT					
Sepsis	30	20,02	20,51	18,12	0,0001
Non-sepsis	30	0,74	1,24	0,25	
3rd day PCT					
Sepsis	30	15,97	18,03	8,64	0,0001
Non-sepsis	30	0,48	0,81	0,17	
5th day PCT					
Sepsis	30	16,82	20,73	8,85	0,0001
Non-sepsis	30	0,36	0,84	0,04	
1st day HDL					
Sepsis	30	18,67	14,03	15	0,0001
Non-sepsis	30	31,63	13,99	31	
3rd day HDL					
Sepsis	30	15,67	7,45	14,50	0,0001
Non-sepsis	30	31,93	14,50	30,50	
5th day HDL					
Sepsis	30	15,10	7,67	14	0,0001
Non-sepsis	30	35,40	16,37	34,50	

Table 3. Correlation of HDL levels with PCT in the sepsis group.

Variable	N	R-value	P value
1st day HDL and 1st day PCT	30	−0,422	0,02
3rd day HDL and 3rd day PCT	30	−0,567	0,001
5th day HDL and 5th day PCT	30	−0,700	0,001

This study also found a significant negative correlation between HDL and PCT with a correlation strength of $r = -0.422$ which shows moderate correlation on the first day, then correlation strength increased on the third day $r = -0.567$ and became stronger on the fifth day $r = -0.7$ (Table 3). This suggests that in the presence of sepsis with elevated PCT the serum HDL level will decrease.

4 DISCUSSION

The results of this study found that the HDL level in the sepsis group was 18.67 ± 14.03, lower than the HDL level in the non-sepsis group of 31.63 ± 13.99. Statistically, there was a significant difference in HDL levels between the sepsis and non-sepsis groups ($p < 0.05$).

In the sepsis group, the mean PCT level at baseline was 20.02 ± 20.51 which decreased from the third day of treatment and increased again on the fifth day of treatment. The mean HDL level at baseline examination was $18.67 \pm 14, 03$ and decreased on third and fifth day of treatments to 15.10 ± 7.67.

Another study conducted by Naresh et al. (2015) using a total of 111 study subjects found that the HDL level on day five increased compared to HDL level at baseline, but among non-survivors, the HDL level was lower than in the initial days.

This study also obtained gram-negative bacteria as the cause of most sepsis. In contrast to conditions that occur in developed countries as well as in the United States where the most gram-positive bacteria are detected, although gram-negative remains high. About half of cases of diagnosed sepsis, unidentified organisms. Gram-positive bacteria continues to increase in incidents associated with increased invasive action and the incidence of nosocomial infections (Artero et al., 2012).

Based on the literature, low levels of HDL in sepsis cases can be explained that during the infection process, significant changes in lipid metabolism and lipoprotein composition occur. Triglycerides (TG) and Very Low-Density Lipoprotein (VLDL) increased concerning several mechanisms, including reduction of hydrolysis of TG. Lipopolysaccharides (LPS) and pro-inflammatory cytokines induce free fatty acid production and TG synthesis in the liver and decrease lipoprotein lipase activity resulting in VLDL clearance and elevated TG levels. Other significant changes are the presence of significant changes in lipoprotein composition and increased levels of acute phase proteins including serum amyloid A (SAA) and secretory phospholipase A (sPLA2), which may contribute to decreased levels of HDL by replacing some of the structural components and functions of HDL (Von, 2007; Pirillo et al., 2013).

Khovidhunkit et al. (2014) found a change in other protein content associated with HDL (Serum paraoxonase (PON1), Platelet-activating Factor Acetylhydrolase (PAF-AH)), resulting in a decrease in antioxidant properties from HDL and enhanced pro-atherogenic lipid content (Cao et al., 1998). Endotoxemia also induces enhancement of some enzymes involved in HDL remodelling, including endothelial lipase [10] and secretory phospholipase A2 and other decreases such as Cholesteryl Protein Transfer Ester (CETP) and Lecithin-Cholesterol Acyltransferase (LCAT) which will eventually decrease the functional properties of HDL (Delaliera et al., 2012).

Low HDL levels are inversely related to the severity of sepsis and are associated with excessive systemic inflammatory responses. As with other plasma lipoproteins, HDL can bind and neutralise gram-negative Lipopolysaccharides (LPS) and gram-positive lipoteichoic acid (LTA), thereby supporting clearance of this product. HDL has several biological functions, but the role of HDL regarding innate immunity emerged in 1970 with the first observation looking for a link between HDL cholesterol (HDL-C) plasma values for protection against sepsis. In the context of infection, HDL and its components have been associated with protection against gram-negative, gram-positive and parasitic bacteria. Furthermore, HDL affects the innate humoral immunity by regulating the activation of the complement and expression systems of Pentraxin 3 (PTX3). HDL is essential not only during sepsis but also in bacterial, parasitic and other viral infections (Von, 2007).

Shor et al. (2008) in their retrospective study in patients at Edith Wolfson Medical Center, Israel, with a total of 204 study subjects, found that very low HDL levels (≤ 20 mg/dl) were associated with sepsis, death and malignant risk. This result is consistent with that obtained by Chien et al. (2005) who found that low HDL levels on day one were significantly associated with increased mortality and poor outcomes.

Van Leeuwen et al. (2003) reported a rapid change that decreased by 50% in lipoprotein levels, especially HDL, which occurred during sepsis. As the HDL sepsis state changes into an acute phase HDL that contains more SAA and less Apo A-I.

Al-Zaidawi et al. (2014) reported low HDL levels in burn patients treated in the ICU room, whose value continued to decrease to <15 mg/dl when sepsis occurred. HDL and triglycerides then begin to rise again when sepsis resolves until it reaches its normal value. Meanwhile, from this study it can be estimated that sepsis occurs when HDL levels are below 17.50 mg/dl.

The differences in these cut-off values may also be attributed to the HDL baseline in each race or demographic and lifestyle. Although the data on HDL values are racially/ethically limited, it is found that people in eastern Asia tend to have low HDL and high TG, whereas those in southern Asia tend to have lower HDL, LDL and TG levels than non-Asians (Morris & Ferdinand, 2009).

The findings also support low HDL levels as a risk factor for sepsis, and it seems that targeting HDL levels can provide efficient and effective sepsis treatment.

5 CONCLUSION

There was a significant negative correlation between HDL with PCT. This suggests that the presence of sepsis with elevated PCT will decrease the serum HDL level. This study also obtained a significant negative correlation between HDL and the severity of sepsis with a correlation strength of $r = -0.586$ showing moderate correlation. This indicates that the increase of the sepsis severity will decrease the value of HDL serum. The cut-off value of non-sepsis HDL was 17.50 mg/dl at baseline with a sensitivity of 80% and a specificity of 73%.

This study also supports the result that HDL value can be used as an assessment to determine the severity of sepsis.

REFERENCES

Arturo, A., Zaragoza, R. & Nogueira, J.M. (2012). *Epidemiology of severe sepsis and septic shock. Severe sepsis and septic shock—Understanding a serious killer.* Retrieved from http://www.intechopen.com/books/severe-sepsis-and-septic-shockunderstanding-a-serious-killer/epidemiology-of-severe-sepsis-and-septic-shock. (18 Mar 2017).

Badellino, K.O., Wolfe, M.L., Reilly, M.P. & Rader, D.J. (2008). Endothelial lipase is increased in vivo by inflammation in humans. *Circulation AHA, 117,* 678685.

Cao, Y., Stafforini, D.M., Zimmerman, G.A., McIntyre, T.M. & Prescott, S.M. (1998). Expression of plasma platelet-activating factor acetylhydrolase is transcriptionally regulated by mediators of inflammation. *The Journal of Biological Chemistry, 273,* 4012–4020.

Christ-Crain, M. & Muller, B. (2005). Procalcitonin in bacterial infections hype, hope, more or less? *Swiss Med, 135,* 451–460.

De la Llera, M.M., McGillicuddy, F.C., Hinkle, C.C., Byrne, M., Joshi, M.R., Nguyen, V., Tabita-Martinez, J., Wolfe, M.L., Badellino, K., Pruscino, L., Mehta, N.N., Asztalos, B.F. & Reilly, M.P. (2012). Inflammation modulates human HDL composition and function in vivo. *Atherosclerosis, 222,* 390–394.

Khovidhunkit, W., Kim, M.S., Memon, R.A., Shigenaga, J.K., Moser, A.H., Feingold, K.R. & Grunfeld, C. (2004). Effects of infection and inflammation on lipid and lipoprotein metabolism: mechanisms and consequences to the host. *Journal of Lipid Research, 4,* 1169–1196.

Morris, A. & Ferdinand, K. (2009). Hyperlipidemia in racial/ethnic minorities: differences in lipid profiles and the impact of statin therapy. *Clin Lipidology, 4*(6), 741–754.

Naresh, M., Vidyasagar, S. & Elagandula, J. (2015). Study of serum HDL levels in severe sepsis patients in medical intensive care unit. *International Journal of Scientific and Research Publication, 5.*

Pirillo, A., Norata, G.D. & Catapano, A.L. (2013). Treating high-density lipoprotein cholesterol (HDL-C): Quantity versus quality. *Current Pharmaceutical Design, 19,* 3841–3857.

Shor, R., Wainstein, J. & Oz, D. Low HDL levels and the risk of death, sepsis, and malignancy. *Clin Res Cardiol, 97*(4), 227–33.

Van Leeuwen, H.J., Heezius, E.C., Dallinga, G.M., VanStrijp, J.A., Verhoef, J. & Van Kessel, K.P. (2003). Lipoprotein metabolism in patients with severe sepsis. *Critical Care Medicine, 31,* 1359–1366.

Von, A. & Kardassis, D. (2007). High-Density Lipoproteins. *Handbook of Experimental Pharmacology.*

Wyllie, D.H., Bowler, I.C. & Peto, T.E. (2005). Bacteraemia prediction in emergency medical admissions: The role of C reactive protein. *Journal of Clinical Pathology, 58,* 352–356.

Zaidawi, A., Sejad, & Hashimi, A. (2014). Pre sepsis biomarker: HDL (high-density lipoproteins). *World Journal of Pharmacy and Pharmaceutical Sciences,* 111–120.

Stem Cell Oncology – Adella (Ed.)
© 2018 Taylor & Francis Group, London, ISBN 978-0-8153-9272-9

Relation of ferritin and nutrition to pulmonary dysfunction in thalassemia major

W. Siregar, B. Lubis & W. Dalimunthe
Department of Pediatrics, Faculty of Medicine, Universitas Sumatera Utara, Medan, North Sumatera, Indonesia

ABSTRACT: Thalassemia major is a chronic disease requiring regular transfusions that may result in iron loading, iron excess complications—such as in heart, liver, endocrine organs, and lung diseases. Restrictive pulmonary dysfunction is known as the dominantly observed. A pulmonary function test was conducted in 50 children aged 6–18 years with TM with no history of chronic respiratory disease. Assessment of nutritional status was based on the anthropometric examination (BW/H and MUAC/A). Among the 50 children, 18 (36%) had restrictive lung function. The mean ferritin levels of the restrictive pulmonary dysfunction group (2096.6 ug/L) was lower than the normal pulmonary function group (2209.6 ug/L). Nine of 18 children were mildly malnourished in the restrictive pulmonary dysfunction group (OR = 6.890; CI95% = 1.152–41.340). There is no significant correlation between serum ferritin level and restrictive pulmonary dysfunction in children with TM. Mild malnutrition increases the risk of restrictive pulmonary dysfunction occurrence in pediatric TM.

Keywords: children, restrictive pulmonary dysfunction, ferritin, malnutrition, thalassemia major

1 INTRODUCTION

Thalassemia is a common genetic blood disorder that is clinically characterised by various degrees of chronic haemolysis anaemia (Permono & Ugraseno, 2010). Chronic anaemia that occurs as a result of ineffective erythropoiesis, haemolysis and reduction of haemoglobin synthesis causes thalassemia patients to require lifelong blood transfusions (Galanello & Origa, 2010; Viprakasit et al., 2014).

Repeated blood transfusions may prolong the life expectancy of major thalassemia patients, but also negatively impact the occurrence of iron overload which can cause damage to various organs, including the lungs (Porter & Garbowski, 2014; Hershko, 2010). Different types of pulmonary function abnormalities have been described in TM patients (Inselman, 2008). However, the precise aetiology of the pulmonary dysfunction remains unknown. Several pathologic mechanisms for the pulmonary dysfunction in thalassemia have been investigated, including iron overload, allergy and correlation with transfusion, but none of these has provided a satisfactory explanation (Prakash, 2005). Examination of serum ferritin levels is the most commonly used method to measure the amount of iron accumulation in the body (Wood, 2015). Malnutrition is thought to be one risk factor for lung problems in thalassemia major.

This study aims to analyse the relationship between serum ferritin levels and nutritional status with lung function impairment in patients with major thalassemia major in our centre.

2 METHODS

This cross-sectional study included 50 patients with TM receiving regular blood transfusion without any history of chronic respiratory disease and had been followed up at Haji

Adam Malik Thalassemia Center. None of the patients had any clinical or echocardiographic evidence of heart failure within six months of the present study. Major thalassemia children with infectious disease and clinical inflammation and a history of chronic lung disease were excluded from the study. Characteristics of the study subjects were also recorded, which included age, sex, weight and height. All subjects were interviewed, and a physical examination, anthropometry, and serum ferritin level and spirometry examinations were performed. A statistical analysis to analyse the variables based on lung function was done using univariate test, Mann-Whitney test and a multivariate test with logistic regression test. The significance is determined based on the value of $p < 0.05$. The ethical research was confirmed by the Research Ethic Committee, Medical Faculty, University of Sumatera Utara.

3 RESULT

A sample of 50 people consisting of 25 boys and 25 girls were recruited. Demographic characteristics based on pulmonary function test results are presented in Table 1. Most of the samples showed normal pulmonary function test results and 18 children (36%) had impaired restrictive lung function. The sample age ranged from 6–18 years with a mean age of sample at 10.2 (SB 2.89) years in children with normal lung function and 12.0 (SB 3.73) years in children with restrictive lung function disorder.

Based on the assessment of nutritional status, 35 children had good nutrition while 15 children had malnutrition, whereas in the group of children with restrictive lung function disorder, nine children (50%) with moderate malnutrition were found.

Of the total sample, 25 children (50%) were of short stature, and in the subgroup of children with restrictive lung function disorder, there were nine children with short stature. Based on serum ferritin level, mean serum ferritin level in the group of children with restrictive lung function disorder was 2096.6 ng/mL, whereas in the group of children without impaired lung function the mean rate of ferritin was 2209.6 ng/mL.

In Table 2, based on the Mann-Whitney test, no difference was found between ferritin levels with normal and restrictive lung function (P = 0.237) in children with thalassemia.

Based on logistic regression multivariate analysis, the risk factors that influence the restrictive lung function in the patient with thalassemia. The analysis showed that only nutri-

Table 1. The demographic characteristics of the sample are based on pulmonary function tests.

Variable	Pulmonary function test	
	Normal (n = 32)	Restrictive (n = 18)
Mean age, years (SD)	10.2 (2.89)	12.0 (3.73)
Sex, n (%)		
Male	14 (43.80)	11 (61.10)
Female	18 (56.30)	7 (38.90)
Body weight, kg (SB)	25.6 (7.71)	29.2 (10.34)
Body height, cm (SB)	126.5 (15.40)	134.7 (17.91)
Nutritional status, n (%)		
Well-nourished	26 (81.30)	9 (50.00)
Moderate malnutrition	6 (18.80)	9 (50.00)
Short stature, n (%)		
Yes	16 (50.00)	9 (50.00)
No	16 (50.00)	9 (50.00)
Ferritin, ng/mL (SD)	2209.6 (327.53)	2096.6 (482.50)
Transfusion amount (SD)	86.6 (40.95)	107.3 (59.14)
FVC, % (SD)	91.5 (8.42)	71.2 (6.64)
FEV1/FVC, % (SD)	89.3 (6.82)	79.6 (3.36)

Table 2. Relation of ferritin levels with impaired lung function.

Pulmonary function	Mean serum ferritin level	SD	Z	CI95%	P
Normal	2209.6	327.53	−1.196	0.228–0.245	0.237
Restrictive	2096.6	482.50			

tional status had an effect on restrictive lung function disorder in children with thalassemia major with a P-value <0.035. Children with thalassemia patients with less nutritional risk 6.89 (CI95% = 1.151–41.340) times higher lung function impairment than patients with thalassemia with normal nutrition.

4 DISCUSSION

Most researchers conclude that restrictive lung function disorder is a major lung function disorder in children with thalassemia major. They believe that early and aggressive use of iron chelation can prevent the impairment of lung function (Sohn et al., 2011; Bourli et al., 2012; Noori et al., 2012). Our results also show that restrictive pulmonary function disorder is a dominant finding based on a lung function test using spirometry, with a result of about 18 (36%) of patients with restrictive lung function disorders and the rest normal. In this study, patients had no complaints of respiratory problems, and all had normal pulmonary patterns based on chest x-rays. It can be concluded that routine lung function tests may be necessary, even in asymptomatic patients.

The study involved 50 children with thalassemia major, in which the proportion of male and female sex was balanced, and the age range was 6–18 years; the mean of children with restrictive lung function disorder is 12 years compared to the mean of children with normal lung function of around 10.2 years. Most of the boys – 11 children (61.1%) were found to have restrictive lung function disorder. Previous studies (Abu Ekhteish et al., 2007; Ozyoruk and Misirlioglu, 2015) found an association between increased age and serum ferritin levels and restrictive lung function disorder, but in this study, age was not associated with restriction lung function disorder.

Assessment of nutritional status based on clinical findings and anthropometry (based on BW/H and MUAC/A) was performed in all patients, and it was found that some children with restrictive lung function had poor nutrition. This moderate malnutrition condition is a risk factor for major thalassemia children who have restrictive pulmonary function compared with thalassemia children with good nutrition, with OR 6.89 (CI95% = 1.151 to 41.340).

Growth disorders are one of the complications of thalassemia that can cause a disproportionate chest cavity (Galanello & Origa, 2010). A disproportionate chest cavity can cause pulmonary volume disturbance resulting in impaired restrictive lung function (Bourli et al., 2012). On anthropometric examination, 25 children (50%) have short stature, while only nine children (36%) have restrictive lung function. Statistical analysis of lung function disorder showed no significant results. The results were consistent with previous studies that performed the logistic regression analysis of factors suspected to cause lung function impairment, in which there was no BH/A relationship to restrictive pulmonary function impairment (Bourli et al., 2012). The outcome may be due to growth disorders not occurring in the chest cavity, other bones. This is indicated by more growth disorders occurring in subjects with normal lung function.

Although the measurement of serum ferritin levels was not the best quantitative estimate of body iron storage (Wood, 2015), thalassemia major patients with serum ferritin serum concentrations ≥3000 ng/dL have been reported to have high lung injury probabilities. Serum ferritin levels >2500 ng/dL have been associated with a mortality risk four times higher (Ozyoruk & Misirlioglu, 2015). The restrictive lung disorder group had a mean serum ferritin level of 2096.60 µg/L, lower than the normal lung function group, with a mean of 2209.60 µg/L. Statistical analysis of serum ferritin levels with lung function impairment showed no significant results. This is in keeping with previous studies which show no association between elevated serum ferritin levels and restrictive lung function disorder in major thalassemia (Parakh et al., 2007; Boddu et al., 2015).

This study has strengths and limitations. The advantages of this research are the first study in North Sumatra. Some limitations of this study are that this study assessed lung function by cross-sectional. An ideal quantitative assessment of iron overload is to measure the liver iron content by biopsy, but this invasive action is not feasible, so it was not performed.

5 CONCLUSION

There is no significant correlation between serum ferritin level and restrictive pulmonary dysfunction in children with TM. Mild malnutrition increases the risk of restrictive pulmonary dysfunction occurrence in paediatric TM.

REFERENCES

Abu-Ekteish, F.M., Al-Rimawi, H.S., Al-Ali, M.K., & Shehabi, I.M. (2007). Pulmonary function tests in children with beta-thalassemia major. *Chronic Respiratory Disease, 4*, 19–22.
Boddu A., Kumble A., Mahalingam S., Baliga B.S., & Achappa B. (2015). Pulmonary dysfunction in children with beta-thalassemia major in relation with iron overload—a cross sectional hospital based study. *AJMS, 6*, 47–50.
Bourli E., Dimitriadou M., Economou M., Vlachaki E., Christoforodis A., & Maratou E., dkk. (2012). Restrictive pulmonary dysfunction and its predictors in young patients with β-thalassemia major. *Ped Pulmo, 21*, 1–7.
Eidani I., Kheikhaei B., Rahim F., & Bagheri A. (2009). Evaluation of pulmonary in β-thalassemia major patients. *Pakistan Journal of Medical Sciences, 25*, 749–54.
Galanello R., & Origa R. (2010). Beta-thalassemia. *Orphanet Journal of Rare Diseases, 5*, 1–15.
Noori N.M., Keshavarz K., & Shariar M. (2012). Cardiac and pulmonary dysfunction in asymptomatic beta-thalassemia major. *Asian Cardio Thorac Annals, 20*, 555–59.
Ozyoruk D., & Misirlioglu E.D. (2015). Pulmonary function in children with thalassemia major. *J Pediatr Hematol Oncol, 37*, 605–10.
Parakh A., Dubey A.P., Chowdhury V., Sethi G.R., Jain S., & Hira H.S. (2007). Study of pulmonary function tests in thalassemic children. *J Pediatr Hematol Oncol, 29*, 151–5.
Permono H.B., Ugrasena IDG. Talasemia. Dalam: Permono H.B., Sutaryo, Ugrasena IDG, Windiastuti E., Abdulsalam M., penyunting. Buku ajar hematologi-onkologi anak. Edisi ke-3. Jakarta: BP IDAI, 2010.h.64–84.
Porter J.B., & Garbowski M. (2014). The pathophysiology of transfusional iron overload. *Hematol Oncol Clin N Am, 28*, 683–701.
Prakash U.B. (2005). Lungs in hemoglobinopathies, erythrocyte disorders, and hemorrhagic diatheses. *Seminars in Respiratory and Critical Care Medicine, 26*, 527–40.
Sohn E.Y., Noetzli L.J., Gera A., Kato R., Coates T.D., & Harmatz P., dkk. (2011). Pulmonary function in thalassemia major and its correlation with body iron stores. *BJH, 155*, 102–5.
Viprakasit V., Origa R., & Fucharoen S. (2014). Genetic basis, pathophysiology, and diagnosis. Dalam: Cappellini, Cohen A, Porter J, Taher A, Viprakasit V, penyunting. *Guidelines for the Management of Transfusion-Dependent Thalassemia (TDT)*. Edisi ke-3. Cyprus: TIF; 2014. h. 14–26.
Wood J.C. (2015). Estimating tissue iron burden: current status and prospects. *British Journal of Haematology, 1*, 15–28.

Stem Cell Oncology – Adella (Ed.)
© 2018 Taylor & Francis Group, London, ISBN 978-0-8153-9272-9

The difference of MMSE and MoCA-Ina scores in brain tumors

S. Bangun, H. Sjahrir & F.I. Fitri
*Department of Neurology, Faculty of Medicine, Universitas Sumatera Utara, Medan,
North Sumatera, Indonesia*

ABSTRACT: The Mini Mental State Examination (MMSE) is the most commonly used screening test for Brain Tumor (BT) patients but relatively insensitive compared to Montreal Cognitive Assessment (MoCA). The aim of this study was to compare the proportion of the MMSE and MoCA-Ina scores in BT patients. A cross sectional study was conducted in 33 patients with BT. All of the subjects were assessed with MMSE and MoCA-Ina. To assess the difference in the proportion of brain tumor patients was used chi-square test or Fisher exact test. In BT patients with group of education 7–9 years presented a significantly higher percentage of abnormal MMSE and MoCA-Ina score than other group. We noticed that over 90.9% was impairment of attention and calculation using MMSE, while delayed recall have been affected on more than 90.9% using MoCA-Ina.

Keywords: Mini Mental State Examination, Montreal Cognitive Assessment, Cognitive Function, Brain Tumor

1 INTRODUCTION

Primary brain tumors are among the top 10 causes of cancer-related deaths in the United States, accounting for approximately 1.4% of all cancers and 2.4% of all cancer related deaths. About 14 per 100,000 people in the United States are diagnosed with a primary brain tumor each year, and 6 to 8 per 100,000 are diagnosed with a primary malignant brain tumor (Berger, M.S. 2005).

In evolution, most patients diagnosed with brain tumors have cognitive decline, but the mechanisms by which these neoplasms may compromise brain function are varied in different patients. It is well known that cognitive tests performances are influenced by patient-related variables (age, level of education) and disease-related variables (the location of the tumor, its growth rate, tumor's size), but was not yet fully explained the nature of interactions between these variables. Cognitive dysfunction is a consequence of neoplastic process but it may be, also, secondary to associated intracranial hypertension or cerebral edema, being evident, at the time of diagnosis, on more than half of patients (Stanca, D, 2011).

There are few studies about cognitive functions at the time of diagnosis in patients with brain tumors. Most of them were conducted to assess post-surgical cognitive function or as a measure for evaluating the effectiveness or adverse effects of treatment (chemo or radio-therapy) (Tucha, O, 2000).

The Mini Mental State Examination (MMSE) was develop by Folstein et al in 1975 (Folstein, M.F., Folstein, S.E., McHugh, P.R. 1975). It has currently been widely used as a standard scoring tools in many countries and translated into various languages, including the Indonesia language (Ong, P.A., 2015).

The MMSE is the most commonly used screening test for patients with brain tumor patients, despite limited validation in this setting. The Montreal Cognitive Assessment (MoCA) has superior sensitivity in part because it does not have a ceiling test effect, likely because it more extensively tests executive functioning, delayed recall, and abstraction (Olson, R.A., 2011; Nasreddine, Z.S., 2005).

The MMSE is best suited to detecting gross cognitive impairment, such as Alzheimer's disease, and has been shown to be relatively insensitive to the cognitive changes that occur in brain tumor patients, especially in detecting impairments in abstract reasoning, executive functioning, and visual perception (Olson, R.A., 2008).

The purpose of our study was to compare two brief and widely used tests (MMSE and MoCA-Ina) for detection of Mild Cognitive Impairment in brain tumor patients. Indonesian version of MoCA test has been validated (Husein, N. 2010).

2 METHOD

The study-group consisted of patients diagnosed with brain tumors in the Haji Adam Malik General Hospital between November 2015 and May 2017. The exclusion criteria of the study were the following:

- Patients with brain tumors that are not confirmed by neuroimaging examination
- Aphasic language disorders
- Previous psychiatric diseases
- Patients who have undergone radiotherapy, chemotherapy, or brain tumor surgery
- Patients with other condition that could influence cognitive function

The location of brain tumors was assessed on the radiological examinations of cranial computed tomography scans with contrast and or Magnetic Resonance Imaging (MRI). The location of the tumor is divided into supratentorial, infratentorial, and both sites. The size of the tumor was assessed on the basis of a radiological examination of head Computed Tomography (CT) scans with contrast and/or MRI. The size of the tumor is divided into large sizes (≥30 mm, there is a mass effect) and small size (<30 mm, no mass effect). The mass effect is midline shift >3 mm and there is minimal cerebral edema to the extent, or the presence of ventricular compression or compression in the basal cisterna.

Cognitive function was assessed using MMSE and MoCA-Ina. A score less than 26 is considered optimal cutoff point for diagnosis of cognitive impairment. This evaluation of cognitive performances was realized at the time of diagnosis.

We compared descriptive data using Chi-square or Fisher exact test. P-value < 0.05 considered statistically significant. All statistical analysis was performed using Statistical Package for the Social Sciences (SPSS).

3 RESULT

The study-group consisted of 33 patients diagnosed with brain tumors. In the distribution by gender, we found a predominance of males (20 cases), representing 60.6% of the total number of cases. the average age of occurrence of brain tumors was 46.48 (SD = 10.78) and mostly, the group of age was 51–60 years. As shown in Table 1, the average score on the MMSE was 23.76 (SD = 4.08), while the average score on the MoCA-Ina was 21.79 (SD = 4.93).

4 DISCUSSION

In this study, we evaluated cognitive function in patients newly diagnosed with brain tumors. Our study demonstrated patients with group of education 7–9 years presented a significantly higher percentage of abnormal MMSE and MoCA-Ina score than other group. The data obtained by us are similar to data obtained by Maharani, patients with brain tumor that education <9 years also more cognitive impairment.

On the other hand, in our study suggest that most patients with tumor located in supratentorial and large tumor was abnormal MMSE and MoCA-Ina score. The Liouta et al show that patients in the large meningioma had poorer performance on language and fine motor

Table 1.   Patient characteristics.

Characteristic	n = 33	%
Age (years), Mean ± SD	46.48 ± 10.78	
Group of Age		
21–30 y	4	12.1
31–40 y	4	12.1
41–50 y	9	27.3
51–60 y	16	48.5
Sex		
Males	20	60.0
Females	13	39.4
Education		
0–6 y	5	15.2
7–9 y	12	36.4
10–12 y	12	36.4
>12 y	4	12.1
Disease duration (month), Mean ± SD	5.94 ± 7.14	
MMSE score, Mean ± SD	23.76 ± 4.08	
MoCA-Ina score, Mean ± SD	21.79 ± 4.93	

Table 2.   Comparison of MMSE and MoCA-Ina score by sex, age, education, and disease duration.

	MMSE		MoCA-Ina	
	Normal	Abnormal	Normal	Abnormal
Sex (%)				
Males	46.2	70.0	44.4	66.7
Females	53.8	30.0	55.6	33.3
p Value	0.276		0.42	
Age (%)				
21–30 y	23.1	5.0	33.3	4.2
31–40 y	15.4	10.0	11.1	12.5
41–50 y	38.5	20.0	22.2	29.2
51–60 y	23.1	65.0	33.3	54.2
p Value	0.104		0.15	
Education (%)				
0–6 y	0	25.0	0	20.8
7–9 y	23.1	45.0	11.1	45.8
10–12 y	53.8	25.0	55.6	29.2
>12 y	23.1	5.0	33.3	4.2
p Value	0.04		0.02	
Disease duration (%)				
<1 y	92.3	80.0	88.9	83.3
1–2 y	7.7	15.0	11.1	12.5
>2 y	0.0	5.0	0	4.2
p Value	0.56		0.81	

testing than patients with small meningioma. According to our results, that either primary and metastatic tumors located more than 1 lobe suffer more cognitive impairment than those located on only 1 lobe. It also explains that the more areas of the brain affected, the impact of cognitive impairment that appears also more real. Cognitive dysfunction may be a direct

Table 3. Comparison of MMSE and MoCA-Ina score by type, location, and size of tumor.

	MMSE		MoCA-Ina	
	Normal	Abnormal	Normal	Abnormal
Type of tumor (%)				
Primary	69.2	55.0	55.6	62.5
Secondary	30.8	45.0	44.4	37.5
p Value	0.485		0.509	
Location tumor	76.9	70.0	77.8	70.8
	15.4	10.0	11.1	12.5
Supratentorial	7.7	20.0	11.1	16.7
	0.598		0.91	
Infratentorial				
Both lesion	84.6	85.0	77.8	87.5
p Value	15.4	15.0	22.2	12.5
Size of tumor	0.669		0.597	
Large				
Small				
p Value				

Table 4. The percentage of MMSE in brain tumor patients impaired in domain-specific cognitive tests.

Domain MMSE	n (%)
Orientation	24 (72.7%)
Registration	2 (6.1%)
Attention and calculation	30 (90.9%)
Recall	26 (78.8%)
Language	27 (81.8%)

Table 5. The percentage of MoCA-Ina in brain tumor patients impaired in domain-sepesific cognitive tests.

Domain MoCA-Ina	n (%)
Visuospatial/Executive function	24 (72.7%)
Naming	4 (12.1%)
Attention	27 (81.8%)
Language	5 (15.2%)
Abstraction	28 (84.8%)
Delayed Recall	30 (90.9%)
Orientation	21 (63.6%)

consequence of the neoplasm growth process or is a secondary outcome such as increased intracranial pressureor cerebral edema found at the time of diagnosis.

We noticed that over 90,9% of patients impairment of attention and calculation using MMSE, while delayed recall have been affected on more than 90.9% of patients using MoCA-Ina. The Stanca et al showed that patients in group A (patients with meninges tumor) most commonly affected cognitive area was attention (66% of patients with meningiomas showing the decline in this area), and in group B (patients with neuroepithelial tumors) over 60% of patients had impaired executive function, memory or attention. A possible hypothesis could be that memory and attention are based on the integrity of widely distributed neural networks and are therefore prone to be affected by nearly any tumor location and histology (Olson, R.A., 2008).

We have some limitations: First, most of patient did not undergo a biopsy so the diagnosis would be difficult to determine. Second, patient with brain tumor were administered the MoCA-Ina and MMSE in the time on the same day, so influence of patient fatigue on test results.

5 CONCLUSION

Our study demonstrated a statistically significant abnormal MMSE and MoCA-Ina score in BT patients with the group of education 7–9 years. The present findings suggest that most patients with tumor located in supratentorial and large size of brain brain tumor demonstrate abnormal MMSE and MoCA-Ina score. Finally, we recommend clinician to evaluate cognitive function in patients newly diagnosed with brain tumors.

REFERENCES

Berger, M.S. and Prados, M.D. 2005. Diagnostic Imaging. *Textbook of Neurooncology.* Elsevier Saunders: Pennsylvania.

Folstein, M.F., Folstein, S.E., McHugh, P.R. 1975. "Mini-mental state". A practical method for grading the cognitive state of patients for the clinician. *J Psychiatr Res.* 12(3): 189–198.

Husein, N., Silvia, L., Yetty, R., & Herqutanto. 2010. Uji Validitas dan Reabilitas Montreal Cognitive Assessment Versi Indonesia (MoCA-Ina) untuk Skirining Gangguan Fungsi Kognitif. *Neurona Neuro Sains.* 27(4): 15–22.

Liouta, E., Koutsarnakis, C., Liakos, F. & Stranjalis, G. 2016. Effects of intracranial meningioma location, size, and surgery on neurocognitive functions: a 3-year prospective study. *J Neurosurg.* 124: 1578–1584.

Maharani, K., Larasari, A., Aninditha, T. & Ramli, Y. 2015. Profil Gangguan Kognitif pada Tumor Intrakranial Primer dan Metastasis. *Journal UI.* 3(2): 107–114.

Margelisch, K., Studer, M., Ritter, B.C., Steinlin, M., Leibundgut, K. & Heinks, T. 2015. Cognitive Dysfunction in Children with Brain Tumors at Diagnosis. *Pediatr Blood Cancer.* 62: 1805–1812.

Nasreddine, Z.S., Phillips, N.A., Bedirian, V., Charbonneau, S., Whitehead, V., Collin, I., et al. 2005. The Montreal Cognitive Assessment, MoCA: A Brief Screening Tool for Mild Cognitive Impairment. *J Am Geriatr Soc.* 53: 695–699.

Olson, R.A., Chhanabhai, T. & Mckenzie, M. 2008. Feasibility Study of the Montreal Cognitive Assessment (MoCA) in Patients with Brain Metastases. *Support Care Cancer.* 16: 1273–1278.

Olson, R.A., Iverson, G.L., Carolan, H., Parkinson, M., Brooks, B.L. & Mckenzie, M. 2011. Prospective Comparison of Two Cognitive Screening Tests: Diagnostic Accuracy and Correlation with Community Integration and Quality of life. *J Neurooncol.* 105: 337–344.

Ong, P.A., Muis, A., Rambe, A.S., Widjojo, F.S., Laksmidewi, A.A. (eds). 2015. *Panduan Praktik klinik Diagnosis dan Penatalaksanaan Demensia.* Perhimpunan Dokter Spesialis Saraf Indonesia: Jakarta.

Stanca, D., Craitoiu, S., Zaharia, C., Tudorica, V., Albu, C., Alexandru, O. et al. 2011. Prospective Study on the Presence of Cognitive Impairments in Patients with Brain Tumors. *Rom J Neurol.* 10(3): 131–135.

Tucha, O., Smely, C., Preier, M. & Lange, K.W. 2000. Cognitive deficits before treatment among patients with brain tumors. *Neurosurgery.* 47: 324–333.

Stem Cell Oncology – Adella (Ed.)
© 2018 Taylor & Francis Group, London, ISBN 978-0-8153-9272-9

Pattern of fungal infections in Chronic Suppurative Otitis Media (CSOM)

M.P.H. Harahap, A. Aboet & T.S.H. Haryuna
Department of Otorhinolaryngology Head and Neck Surgery, Faculty of Medicine,
Universitas Sumatera Utara, Medan, North Sumatera, Indonesia

ABSTRACT: Organisms that can be found in CSOM can be either aerobic or anaerobic fungi or a combination of both. Chronic secretions and the use of irrational and excessive otic topical antibiotics encourage the growth of fungal infections in CSOM. *Aspergillus* and *Candida sp* are fungi which are commonly found in CSOM. To understand the pattern of fungal infections of patients with CSOM at the ORL-HNS Department, Faculty of Medicine, Universitas Sumatera Utara/Haji Adam Malik General Hospital Medan, a descriptive study with case series approach was conducted. Positive fungal cultures with as many as four specimens (13.33%) were found from 30 aural discharges. The types of fungi were *Aspergillus sp.* (75%) and *Candida sp.* (25%). From the results conducted a positive fungal culture, so the fungal infection is still considered on CSOM especially from the patients who do not respond to treatment.

Keywords: CSOM, fungal infections, fungal culture

1 INTRODUCTION

Chronic Suppurative Otitis Media (CSOM) is a chronic inflammation of the middle ear with perforation of the tympanic membrane and a history of secretion from the ear (otorrhoea) over three months, either continuous or disappearing. Secretions may be watery or thick, clear or pus (Helmi, 2005; Chole & Nason 2009).

CSOM can cause extracranial and intracranial complications in order to increase high morbidity. In developing countries the problem of poverty, little knowledge, lack of specialist personnel and limited access to health services exacerbate the course of illness and complications of CSOM (Geeta, 2014; Orji, 2013).

Otomycosis is a fungal infection of the ear that is usually an infection of the outer ear canal; in some cases this fungal infection may affect the middle ear in the case of perforation of the tympanic membrane (Chao et al., 2011). Chronicity of the discharge plays an important role in the causation of fungal otitis media as it causes humid conditions in the ear and alters the pH of the media to alkaline epithelial debris. Both these factors help in the growth of fungus (Dhingra et al., 2014). However, the disease is still a challenge and can even lead to frustration in both patients and ENT specialists because of prolonged treatment due to high recurrence (Chao et al., 2011; Ozturkcan, 2014).

The use of irrational topical antibiotics and excessive ear drops encourages the growth of fungal infections in CSOM (Mittal, 1997; Mungia, 2008; Wolk, 2016). Common fungi in CSOM are *Aspergillus* and *Candida Sp.* Fungi spores are easily found in the middle ear as it has a warm and humid environment (Ashok, 1997). Organisms that can be found in CSOM can be aerobic, anaerobic or a combination of both fungi. However, many cases of CSOM in the administration of medication that do not use proper antibiotics could lead to therapeutic failure, other hazards that can arise are the occurrence of resistance to microorganisms, sustained infection and ultimately complications that cause suffering to patients and require large medical expenses (Mungia & Daniel, 2008; Saraswati et al., 2013; Lubis, 2010).

According to Lubis' study (2010) from 75 secretion samples of CSOM patients who went to H. Adam Malik General Hospital Medan found that positive fungal culture were 54.7% and negative fungal culture were 45.3% with the most commonly results were *Aspergillus sp.* (Lubis, 2010).

Research on the pattern of these fungal infections is still to be renewed again, considering many cases of CSOM with chronic aural discharge and irrational uses of antibiotic so it needs to examined changes in the pattern of fungal infections in CSOM patients in H. Adam Malik General Hospital Medan. Therefore it is important to know how the role of fungal infections to CSOM patients especially in Department of ORL-HNS Faculty of Medicine USU/H. Adam Malik General Hospital Medan.

2 METHOD

The type of research is descriptive using a case series approach. The research was conducted in the Department of ORL-HNS Faculty of Medicine USU/H. Adam Malik General Hospital Medan. Specimens from the middle ear were collected from December 2014 to September 2015. Examination of fungal patterns was conducted at the Department of Microbiology Faculty of Medicine USU/Haji Adam Malik General Hospital Medan.

The population of this study consists of CSOM patients who went to the Department of ORL-HNS Faculty of Medicine USU/H. Adam Malik General Hospital Medan during the period December 2014–September 2015. Diagnosis of CSOM is established based on history, physical examination and investigation.

The sample in this study is the entire population that meets the inclusion and exclusion criteria. Inclusion criteria: New/old CSOM patients with active aural discharge, willing to participate in research, subtotal and total tympanic membrane perforation, the not administered any ear drops for the last seven days. Exclusion criteria: The anatomic conditions of the ear canal and the tympanic membrane cause specimen could not be taken.

The sample of the study that fulfilled both inclusion and exclusion criteria comprised 26 people. The research sampling approach used is non-probability. The samples were taken purposively, that is from all patients who came to Department of ORL-HNS Faculty of Medicine USU/H. Adam Malik General Hospital Medan who met the inclusion and exclusion criteria.

3 RESULTS

This research is descriptive conducted in Department of ORL-HNS Faculty of Medicine USU/H. Adam Malik General Hospital Medan in the period December 2014–September 2015. From 26 patients collected 30 samples from unilateral ears both right and left were 22 samples while bilateral were four samples.

From Figure 1 it can be seen that from 30 secretions from middle ear, four (13.33%) are positive for fungal culture, while the negative culture was 26 (86.67%).

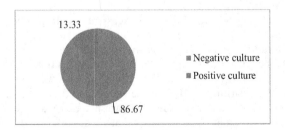

Figure 1.   Distribution of the results of the secretions culture of CSOM patients (in percent).

Table 1. Distribution of the type of fungus on CSOM patients.

Fungal	Number (n)	%
Aspergillus fumigatus	3	75
Candida sp	1	25
Total	4	100

Based on Table 1 it can be seen that from fungal culture result obtained four fungal infection. The most common fungi are *Aspergillus fumigatus* with three (75%) followed by *Candida sp.* as the remainder (25%).

4 DISCUSSION

This study was conducted on 26 CSOM patients in H. Adam Malik General Hospital Medan over the period December 2014–September 2015, and the results found that from 30 samples of secretions from middle ear were positive fungus culture as many as four (13.33%), whereas negative culture was 26 (86.67%) where *Aspergillus fumigatus* was obtained by 75% followed by *Candida sp.* as many as 25%.

The results of this research are similar to those of Prakash (2003) which obtained 12.25% of the fungal culture from 204 CSOM patients, where *Aspergillus sp.* obtained the highest of 70.83%, while *Candida sp.* amounted to 29.17%. Vishwanath (2012) out of the 115 fungal cultures obtained found only 11 (9.6%) where *Aspergillus sp.* was obtained by 22.7% while *Candida sp.* was 27.27%. Aquino (2009) in 160 CSOM patients obtained fungi by 15.6% (Vishwanatha et al., 2012; Prakash et al., 2013; Aquino et al., 2009).

The results of Kumar and Seth's (2011) study obtained from 100 cases of CSOM found *Candida albicans* to be the most common fungus with as many as nine (60%), followed by *Aspergillus fumigatus* with as many as three (20%), *Aspergillus niger* as many as two (13.3%) and *Aspergillus flavus* as many as one (6.7%) (Kumar, 2013).

This is slightly different from Geeta's research (2014) which obtained a positive fungal culture of 25.6% where *Aspergillus sp.* is 16% while *Candida sp.* is 4% (Geeta, 2014).

A previous study conducted at the H. Adam Malik General Hospital Medan by Lubis in 2010 found a positive culture result of fungi in 41 of 75 samples or 54.7%. The most common types of fungi are *Aspergillus sp.*, which consists of *Aspergillus niger* with as many as 14 samples (43.9%), *Aspergillus fumigatus* with as many as five samples (8.7%) and *Aspergillus flavus* with as many as three samples. This is followed by *Candida sp.* with as many as 18 samples (43.9%), consisting of *Candida albicans,* as many as nine samples (21.9%), *Candida tropicalis* six samples (14.6%), *Candida parapsilosis* as many as two samples (4.8%), *Candida krusei* as many as one sample (1.3%) and *Penicillium sp.* as many as one sample (1.3%). From this it can be seen that the frequency of fungal infections in CSOM at H. Adam Malik General Hospital Medan has decreased from 54.7% in 2010 (Lubis, 2010) to 13.33% in this study (December 2014–September 2015). Specimen collection methods and inclusion criteria in both studies are relatively similar, but in our study we did not include the patients that have previously used ear drops. The use of irrational topical antibiotics and excessive use of ear drops encourage the growth of fungal infections in CSOM (Mittal et al., 1997).

Fungal infections of the middle ear generally develop well in moist and otorrhoea (Sauders et al., 2011). Chronic secretions play an important role as a cause of fungal infections in CSOM because they cause a moist condition in the ear and alter the middle ear pH to a base (Dhingra et al., 2014). The most common fungi found in CSOM are the *Candida* and *Aspergillus* species. In this study 75% *Aspergillus fumigatus* and 25% *Candida sp.* were found.

The likelihood of this is due to the type of fungus that often grows in the ear, when conditions that support the influence of fungal infection become opportunistic. One theory states that *Aspergillus* and *Candida* are the opportunistic fungi. Pradhan's (2003) findings in his study in India suggest the most common types of *Aspergillus sp.* were *Aspergillus flavus, Aspergillus niger and Aspergillus fumigatus. Candida albicans* is another fungal cause of ear infections that are endogenous microorganisms that often interfere with the gastrointestinal tract and urinary tract (Levinson, 2008; Pradhan et al., 2003).

5 CONCLUSION

There were positive fungal cultures in as many as four specimens (13.33%) from 30 ear secretions, which consist of *Aspergillus fumigatus* and *Candida sp.*

REFERENCES

Aquino, J.E., Pererira, S.H., Aquino, J.N., Neto, R.G., Carvalho, M.R., & Filho, N.A. (2009). Bacterial finding found in the Chronic Otitis Media Secretion: Comparative study between Cholesteatoma (OMCC) and Simple Chronic Otitis Media (SCOM). *Intl. Arch. Otorhinolaryngol*, 287–292.

Ashok, M., Mann, S.B., Naresh, K.P., Menhra, & Taiwar, P. (1997). Secondary fungal infectionin Chronic Suppurative Otitis Media, *IJO & HNS*, *49*(2).

Chao, L.H., Chen, W.C., & Wang, K.H. (2011). Iatrogenic Invasive Otomycosis. *Tzu Chi Medical Journal*.

Chole, R.A. & Nason, R., (2009). Chronic Otitis Media and Cholesteatoma In ****. *Ballenger's manual of otorhinology head and neck surgery* (pp. 217–27). Connecticut: BC Decker.

Dhingra, R., Monga, S., Kaur, M., Brar, R., Rupali, & Arora, H. (2014). Role of fungal infections in CSOM: Prospective study. *Indian Journal of Basic and Applied Medical Research*, *3*(2), 598–608.

Geeta, S.H. (2014). Study of aerob, anaerobs and fungi in CSOM in a referral hospital of Bangalore rural. *Journal of Evolution of Medical and Dental Sciences, 3*(23), 6297–6303.

Helmi, (2005). Chronic Suppurative Otitis Media, in Chronic Suppurative Otitis Media: Basic Knowledge, Mastoidectomy Medical Therapy. Publisher Hall FK UI. Jakarta. 55–72.

Kumar, H. & Seth, S. (2011). Bacterial and fungal study of 100 cases of Chronic Suppurative Otitis Media. *Journal of Clinical and Diagnostic Research*, *5*(6), 1224–7.

Levinson, W. (2008). Antimicrobial drugs, mechanism of action. *Review of medical microbiology and immunology* (10th Ed). New York: Mc Graw Hill.

Lubis, Y.M. (2010). *Profile of fungi in CSOM patients in Haji Adam Malik General Hospital Medan.* Thesis. Medan.

Mittal, A., Mann, S., Panda, N., Mehra, Y., & Talwar, P. (1997). Secondary fungal infections in chronic suppurative otitis media. *Indian Journal Otorhinolaryngology-Head and Neck Surgery*, *49*(2).

Mungia, R. & Daniel, S. (2008). Ototopical antifungals and otomycosis: A review. *72*, 453–459.

Orji, F.T. (2013). A survey of the burden of management of chronic suppurative otitis media in developing country. *Annals of Medical and Health Sciences Research*, *3*(4).

Ozturkcan, S. (2014). Dermatologic diseases of the external ear. *Clinics in Dermatology*, *32*, 141–152.

Pradhan, B.,Tuladhar, N.R., & Amatya, R.M. (2003). Prevalence of otomycosis in outpatient department of otolaryngology in Tribhuvan University Teaching Hospital, Kathmandu, Nepal. *The Annals of Otology, Rhinology & Laryngology*, *112*(4), 384–387.

Prakash, M., Lakshmi, K., Anuradha, S. & Swathi, G.N. (2013). Bacteriological profile and their antibiotic susceptibility pattern of cases of Chronic Suppurative Otitis Media. *Asian Journal of Pharmaceutical and Clinical Research* (Chennai. June-July), *6*(3).

Saraswati, J., Venkatesh, R., & Jeya, M. (2013). Study of areboic bacterial and fungal etiology of chronic suppurative otitis media in tertiary care hospital in out skirts of Chennai, India. *International Journal of Research in Health, 1*(3).

Sauders, J., Raju, R., Boone, J., Hales, N., & Berryhill, W. (2011). Antiviotic resistance and otomycosis in the draining ear: Culture results by diagnosis. *American Journal of Otolaryngology*, *32*, 470–476.

Vishwanath, S., Mukhopadhyay, C., Mukhopadhyay, Prakash, R., Pillai, S., & Pujary, K. (2012). Chronic Suppurative Otitis Media: Optimizing initial antibiotic therapy in a tertiary care setup. *Indian Journal Otolaryngol Head Neck Surgery, 64*(3), 285–289.

Wolk, D. (2016). Microbiology of middle ear infections: Do you hear what I hear? *Clinical Microbiology Newsletter*, *38*(11), 87–93.

Stem Cell Oncology – Adella (Ed.)
© 2018 Taylor & Francis Group, London, ISBN 978-0-8153-9272-9

Correlation of TNF-α expression to clinical stadium in Nasopharyngeal Carcinoma (NPC)

Farhat, R.A. Asnir, A. Yudhistira & R.R. Susilo
Department of Otorhinolaryngology Head and Neck Surgery, Faculty of Medicine, Universitas Sumatera Utara, Medan, North Sumatera, Indonesia

E.R. Daulay
Department of Radiology, Faculty of Medicine, Universitas Sumatera Utara, Medan, North Sumatera, Indonesia

J. Chrestella
Department of Anatomic Pathology, Faculty of Medicine, Universitas Sumatera Utara, Medan, North Sumatera, Indonesia

ABSTRACT: Nasopharyngeal Carcinoma (NPC) is one of the most common malignancies in Indonesia with over 13,000 new cases reported yearly, especially in males. TNF-α serum is reported as a new biomarker to predict bone invasion, post-therapy distant metastasis and poor life sustainability in NPC. To identify the expression of TNF-α in regard to clinical stage of NPC. This is an analytic study with 126 NPC samples of patients in Haji Adam Malik General Hospital. NPC was mostly found in the age group 41–60 years (57.1%), males (71.4%), non-keratinising SCC (79.4%), and stage IV group (54.8%). In immunohistochemistry evaluation, most TNF-α is overexpressed in non-keratinising SCC (68.0%), T3-T4 (50.8%), N2-N3 (62.7%) and clinical stage III–IV (69.9%). Spearman's test for categorical correlation yields a p value of <0,001. Conclusion: There is a significant correlation between TNF-α expression and the stage of NPC.

Keywords: Nasopharyngeal carcinoma, TNF-α, overexpression

1 INTRODUCTION

Nasopharyngeal carcinoma (NPC) is a squamous cell carcinoma that grows on the lateral wall surface of nasopharynx (Adham et al., 2012; Tualalamba, 2012). In Asia, especially China, NPC is the 11th most common malignancy with an average incidence of nearly 25 cases per 100,000 (Patel et al., 2017; Chan et al., 2012). In Indonesia, more than 13,000 new cases are reported yearly, especially in men, and this is associated with a high mortality rate (Cao et al., 2011; Dhingra, 2014; Fles et al., 2017).

Cytokines play an important role in the pathogenesis and maintenance of cancer with different ways which include TNF-α, TRAIL, IL-6, IL-10, IL-12, IL-17 dan IL-23 (Kabel, 2014). TNF-α as a main pro-inflammatory cytokine is capable as an endogenous tumour promoter in bridging inflammation and carcinogenesis. New studies have shown the role of TNF-α in all carcinogenesis aspects such as cellular transformation, proliferation, invasion, angiogenesis and metastasis (Wang & Lin, 2008).

TNF-α serum is reported as a new biomarker to predict bone invasion, post-therapy distant metastasis and poor life sustainability in NPC, which shows that TNF-α has biological significance in NPC (Song et al., 2013; Lu et al., 2011; Lu et al., 2012).

Signal pathway and the transcription factor activated by TNF-α are considered important in invasion and metastasis of cancer cells. Cancer cells are more dependent on transcription factors compared to normal cells. The development of cancer cells is inhibited and apoptosis is promoted through the inhibition of the transcription factor and targeted signal pathway (Tang et al., 2017).

Considering the importance of TNF-α, the correlation of TNF-α expression to clinical stadium of NPC patients is studied.

2 METHODS

Research was conducted over the period July–October 2017 in the Adam Malik General Hospital, Medan, recruiting 126 samples of patients diagnosed with NPC based on history taking, physical examination and histopathological biopsy during the period 2015–2016.

The inclusion criteria includes patients diagnosed with NPC based on histopathological reports and who have not received radiotherapy, chemotherapy or a combination of both.

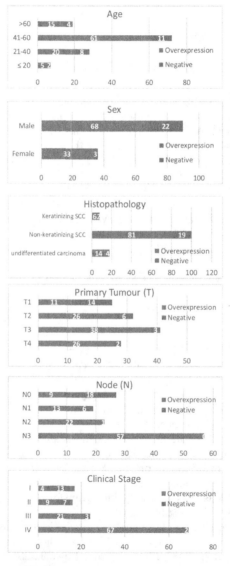

Figure 1. Frequency of Age, Sex, Histopathology, Primary Tumour (T), Nodes (S) and Clinical Staging results based on TNF-α expression.

By using the sampling formula, a minimal of 68 patients was required for the research. The samples were collected using non-probability consecutive sampling.

The tissues were examined using immunohistochemistry under a fluorescent microscope evaluating the immunoreaction of the TNF-α antibody. The results were evaluated based on the immunoreactivity score (≥ 4 is considered positive or overexpressed TNF-α) (Fedchenko & Reifenrath, 2014). All data is presented in the figure.

3 RESULTS

This study involved 126 samples with the highest frequency of patients found in the age group 41–60 years (57.1%). With regard to gender, males are the largest population of NPC patients with 90 samples (71.4%). The non-keratinising squamous cell carcinoma (79.4%), and stage IV group (54.8%) is the most frequent regarding the histopathology characteristic. In immunohistochemistry evaluation, most TNF-α overexpressed in non-keratinising squamous cell carcinoma (64.3%), T3-T4 primary tumour size (50.8%), neck nodes enlargement in the N2–N3 group (62.7%) and clinical stage in the III–IV group (69.9%).

Correlation analysis using Spearman's test for categorical correlation yielded a p value of < 0,001, which indicates that there is a statistically significance correlation of clinical staging and the expression of TNF-α.

4 DISCUSSION

In this study, the largest age group in nasopharyngeal carcinoma is in the age group of 41–60 years (57.1%). Similar to Adham's (2012) study, the peak of most NPC patients was found to be 40–49 years old. This has happened because the DNA repair mechanism function and immune system have decreased as they undergo mutation after the age of 40 years. (Soehartono et al., 2007).

In our study, we found a similar predominance, with 71.4% male and 28.6% female cases yielding a 2.5:1 ratio. The male:female ratio was relatively stable over the years. Cao's study (2011) also found the incidence rate of NPC in men to be higher than in women, with a ratio of 2–3:1. The exposure to environmental pollution from occupation and lifestyle caused males to have a higher ratio than females diagnosed with NPC (Lara, 2016).

In our study, non-keratinising squamous cell carcinoma (79.4%) was the most common form of NPC, consistent with studies conducted in other high-risk countries. More than 90% of NPC in endemic area is non-keratinising squamous cell carcinoma (Cao, 2011).

Tumour Necrosis Factor Alpha (TNF-α) is a kind of pro-inflammatory cytokine mainly secreted by tumour cells and macrophages. TNF-α can not only take part in the mechanisms of apoptosis induction, but also accelerates tumour growth in the process of tumour progression. And increasing evidence shows that TNF-α participates in many key processes of tumour progression including activation of the cancer gene, DNA damage and tumour metastasis. High expression of TNF-α is closely related to tumour recurrence and lymph node metastasis (Wang & Lin, 2008). In this study, we found TNF-α overexpression is most common in T3 primary tumours (30.2%). In regional metastasis, TNF-α overexpression was found most frequently in the N3 lymph node (45.3%), and the lowest in N0 (7.1%). Elevated TNF-α expression was most common in stage IV (70%) and the highest TNF-α expression was found in non-keratinising squamous cell carcinoma type (64.3%).

The result of this study showed that there is a significant correlation of NPC clinical stage and the expression of TNF-α. Jin et al. (2017) reported a significant reduction of TNF-α expression after treatment of NPC, indicating that TNF-α expression may be used for clinical staging of NPC. Andersson et al. (2014) also found that the upregulation of CRP and TNF-α in the NPC patient plasma was significantly related to shorter patient survival.

5 CONCLUSION

Our study suggests that there is a significant relationship between TNF-α expression and NPC clinical stage. Therefore, a further study with larger samples is warranted, which could contribute to fully understanding the association of TNF-α and NPC, and to establish a new approach in screening and surveillance of NPC using TNF-α.

REFERENCES

Adham, M., Kurniawan, A.N., Muhtadi, A.I. et al. (2012). Nasopharyngeal carcinoma in Indonesia: Epidemiology, incidence, signs and symptoms at presentation. *Chinese Journal of Cancer, 31*(4), 185–196.

Andersson, B.Å., Lewin, F., Lundgren, J., Nilsson, M., Rutqvist, L.E., Löfgren, S. & Laytragoon-Lewin, N. (2014). Plasma tumor necrosis factor-α and C-reactive protein as biomarker for survival in head and neck squamous cell carcinoma. *Journal of Cancer Research and Clinical Oncology, 140*(3), 515–519.

Cao, S., Simons, M.J., & Qian, C. (2011). The prevalence and prevention of nasopharyngeal carcinoma in China. *Chinese Journal of Cancer, 30*(2), 114–119.

Chan, A.T., Gregoire, V., Lefebvre, J.L. et al. (2012). Nasopharyngeal cancer: EHNS-ESMO-ESTRO clinical practice guidelines for diagnosis, treatment and follow-up. *Annals of Oncology, 7*, vii83–vii85.

Dhingra, P.L. (2014). Tumours of Nasopharynx. In *Disease of Ear, Nose and Throat & Head and Neck Surgery* (p. 49 & pp. 250–252). New Delhi: Elsevier.

Fedchenko, N., & Reifenrath, J. (2014). Different approaches for interpretation and reporting of immunohistochemistry analysis results in the bone tissue – a review. *Diagnostic Pathology, 9*, 221.

Fles, R., Bos, A.C., Supriyati et al. (2017). The role of Indonesian patients' health behaviors in delaying the diagnosis of nasopharyngeal carcinoma. *BMC Public Health*, 17, 510.

Jin, Y.B., Zhang, G.Y., Lin, K.R., Chen, X.P., Cui, J.H., Wang, Y.J. & Luo, W. (2017). Changes of plasma cytokines and chemokines expression level in nasopharyngeal carcinoma patients after treatment with definitive intensity-modulated radiotherapy (IMRT). *PloS One, 12*(2), p.e0172264.

Kabel, A.M. (2014). Relationship between cancer and cytokines. *Journal of Cancer Research and Treatment, 2*(2), 41–43.

Lara, H.H.R, & Monroy, A. (2016). Prevalence of nasopharyngeal carcinoma among patients with nasopharyngeal mass in a Philippine tertiary training hospital. *Philippine Journal of Otolaryngology-Head and Neck Surgery, 31*(1), 35–38.

Lu, K., Feng, X., Deng, Q. et al. (2012). Prognostic role of serum cytokines in patients with nasopharyngeal carcinoma. *Onkologie*, 35, 494–498.

Lu, X., Qian, C.N., Mu, Y.G. et al. (2011). Serum CCL2 and serum TNF-α – Two new biomarkers predict bone invasion, post-treatment distant metastasis and poor overall survival in nasopharyngeal carcinoma. *European Journal of Cancer*, 47, 339–346.

Patel, V.J., Chen, N.W., & Resto, V.A. (2017). Racial and ethnic disparities in nasopharyngeal cancer survival in the United States: A SEER study. *Otolaryngology-Head and Neck Surgery, 156*(1), 122–131.

Song, Q., Wang, G., Chu, Y et al. (2013). TNF-α up-regulates cellular inhibitor of apoptosis protein 2 (c-IAP2) via c-Jun N-terminal kinase (JNK) pathway in nasopharyngeal carcinoma. *International Immunopharmacology*, 16, 148–153.

Soehartono, Rahaju, P. & Kentjono, W.A. (2007). Hubungan antara ekspresi latent membrane protein-1 dengan peningkatan ekspresi epidermal growth factor receptor pada karsinoma nasofaring jenis undifferentiated. *Otorhinolaryngologica Indonesia, 31*(3), 1–35.

Tang, D., Tao, D., Fang, Y. et al. (2017). TNF-α promotes invasion and metastasis via NF-κB pathway in oral squamous cell carcinoma. *Med Sci Monit Basic Res*, 23, 141–149.

Tualalamba, W., & Janvilisri, T. (2012). Nasopharyngeal carcinoma signaling pathway: An update on molecular biomarkers. *International Journal of Cell Biology*, 2012. 1–10.

Wang, X. & Lin, Y. (2008). Tumor necrosis factor and cancer, buddies or foes?. *Acta Pharmacol Sin, 29*(11), 1275–1288.

Wu, Y., & Zhou, B. (2010). TNF-α/NF-κB/Snail pathway in cancer cell migration and invasion. *British Journal of Cancer, 102*(4), 639–644.

Stem Cell Oncology – Adella (Ed.)
© 2018 Taylor & Francis Group, London, ISBN 978-0-8153-9272-9

Immunohistochemical evaluation in Nasopharyngeal Carcinoma (NPC); microvessel density expressions

Farhat, R.A. Asnir, A. Yudhistira, N.R. Hasibuan & S. Yulius
Department of Otorhinolaryngology Head and Neck Surgery, Faculty of Medicine, Universitas Sumatera Utara, Medan, North Sumatera, Indonesia

E.R. Daulay
Department of Radiology, Faculty of Medicine, Universitas Sumatera Utara, Medan, North Sumatera, Indonesia

ABSTRACT: To determine the expression of microvessel density in primary tumour size (T), lymph node (N) and clinical stage in nasopharyngeal carcinoma this descriptive study involved 30 samples in Haji Adam Malik General Hospital Medan. Nasopharyngeal carcinoma was mostly found in males (73.3%); 41–60 years old (60%); T4 primary tumour (36.7%), N3 lymph node (43.3%), and non-keratinising squamous cell carcinoma (53.3%). High microvessel density (>45 MV/LP) was found in 56.7%; non-keratinising squamous cell carcinoma (58.8%), T4 primary tumour (35.3%), N3 lymph node (47.1%); and stage 4 (76.4%). Microvessel density mostly overexpressed in non-keratinising squamous cell carcinoma, primary tumour size (T4), lymph node size (N3) and clinical stage 4.

Keywords: Nasopharyngeal carcinoma, microvessel density, immunohistochemistry

1 INTRODUCTION

Nasopharyngeal Carcinoma (NPC) is the most common malignancy in Asia, with a men to women ratio of 2:1. In Indonesia, the incidence of NPC is 3.9 cases per 100,000 people. In 2006–2010 there were 335 new cases of NPC who came to the oncology division of the ENT department (Cho, 2007; Fachiroh et al., 2004; Puspitasari, 2011).

The process of formation of new blood vessels or angiogenesis plays an important role in the proliferation of cancer cells that are highly dependent on oxygen and nutrients. In addition, angiogenesis plays an important role in the spread of cancer cells. Cancer cells are able to penetrate into the blood vessels or lymph, circulate through the intravascular flow, and then proliferate elsewhere, known as metastases, as well as induce angiogenesis. Therefore, the increased density of newly formed blood vessels in a tumour is closely related to an increase in the number of tumour cells (Nishida et al., 2006; Poon et al., 2002). The pathological approach to estimating an angiogenesis is through microscopic estimation of blood vessel density or Microvessel Density (MVD) through immunohistochemical examination. Increased MVD was also associated with survival rates and metastatic spread in patients with NPC (Choi et al., 2005; Roychowdhury et al., 1996).

2 MATERIALS AND METHOD

This descriptive study was conducted at Haji Adam Malik General Hospital and Pathology Anatomy Department Medan, Indonesia. The study sample was NPC patients diagnosed with histopathologic examination (WHO, 2012) who came to the oncology division of ENT department during the period December 2011–May 2012. A total of 30 samples were included in this study and grouped according to histopathology type, primary tumour size (T), size of enlarged lymph node (KGB), and clinical stage. This study has obtained approval from the ethics commission Medical Faculty of Universitas Sumatera Utara. Histopathologic preparations are examined under in pathology anatomy of the Medical Faculty of Universitas Sumatera Utara for immunohistochemical staining in order to demonstrate MVD expression.

Immunohistochemical MVD was examined using a Monoclonal Mouse anti-Human CD31 Endothelial cell with a low (< 45 MV / LP) or high (> 45 MV/LP) measurement. Histopathologic examination was performed by three pathologists without knowing the clinical data of the sample. All data were collected and presented in tabulation form.

3 RESULTS

Thirty samples with various histopathologic types were then examined with CD31 immunohistochemical immersion to assess MVD expression. In this study high MVD expression as much as 58.8% was found in NPC-type non-keratinising squamous cell carcinoma. Along with increasing tumour size (T), high expression of MVD was more common, T4 as much as 35.3%. High MVD expression was most prevalent in clinical stage 4, at 76.4%. On the size of node grade 3 is the highest group with high MVD (47.1%).

Table 1. Frequency distribution of MVD expression with histopathological type, primary tumour size (T), lymph neck enlargement (N) and clinical stage in nasopharyngeal carcinoma.

| | Microvessel density (MV/LP) | | | |
| | Overexpression | | Negative | |
	N	%	N	%
Histopathological Type				
Keratinising squamous cell carcinoma	1	5,9	0	0
Non-keratinising squamous cell carcinoma	10	58,8	6	46,2
Undifferentiated carcinoma	6	35,3	7	53,8
Grade of Primary Tumour (T)				
T1	3	17,6	4	30,7
T2	3	17,6	2	15,4
T3	5	29,5	2	15,4
T4	6	35,3	5	38,5
Lymph Node Enlargement (N)				
N0	0	0	1	7,7
N1	5	29,4	3	23,1
N2	4	23,5	4	30,
N3	8	47,1	5	38,5
Clinical Stage				
1	0	0	0	0
2	2	11,8	1	7,7
3	2	11,8	5	38,5
4	13	76,4	7	53,8

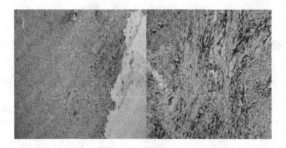

Figure 1. Examination of MVD expression using immunohistochemical CD 31 staining on NPC tissue; Left: low MVD, Right: High MVD expression (200x magnification).

4 DISCUSSION

In this study, high MVD values were mostly found in non-keratinising squamous cell carcinoma (58.8%). NPC, especially non-keratinising squamous cell carcinoma, is often associated with Epstein-Barr virus (Lutzky et al., 2008). In addition, an increase of MVD is often encountered simultaneously with Latent Membrane Protein-1 (LMP-1). LMP-1 is the main oncoprotein of the Epstein-Barr virus. Therefore, it causes a high MVD expression tendency to be found in certain types of NPC non-keratinising squamous cell carcinoma (Hardianti et al., 2010). Choi (2005) found a significant association between histopathologic type and MVD expression in breast cancer ($p < 0.01$) by using the cytometry method.

High MVD expression was found in T4 (35.3%). Sari et al. (2004) found a high MVD expression in all primary tumour sizes T3 and T4, while 76.75% of samples with T1 and T2 showed a low MVD expression (Sari, 2004). Increased tumour size (about 10^6 cells), the expansion of tumour cell populations requires vascular induction new capillaries (Weidner et al, 1991). Mohanad and Mohammed (2010) found significant increases in MVD in colorectal adenocarcinoma with a size > 3 mm3 compared with the size <3 mm3.

A total of eight samples (47.1%) with N3 KGB neck size had high MVD expression, whereas only 1 sample (7.7%) was present with low MVD expression at N0. Angiogenesis of tumours quantified by MVD measurement is currently believed to be one of the most important factors in tumour growth and metastasis (Zhao et al, 2006). The increased density of the newly formed microvessel is related to the number of cells entering the blood vessels (Weidner, 1995). This explains the increase in MVD expression in groups of N1, N2, N3 compared to N0. The highest MVD expression which was 13 samples (76.7%) was also found in clinical stage 4. No NPC with clinical stage 1 samples were found because generally patients with KNF came at an advanced stage (Taweevisit et al., 2010).

5 CONCLUSIONS

Microvessel high density (> 45 MV/LP) was encountered in 17 tissues of tissues throughout the entire tissue (56.7%). Overexpression of MVD was mostly found in non-keratinising squamous cell carcinoma, primary tumour T4, lymph neck enlargement N3 and clinical stage 4. In this study, there was an increasing trend of MVD proportional to the increase in tumour size, lymph nodes and clinical stage. These three indicators influence the management and prognosis of NPC. Therefore, further research is needed on the role of MVD in the management and prognosis of patients.

REFERENCES

Cho, W.C. (2007). Nasopharyngeal carcinoma: Molecular biomarker discovery and progress. *Molecular Cancer, 6*(1), 1–9.

Choi, W.W.L., et al. (2005). Angiogenic and lymphangiogenicmicrovessel density in breast carcinoma: Correlation with clinicopathologic parameters and VEGF family gene expression. *Modern Pathology, 18*, 143–152.

Fachiroh, J., et al. (2004). Molecular diversity of Epstein-Barr virus IgG and IgA antibody responses in nasopharyngeal carcinoma: A comparison of Indonesian, Chinese, and European subjects. *The Journal of Infectious Diseases, 190*, 53–62.

Hardianti, M.H., et al. (2010). Epstein-Barr virus latent membrane protein-1 (LMP-1) expression and angiogenesis in Indonesian nasopharyngeal carcinoma (NPC). *Journal of Cancer Research and Experimental Oncology, 2*(4), 47–53.

Lutzky, V.P., et al. (2008). biomarkers for cancers of the head and neck. *Clinical Medicine: Ear, Nose and Throat, 1*, 5–15.

Mohanad M.A. & Mohammed, S.H. (2010). Significance of intratumoralmicrovessel density quantification based on immunohistochemical detection of PECAM-1 and vWF in colorectal carcinoma from Iraqi patients. *Indian J Pathol Microbiol, 53*, 439–46.

Nishida, N., et al. (2006). Angiogenesis in cancer. *Vascular Health and Risk Management, 2*(3), 213–219.

Poon, R.T., et al. (2002). Tumor microvessel density as a predictor recurrence after resection of hepatocellular carcinoma: A prospective study. *Journal of Clinical Oncology, 20*(7), 1775–1785.

Puspitasari, D. (2011). *Gambaran Karsinoma Nasofaring di RSUP H. Adam Malik Medan Tahun 2006–2010*. Tesis. Universitas Sumatera Utara.

Roychowdhury, D.F., Tseng, A., Fu, K.K., Weinberg, V., & Weidner, N. (1996). New prognostic factors in nasopharyngeal carcinoma. *American Cancer Society, 77*(8), 1419–1426.

Sari, V.A. (2004). Korelasi tingkat ekspresi cyclooxygenase-2 dan gambaran angiogenesis pada karsinoma nasofaring tak berdiferensiasi. Tesis. Program Pendidikan Dokter Spesialis Ilmu Penyakit THT FKUI. Jakarta.

Taweevisit, M., Keelawat, S., & Thoner P.S. (2010). Correlation of microvascular density and proliferation index in undifferentiated nasopharyngeal carcinoma. *Asian Biomedicine, 4*(2), 315–321.

Weidner, N. (1995). Intratumormicrovessel density as a prognostic factor in cancer. *America Journal of Pathology, 147*(1), 9–19.

Weidner N., Semple J.P., Welch W.R., & Folkman J. (1991). Tumor angiogenesis and metastasis-correlation in invasive breast carcinoma. *The New England Journal of Medicine, 324*(1), 1–7.

Zhao, H.C., et al. (2006). Microvessel density is a prognostic marker of human gastric cancer. *World Journals of Gastroenterology, 12*(47),7598–7603.

Stem Cell Oncology – Adella (Ed.)
© 2018 Taylor & Francis Group, London, ISBN 978-0-8153-9272-9

Overexpression of Cyclooxygenase-2 in advanced stages of nasopharyngeal carcinoma

Farhat, R.A. Asnir, A. Yudhistira, F. Nurdiansyah & S. Yulius
Department of Otorhinolaryngology Head and Neck Surgery, Faculty of Medicine, Universitas Sumatera Utara, Medan, North Sumatera, Indonesia

E.R. Daulay
Department of Radiology, Faculty of Medicine, Universitas Sumatera Utara, Medan, North Sumatera, Indonesia

ABSTRACT: Nasopharyngeal Carcinoma (NPC) is one of the most dominant cancers in Southern China and Southeast Asia. The prevalence of NPC in Indonesia is 3.9 per 100,000 population every year. Cyclooxygenase (COX) is an enzyme in biosynthetic pathways of Prostaglandins (PG), thromboxane and prostacyclin of arachidonic acid. Expression of COX-2 increases in the early stages of carcinogenesis, and during the development and invasive growth of tumours. To find out the expression of COX-2 in nasopharyngeal carcinoma patients this descriptive study was undertaken with 30 NPC samples of patients in Haji Adam Malik General Hospital Medan. NPC was mostly found in the group 41–60 years (60%), males (73.3%), and non-keratinising squamous cell carcinoma (53.3%). Positive COX-2 expression in non-keratinising squamous cell carcinoma (54.5%), T3-T4 primary tumour size (68.2%), neck enlargement of N2-N3 (68.3%) and clinical stage of III–IV (90.9%). There is an increase of COX-2 expression in the advanced stages of nasopharyngeal carcinoma.

Keywords: Nasopharyngeal carcinoma, COX-2, immunohistochemistry

1 INTRODUCTION

The main therapy for nasopharyngeal carcinoma (NPC) is radiotherapy. Considerations of radiotherapy selection are based on the fact that histopathologically most NPCs are undifferentiated carcinoma (75–95%) and radiosensitive non-keratinised carcinomas (Wei, 2006; Jeyakumar, 2006). Recent meta-analysis studies suggest the need for additional chemotherapy to radiotherapy. Concomitant chemoradiotherapy is considered better than single radiotherapy and in 2006 it was started as standard therapy in patients at an advanced stage (T2B or more and/or N+) (Guigay et al., 2006; NCCN, 2010).

Cyclooxygenase (COX) is an enzyme in the biosynthetic pathway of Prostaglandin (PG), thromboxane and prostacyclin from arachidonic acid. There are two forms of COX, namely COX-1 and COX-2. Cellular expression of COX-2 increases in early stages of carcinogenesis, and during the development and invasive growth of the tumour (Murono et al., 2001; Gallo et al., 2001; Choi & Milas, 2003). COX-2 expressed on several tumours and in its development proved to be a cause of carcinogenesis (Murono et al., 2001; Levita et al., 2009).

2 METHOD

This is a descriptive study conducted at **RSUP Haji Adam Malik** and Anatomy Pathology Department of **FK USU**. The sample of the study was NPC patients who had been diagnosed by anamnesis, physical examination, radiology examination and histopathology examination. Exclusion criteria in this study were patients who had received treatment with radiotherapy, chemotherapy or both. Samples were grouped according to gender, age, histopathology type and clinical stage. COX-2 expression was assessed using histopathologic tests based on immunoreactivity (negative = 0–3, positive/overexpression = 4–9). All data is presented in table.

3 RESULTS

This study involved 30 samples with the most being aged 41–60 years (60.0%), while in the gender category it was found that the male group is the largest population of NPC patients with as many as 22 samples (73.3%). In the histopathologic group, the non-keratinising squamous cell carcinoma (53.3%), and stage in stage IV group (70%) were the highest categories. In immunohistochemistry evaluation, most COX-2 overexpressed in non-keratinising squamous cell carcinoma (54.5%), T3–T4 primary tumour size (68.2%), neck enlargement in the N2–N3 group (68.3%) and clinical stage in the III–IV group (90.9%).

Table 1. Frequency of Histopathology, Primary Tumour (T), Nodes (S) and Clinical Staging results based on COX-2 expression.

Characteristic	COX-2 Expression			
	Over-reactive	%	Negative	%
Age (y)				
≤ 20	0	0,0	1	12,5
21–40	6	27,3	0	0,0
41–60	12	54,5	6	75
> 60	4	18,2	1	12,5
Sex				
Male	16	72,7	6	75
Female	6	27,3	2	25
Primary Tumour (T)				
T1	5	22,7	2	25,0
T2	2	9,1	3	37,5
T3	6	27,3	1	12,5
T4	9	40,9	2	25,0
Nodes (N)				
N0	1	4,5	0	0,0
N1	6	27,3	2	25,0
N2	5	22,7	3	37,5
N3	10	45,6	3	37,5
Clinical Staging				
I	0	0,0	0	0,0
II	2	9,1	1	12,5
III	3	13,6	3	37,5
IV	17	77,3	4	50,0
Histopathology				
Keratinising SCC	1	4,5	0	0
Non-keratinising SCC	12	54,5	4	50
Undifferentiated carcinoma	9	41,0	4	50

4 DISCUSSION

In this study, we found the largest group in nasopharyngeal carcinoma were aged 41–60 years (60.0%). Chew (1997) in his study found that most NPC patients were aged over 20 years, with the biggest group between 50–70 years. In China, NPC started to appear from 15–19 years old, most often found at 15–34 years with peak age 35–64 years after which there is a decline (Chew, 1997).

This study found the gender of patients with nasopharyngeal carcinoma is mostly men with as many as 22 people with a ratio to women of 2.7: 1. This is allegedly as a result of the work and life habits of men who are often exposed to carcinogenic substances such as exposure to steam, dust smoke, chemical gases, and exposure to formaldehyde and wood vapour in the workplace (Chang & Adami, 2006).

The histopathological type found in patients in this study is non-keratinising squamous cell carcinoma of 16 tissues (53.3%), followed by WHO type 3 (undifferentiated carcinoma, 43.4%) and WHO type 1 (keratinising squamous cell carcinoma, 3.3%). This result is consistent with the Harahap (2009) study which found the most histopathologic type in NPC patients was WHO type 2 (non-keratinising squamous cell carcinoma) by 50.0%. Non-keratinising squamous cell carcinoma and undifferentiated carcinoma are the most common in NPC endemic areas, such as South China, Southeast Asia and North Africa, while the NPC type keratinising squamous cell carcinoma is more common in Europe (Guigay et al., 2006).

Increased COX-2 expression has been reported in various types of cancer in humans, including at least 80% of breast, colon, oesophageal, liver, lung, pancreatic, prostate, cervical and head and neck cancers (Choy & Milas, 2003). COX-2 overexpression is most common in T4 primary tumours (40.9%). The difference in the rate of proliferation with apoptosis rate when the greater the value, the greater the growth. Decreasing levels of COX-2 expression also reduce the rate of proliferation and apoptosis, which means lower tumour growth rates (Wu et al., 2003; Irianiwati, 2006). This is seen in the use of selective COX-2 inhibitors (Gandamihardja, 2010). High COX-2 expression will also increase proliferative markup expression such as Ki-67. In addition, the larger the size of the tumour the lower the expression of kaspase-3. This explains that COX-2 is involved in maintaining proliferation and inhibiting apoptosis thus accelerating tumour growth. Appropriate results were also proposed by Gandamihardja (2010) that selective COX-2 inhibitors resulted in a significant decrease in COX-2 expression, specifically 10% in the control group and 42% in the treatment group.

In regional metastasis, COX-2 overexpression was found most frequently in N3 lymph node (45.6%), with the lowest in N0 (4.5%). Kardinan (2003) in his study in colon carcinoma suspected COX-2 involvement in lymph node metastasis.

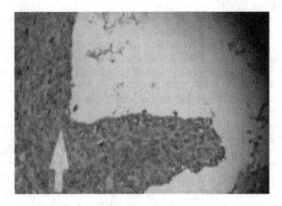

Figure 1. Immunohistochemical COX-2 staining (100x magnification) Left: weak intensity; Right: strong intensity.

Elevated COX-2 expression was most common in stage 4 of 21 tissues (70%), and the lowest was found in stage 2, in three tissues of nasopharyngeal carcinoma (10.0%). Tan and Putti (2005) conducted a study to assess COX-2 expression in NPC. Their research shows that there is a high proportion (60 out of 85 cases of NPC, 71%) expressing COX-2. Soo (2005) found an increase in COX-2 expression in 33 of 42 cases of NPC (79%) using immunohistochemical methods. Although in the last two decades progress has been made in the methods of health screening and education, only a few changes have been made in establishing early diagnosis of NPC. Stage I still ranges from less than 10% of all cases (Chew, 1997).

The highest COX-2 expression was found in non-keratinising squamous cell carcinoma type of 12 samples (54.5%). Tan (2008) in his study found the same result. Another study found that COX-2 is associated with inflammatory responses, cell differentiation, cell cycle resting phases, apoptosis, cytokine production and RNA-related separation settings associated with EBV infection. Non-keratinising squamous cell carcinoma and undifferentiated carcinoma are most associated with EBV infection (Yenita & Asri, 2012).

5 CONCLUSION

In this study, we found an elevated of COX-2 expression in non-keratinising squamous cell carcinoma type, primary tumour T3-T4, nodes N2–N3 and clinical staging III–IV. Further research is required to understand the role of Cyclooxygenase-2 in the progression and prognosis of disease in nasopharyngeal carcinoma patients that can be used to provide optimal therapy.

REFERENCES

Chang, E.T & Adami, H.O. (2006).The enigmatic epidemiology of NPC. *Cancer Epidemiol Biomarkers Prev, 15,* 1765–77.

Chew, C.T. (1997). Nasopharynx (the post nasal space). In A.G. Kerr (Ed.), *Scott-Brown's Otolaryngology, Volume 5* (6th ed.) pp. 5/13/1–30. Oxford: Butterworth Heinemann.

Choy, H. & Milas, L. (2003). Enhancing radiotherapy with cyclooxygenase-2 enzyme inhibitors: A rational advance? *Journal of the National Cancer Institute, 95*(19), 1440–52.

Gallo, O., Franchi, A, Magnelli, L., Sardi, I, Vannacci, A., Boddi V., et al. (2001). Cyclooxygenase-2 pathway correlates with VEGF expression in head and neck cancer. Implications for tumor angiogenesis and metastasis. *Neoplasia, 3*(1), 53–61.

Gandamihardja, S., Firman, et al. (2010). Peran Siklooksigenase dalam Pertumbuhan Kanker Leher Rahim, Departemen Obstetri dan Ginekologi, Departemen Biokimia, Departemen. Farmakologi Klinik Fakultas Kedokteran Universitas Padjdjaran, Bagian Obsteri dan Ginekologi Klinik Universitas Indonesia. *Jurnal MKB, 42*(4).

Guigay, J., Temam S., Bourhis, J., Pignon, J.P. & Armand, J.P. (2006). Nasopharyngeal carcinoma and therapeutic management: The place of chemotherapy. *Annals of Oncology, 17*(10), 304–7.

Harahap, M.P.H. (2009). Ekspresi Vascular Endothelial Growth Factor pada Karsinoma Nasofaring. *Tesis*. Program Pendidikan Dokter Spesialis Bidang, Ilmu Kesehatan Telinga HidungTenggorok, Bedah Kepala Leher, Fakultas Kedokteran, Universitas Sumatera Utara, Medan.

Irianiwati, A., Ghozali & Yoan, I. (2006). Hubungan antara ekspresi cyclooxygenase-2 dan reseptor dengan derajat histologis dan stadium karsinoma pada payudara. *Berkala Ilmu Kedokteran, 38*(4), 183–188.

Jeyakumar, A., Brickman, T.M., Jeyakumar, A. & Doerr, T. (2006). Review of nasopharyngeal carcinoma. *Ear, Nose and Throat Journal, 85*(3), 168–184.

Kardinan A. & Azmi D. (2003). *Pegagan (cantellasiatica) Tanaman Multimanfaat*: Balai Penelitian Tanaman Rempah dan Obat.

Levita, J., Istyastono, E.P., Nawawi, A., Mutholib, A., Esch, I.J.P. & Ibrahim, S. (2009). Analyzing the interaction of andrographolide and neoandrographolide, diterpenoid compounds from *Andrographis Paniculata* (Burm.F) nees, to cyclooxygenase-2 enzyme by docking simulation. *ITB J. Sci, 41 A*(2), 110–9.

Murono, S., Inoue, H., Tanabe, T., Joab, I., Yoshizaki, T., Furukawa, M., et al. (2001). Induction of cyclooxygenase-2 by Epstein-Barr virus latent membrane protein 1 is involved in vascular endothelial growth factor production in nasopharyngeal carcinoma cells. *PNAS, 98*(12), 6905–10.

National Comprehensive Cancer Network. (2010). Practice guidelines in oncology head and neck cancers. In *Head and Neck Cancer.*

Soo, R., Putti, T., Tao, Q., Goh, B.C., Lee, K.H., Seng, L.K., et al. (2005). Overexpression of cyclooxygenase-2 in nasopharyngeal carcinoma and association with epidermal growth factor receptor expression. *Arch Otolaryngol Head Neck Surg, 131*, 147–52.

Tan, B., Hammound, Z., Badve & S, Bigsby. (2008). In: *Estrogen promotor tumor progression in a genetically defined model of lung adenocarcinoma: Endocrine-Related cancer, 15*, 475–483.

Tan, K.B. & Putti, T.C. (2005). Cyclooxygenase-2 expression in nasopharyngeal carcinoma: Immunohistochemical findings and potential implications. *Journal of Clinical Pathology, 58*, 535–8.

Wei, W.I. (2006). Nasopharyngeal cancer. In B.J. Bailey, J.T. Johnson, S.D, Newland (Eds.), *Head and Neck Surgery Otolaryngology, vol. 2* (4th ed.) (pp. 1657–71). Philadelphia: Lippincot Williams and Wilkins.

Wu, A.W.,Gu, J., Ji, F.J., Li, F.Z. & Xu, G.W. (2003). Role of COX-2 carcinogenesis of colorectal cancer and its relationship with tumor biological characteristic and patients prognosis. *World J. Gastroenterol, 14*(10), 256–265.

Yenita & Asri A. (2012). Korelasi antara latent membrane protein-1 virus Epstein-Barr dengan p53 pada karsinoma nasofaring. *Jurnal Kesehatan Andalas, 1*(1).

Stem Cell Oncology – Adella (Ed.)
© *2018 Taylor & Francis Group, London, ISBN 978-0-8153-9272-9*

Primary Squamous Cell Carcinoma (SCC) of the parotid gland

F.M. Farhat & M.Z.B.A. Bakar
*Department of Otorhinolaryngology, Faculty of Medicine, University of Malaya,
Kuala Lumpur, Malaysia*

ABSTRACT: Parotid glands Squamous Cell Carcinoma (SCC) are extremely uncommon. Most of the parotid SCC are metastases from the skin squamous cell carcinomas. Diagnosis of primary SCC of the parotid gland can be made by excluding the high-grade mucoepidermoid carcinoma or metastatic SCC to the parotid gland. Combined modality treatment with surgery, facial nerve sparing and adjunctive radiotherapy is the treatment recommended by most of the researchers.

Keywords: squamous cell carcinoma, parotid gland.

1 INTRODUCTION

Parotid glands carcinoma are considered uncommon with an overall incidence of 3–5% of all head and neck cancers (DeVita et al., 2011; Edge, 2010). Mucoepidermoid carcinoma is the most common salivary malignancy, of which 50–70% arise in the parotid gland. On the other hand, most of the squamous cell carcinomas (PSCC) of the parotid glands are metastases from the skin squamous cell carcinomas. Occasionally, the primary site cannot be found. Primary parotid gland SCC is an aggressive tumour with an incidence 0.1–3, 4% of all parotid malignancy (Flynn et al., 1999). It is unknown whether or not such cases represent true primary parotid squamous cell carcinoma. We are reporting here a case of primary squamous cell carcinoma of the left parotid gland that means squamous cell carcinoma of parotid may not be metastases from another site.

2 CASE REPORT

A 74-year-old Malay female was presented to our otorhinolaryngology clinic at University Malaya Medical Center one and half years ago with painless left side facial swelling. The mass gradually increased in size with no facial asymmetry. The overlying skin and oral mucosa were found to be normal in colour and not swollen. Fine needle aspiration was done which reported that neoplastic squamous epithelium was present; and the patient refused surgical intervention.

After a few months she returned back to the clinic with worsening facial swelling of about 5 × 5 cm. It was firm, non-tender and extended from the annular area to retro mandibular area with a raised pinna lobule. No remarkable change was noted either on the surface of the buccal mucosa or on the skin of the cheek. A repeated FNAC resulted in SCC of the parotid gland. A whole body scanning and a Computed Tomography (CT) scan revealed a solid mass measuring 3.3 × 4.5 × 5.9 cm with area of rim enhancing hypo density seen within the gland as in Figure 1.

The patient underwent a preservative total parotidectomy. Intraoperative frozen section showed SCC of parotid gland. The tumour was extensive and the facial nerve ran through the tumour itself as in Figure 2. To excise the whole tumour we had to sacrifice the facial nerve. The histopathology report came out as moderately differentiated SCC and she was referred to oncology for post-operative radiation.

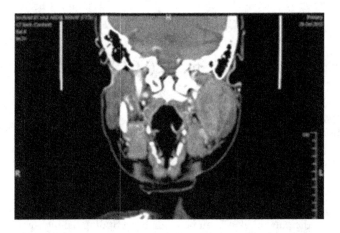

Figure 1.   Shows left parotid gland enlargement and heterogeneously enhancing.

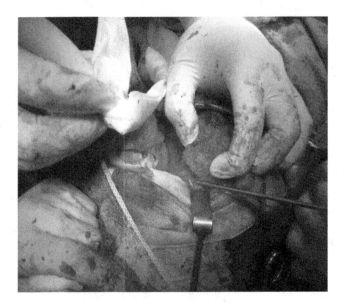

Figure 2.   Shows intraoperative facial nerve runs through parotid tumour.

3   DISCUSSION

Primary parotid gland SCC is an uncommon and highly malignant potential tumour that occasionally occurs in the major salivary glands (Ellis & Auclair, 1996; Wenig, 1993). Among various pathologic subtypes of parotid gland malignancy, the primary parotid gland SCC accounts for approximately 0.3–9.8% of all parotid gland malignant tumours (Bataskis et al., 1976; Shemen et al., 1987). The frequency of PSCC is about nine times greater in the parotid gland than in the submandibular gland (Ellis & Auclair, 1996). Diagnosis of primary SCC of the parotid gland can be made by excluding the high-grade mucoepidermoid carcinoma or metastatic SCC to the parotid gland (Bataskis et al., 1976; Shemen et al., 1987) and it has been reported that the incidence of primary SCC of parotid is lower than that of metastatic SCC to the parotid glands (Bataskis et al., 1976; Shemen et al., 1987). It is proved that in parotid malignancy that histology is an important factor in survival. But because of the rarity of this disease and it usually being categorised under parotid malignancies (Friedman et al., 1986), clinical features and modality of treatment for primary SCC of the parotid gland are not yet fully understood (Friedman et al., 1986).

Primary SCC of the parotid gland has been accepted in case the high-grade mucoepidermoid or metastatic carcinoma are excluded. The incidence of primary SCC is much lower than that of SCC metastatic to the parotid glands (Bataskis et al., 1976; Shemen et al., 1987).

Marks et al. (1987) stated that "of 30 patients with parotid gland SCC, majority 24 patients had experienced intra-parotid nodal metastasis from other areas of cancer, three patients had direct invasion into the gland from skin cancer overlying the parotid gland, whereas only three patients were diagnosed as a primary SCC of the parotid gland".

In literature it has been established that the surgical resection is the major treatment modality for primary parotid gland malignancies. However several factors such as such as tumour size, extent of tumour, presence of metastasis and facial nerve involvement have an influence in management decision (Woods et al., 1975; Zbaren et al., 2005).

The clinically negative (N0) neck management is still challenging. It's well established that presence of regional metastasis is an indication for therapeutic neck dissection; however most experts strongly recommend elective neck dissection (END) in the management of clinically negative (N0) neck (Armstrong et al., 1992) although the effectiveness of the elective neck treatment (radiotherapy or neck dissection) are limited on survival rate (Zbaren et al., 2005; Armstrong et al., 1992).

Zbaren et al. report that "routine END should be performed to all primary SCC of parotid gland" [12], whereas Kelley and Spiro state that "END is an appropriate management for patient with facial nerve paralysis, extra parotid tumour extension, old age, perilymphatic invasion and the high tumour grade" (Kelley & Spiro, 1996).

In term of 5-year survival rate the parotid gland SCC has a poor prognosis being less than 50% (Woods et al., 1975; Armstrong et al., 1992). While Lee et al. (2001) put forth that "a 5-year DSS of 31.3% for primary parotid SCC" and Michael J et al. (2014) found out that a 5-year DSS of 54.4% for primary parotid SCC.

Michael J. P. Fisterer et al. conducted a population-based analysis of 2,545 cases and discovered that parotid SCC was predominant in males (79.8%), whites (92.9%), and age group ≥ 75 years. The poor prognostic factors were black race, age ≥ 75 years and clinical stages T3 or greater. Patients with negative neck (N0) who underwent elective neck dissection (END) were associated with higher DSS (78.3% versus 51.1%, $p < 0.0001$) (Michael et al., 2014) whereas patients who did not receive END had a DSS of 51.1%. In terms of the histological grades they claim that "parotid gland SCC with histologic grade III has a 1.4-fold greater hazard of death than relative to grade I". Patients with positive neck disease and did not undergo a neck dissection had poor prognosis with a 2.8-fold hazard of death compared to patients who received a TND.

4   CONCLUSION

Primary parotid gland SCC is a rare entity, and it is concluded that SSC of the parotid glands are mostly metastatic rather than primary tumours. The objective of reporting this case is to provide information in the field of primary parotid gland SCC management to deal with reporting the tumour's behaviour and its management. Most authors recommend that combined modality treatment with surgery, facial nerve sparing, and adjunctive radiotherapy is the treatment.

REFERENCES

Armstrong, J.G., Harrison, L.B., Thaler, H.T., et al. (1992). The indications for elective treatment of the neck in cancer of the major salivary glands. *Cancer, 69*, 615–9.

Barren, P., Schupbach, J., Nuyens, M., et al. (2005). Elective neck dissection versus observation in primary parotid carcinoma. *Otolaryngol Head Neck Surg, 132*, 387–91.

Batsakis, J.G., McClatchey, K.D., Johns, M., et al. (1976). Primary squamous cell carcinoma of the parotid gland. *Arch Otolaryngol, 102*, 355–357.

DeVita, V.T., Lawrence, T.S., Rosenberg, S.A. (2011). *DeVita, Hellman, and Rosenberg's cancer: Principles & practice of oncology.* Philadelphia: Wolters Kluwer Health/Lippincott Williams & Wilkins.

Edge, S.B. & American Joint Committee on Cancer. (2010). *AJCC cancer staging manual.* New York: Springer.

Ellis, G.L., Auclair, P.L. (1996). Tumors of the salivary glands. In *Atlas of tumour pathology (3rd series, Fasc. 17)* (pp. 251–7). Washington, DC: Armed Forces Institute of Pathology.

Flynn, M.B., Maguire, S., Martinez, S., et al. (1999). Primary squamous cell carcinoma of the parotid gland: the importance of correct histological diagnosis. *Ann Surg Oncol, 6*, 768–70.

Friedman, M., Levin, B., Grybauskas, V., et al. (1986). Malignant tumors of the major salivary glands. *Otolarygol Clin North Am, 19*, 625–636.

Kelley, D.J., Spiro, R.H. (1996). Management of the neck in parotid carcinoma. *Am J Surg, 172*, 695–7.

Lee, S., Kim, G.E., Park, C.S., et al. (2001). Primary squamous cell carcinoma of the parotid gland. *Am J Otolaryngol, 22*, 400–6.

Marks, M.W., Ryan, R.F., Litwin, M.S., et al. (1987). Primary squamous cell carcinoma of the parotid gland. *Plast Reconstr Surg, 79*, 550–554.

Michael, J., Pfisterer, M.D., et al. (2014). Squamous cell carcinoma of the parotid gland: A population-based analysis of 2545 cases. *American Journal of Otolaryngology-Head and Neck Medicine and Surgery, 35*, 469–475.

Sang-wook Lee, M.D., et al. (2001). Primary squamous cell carcinoma of the parotid gland. *Am J Otolaryngol, 22*:400–406.

Shemen, L.J., Huvos, A.G., Spiro, R.H. (1987). Squamous cell carcinoma of salivary gland origin. *Head Neck Surg, 9*, 235–240.

Spitz, M.R. & Batsakis, J.G. (1984). Major salivary gland carcinoma – descriptive epidemiology and survival of 498 patients. *Arch Otolaryngol, 110*, 45–49.

Wenig, B.M (1993). *Atlas of head and neck pathology.* Philadelphia: W.B. Sannders.

Woods, J.E., Chong, G.C., & Beahrs, O.H. (1975). Experience with 1,360 primary parotid tumors. *Am J Surg, 130*, 460–2.

Ying, Y.L., Johnson, J.T., & Myers, E.N. (2006). Squamous cell carcinoma of the parotid gland. *Head Neck, 28*, 626–32.

Stem Cell Oncology – Adella (Ed.)
© 2018 Taylor & Francis Group, London, ISBN 978-0-8153-9272-9

Influence of smoking on proximal femur bone density in Haji Adam Malik Hospital, Medan

S. Ibrahim
Department of Orthopaedics and Traumatology, Faculty of Medicine, Universiti Kebangsaan, Selangor, Malaysia

M.B. Rizaldy & H. Hanafiah
Department of Orthopaedics and Traumatology, Faculty of Medicine, Universitas Sumatera Utara, Medan, North Sumatera, Indonesia

ABSTRACT: The Singh index is the classification of trabecular patterns on the proximal femur, which can be seen with the use of X-rays. Since 1976, smoking has been linked to a decrease in bone density. This cross-sectional study was performed at the Haji Adam Malik Medan Hospital, Medan, Indonesia. Samples were divided into two groups of smokers and non-smokers, with 43 persons in each group. The Singh index value was evaluated from pelvic X-rays undertaken within both samples. There was a significant correlation between smoking and the Singh index value ($p = 0.002$). The duration of smoking directly affected the Singh index ($p = 0.001$), but there was no correlation between the cigarette type ($p = 0.932$) and the frequency of smoking ($p = 0.259$) with the Singh index. It was found that smoking has a significant correlation with the Singh index value, where the smoking group had a lower Singh index value compared to the non-smoking group.

Keywords: osteoporosis, Singh index, smoking

1 INTRODUCTION

Osteoporosis is now viewed as a metabolic disease of the bone that is quite often found daily (World Health Organisation, 2004). In 2005, it was noted by the Center for Research and Development of Nutrition and Maintenance that as many as 10.3% of the entire Indonesian population suffered with osteoporosis. According to PEROSI data in 2006, of the total number of patients who came for bone mineral density examination in Makmal integrated FK UI, as much as 14.7% had osteoporosis. This amount will certainly increase every year, which will bring high morbidity with the occurrence of fractures. The more obvious problems in the Indonesian population are the low level of awareness and the high 'undiagnosed' rate in patients, due to the lack of both material and expert facilities needed to detect osteoporosis (Roeshadi, 2008).

The most feared and often occurs Battery process osteoporosis is a fracture. Fractures will greatly increase the morbidity and mortality of patients with osteoporosis, and the most common incidence of fractures is in the spine and wrist (Lucas et al., 1993). Therefore the examination detects.

Osteoporosis within the pelvic bone (proximal femur), spine (lumbar spine) and wrist (distal radius) was focused on within this study.

The Singh index is a trabecular image of the proximal femur that can be assessed using X-rays. This method has long been used in the screening as well as grading of the presence of osteoporosis in a patient. Much research has been done to assess the reliability of the Singh index, especially its comparison with the DEXA scan method, that has been determined as the 'gold standard' for diagnosing osteoporosis. But there are still some modern-day

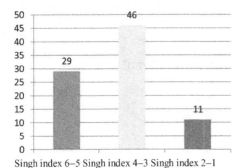

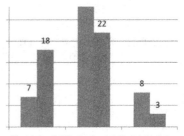

Figure 1. Distribution of Singh index value in the total population.

Figure 2. Distribution of Singh index value in each proportion.

advantages of the Singh index method, especially regarding cost-effectiveness when compared with other methods (Greenspan, 2004; Jergas, 2000). A meta-analysis study has attempted to find a direct link between smoking behaviour and bone health. It has been shown that there is a significantly proportional and significant effect of smoking behaviour on the risk of fracture, especially in the pelvis, spine and heel bone. For the smoking population, there is an increased risk in the occurrence of osteoporosis fractures; as much as 25% increasing to 40–80% in the hip bone. The risk of an osteoporosis related fracture reaches 90% in smoking populations aged over 85 years.

2 METHOD

This research used a descriptive-analytic (cross-sectional) method. The population in this study were Indonesian men aged 60 years or older who came to Haji Adam Malik Hospital in Medan. The inclusion criteria was defined as: 1) male; 2) aged 50 years or more; 3) an X-ray taken in the Department of Radiology at the Haji Adam Malik Hospital; and 4) the patient was willing to participate in the study. The exclusion criteria was defined as: 1) a history of trauma to the pelvic bone or pelvis for longer than two weeks; 2) a history of taking corticosteroid drugs and anti-osteoporosis medications; 3) a history of intestinal surgery or thyroid surgery; 4) a history of cancer; and 5) a history of mumps.

3 RESULTS

In this research, the study population came from the patient population of Haji Adam Malik Hospital. As many as 86 people fulfilled the inclusion and exclusion criteria, and consisted of 43 people who smoked and 43 people who did not smoke.

Figure 1 shows most of the sample population (46) had a Singh index of 4–3 which is categorised as light osteoporosis (59.3%).

From Figure 2, it can be seen that the non-smoking population mostly had a Singh index of 6–5 (in 18 samples), which is classified as normal and corresponds to 20.9% of the total sample population. While the smoking population, mostly had a Singh index of 4–3 (in 35 samples) which equates to mild osteoporosis in 40.6% of the total sample population.

4 DISCUSSION

Since it was first publicised in 1976 that there is a relationship between smoking and the occurrence of osteoporosis, more research has been done, including those seeking a link between smoking and the incidence of pathologic fracture in the pelvis. A meta-analysis study published by Vestergaard et al., stated that smoking significantly increases the risk of osteoporotic fractures in each region of the body, especially in the lumbar and proximal bone of the femur (Hoidrup, et al., 2000).

In the population who smoked, 35 samples (40.6%) were categorised as having mild osteoporosis (Singh index of 4–3) and four samples (6%) were categorised as having severe osteoporosis (Singh index of 2–1).

REFERENCES

Greenspan, A. (2004). Osteoporosis. In A. Greenspan (Ed.), *Orthopaedic imaging: A practical approach* (4th ed.). USA: Lippincott Williams & Wilkins.

Hoidrup, S., et al. (2000). Tobacco smoking and risk of hip fracture in men and women. *International Journal of Epidemiology, 29*, 253–9.

Jergas, M. (2000). Radiology of osteoporosis. In S. Grampp (Ed.). *Radiology of osteoporosis* (pp. 77–104). Austria: Springer.

Lucas, T.S., et al. (1993). Osteoporosis: The role of the orthopaedist. *Journal of the American Academy of Orthopaedic Surgeons, 1*, 48–56.

Roeshadi, J. (2008). *The incidence of hip fracture, vertebrae and wrist fracture at Dr. Soetomo Hospital Surabaya 2001–2005*. Surabaya, Indonesia: Anonymous Publisher.

World Health Organization. (2004). *Scientific group on the assessment of osteoporosis at primary health care level*. Brussels, Belgium: Author.

Stem Cell Oncology – Adella (Ed.)
© 2018 Taylor & Francis Group, London, ISBN 978-0-8153-9272-9

Association between nutritional and serum zinc levels amongst children aged six months to five years old

W. Agusthin, T. Sembiring & P. Sianturi
Department of Child Health, Faculty of Medicine, Universitas Sumatera Utara, Medan, North Sumatera, Indonesia

ABSTRACT: Malnutrition is still a health problem that affects a child's development and survival rate in developing countries. Malnutrition may cause lower serum zinc levels than normal children. Albumin is an important protein transport for zinc because 80% of zinc is bound to the albumin. A cross-sectional study was conducted in H. Adam Malik Hospital, Pirngadi Hospital and the University of Sumatera Utara Hospital, Indonesia, between July and November 2016. The study sample was children aged six months to five years old who had no liver function disturbances, kidney disease, were not obese or overweight, and did not take any zinc supplements. Anthropometric, serum zinc, and albumin level measurements were taken along with demographic information. Fifty-one samples were obtained and divided into normal nutrition status, moderate malnutrition, and severe malnutrition groups, equally. Significant associations between malnutrition and serum zinc, and also malnutrition and albumin were found. There was a significant correlation between serum zinc and albumin level.

Keywords: albumin, children, malnutrition, zinc

1 INTRODUCTION

Malnutrition is still a health problem that affects a child's development and survival in developing countries (Nolla, 2014). Data from the World Health Organization shows that for under-fives, approximately 150 million suffer with low weight and around 182 million have short stature (World Health Organization, 2007). Riset (2013), reported that work completed by Badan Penelitian dan Pengembangan Kesehatan Kementerian Kesehatan of Indonesia between 2007 and 2010, found that 18.4% of under-fives had mild to moderate malnutrition. This number increased to 19.6% in 2013.

Zinc is one of the trace elements which plays an important role in nutritional requirements. A case-control study amongst children with marasmus, kwashiorkor and marasmic-kwashiorkor, stated that zinc serum levels in malnutritioned children was lower than that of healthy ones (Khubchandani, 2003). In a prospective study, the prevalence of zinc deficiency was found to be 50% (Gatto, 2015).

2 METHOD

This cross-sectional study was conducted at Haji Adam Malik Hospital, Pirngadi Hospital and the University of Sumatera Utara Hospital, Indonesia, between July and November 2016. Study samples were hospitalised children aged six months to 5 years old who had no liver function disturbances and kidney disease. Samples were also not overweight or obese and did not consume zinc supplements two weeks prior to the study. Samples were obtained by using a consecutive sampling method. Demographic and anthropometric data were obtained by questionnaire and physical examination. Blood samples were collected and analysed for zinc and albumin serum levels. Data analysis was undertaken using statistical software, and the results are presented in Tables 1–4. Informed parental consent was obtained before the child was enrolled onto the study. This study was approved by the Health Research Ethical Committee at the Medical School of the University of Sumatera Utara.

Normality tests were conducted using the Kolmogorov-Smirnov test. A Kruskal-Wallis test was performed in order to determine the association between nutritional status, and

Table 1.   Sample characteristics distribution.

Characteristics	Normoweight n = 17	Mild to moderate malnutrition n = 17	Severe malnutrition n = 17
Sex, n (%)			
Male	9 (52,9)	11 (64,7)	7 (41,2)
Female	8 (47,1)	6 (35,3)	10 (58,8)
Age, n (%)			
6–12 months	5 (29,4)	5 (31,2)	7 (41,2)
12–24 months	5 (29,4)	4 (25,0)	5 (29,4)
24–60 months	7 (41,2)	7 (43,8)	5 (29,4)
Monthly income, n (%)			
<500.000	2 (11,8)	4 (23,5)	9 (52,9)
500.000–1.000.000	11 (64,7)	12 (70,6)	7 (41,2)
>1.000.000	4 (23,5)	1 (5,9)	1 (5,9)
Mean of body weight, kg (SD)	10,2 (2,80)	9,4 (2,46)	6,9 (2,33)
Mean of height, cm (SD)	80,6 (12,38)	82,6 (15,00)	79,0 (12,58)
Mean of age, months (SD)	22,7 (14,16)	24,3 (16,98)	20,6 (14,13)

Table 2.   Association between nutritional status and mean serum zinc level.

Nutritional status	Mean serum zinc level (mcg/dL)	Standard deviation (SD)	p*
Normoweight	40,0	3,03	0,026
Mild to moderate malnutrition	29,9	2,10	
Severe malnutrition	6,9	0,56	

*Kruskal-Wallis test.

Table 3.   Association between nutritional status and mean serum albumin level.

Nutritional status	Mean serum albumin level (g/dL)	Standard deviation (SD)	p*
Normoweight	3,7	0,12	0,007
Mild to moderate malnutrition	3,4	0,06	
Severe malnutrition	3,0	0,19	

*Kruskal-Wallis test.

Table 4.   Correlation between serum albumin and serum zinc level.

Variable	Mean	Standard deviation (SD)	R	p*
Zinc	33,3	1,48	0,371	0,007
Albumin	3,4	0,08		

*Spearman test.

serum albumin and zinc levels. To determine the correlation between serum albumin and zinc levels, the Spearman test was used. A 95% confidence interval was chosen and p < 0.05 was considered significant.

3 RESULTS

A total of 51 children were enrolled onto this study and divided into three groups which were equally based on nutritional status. Of 51 children, 23 were from North Sumatera province, and the rest were from other provinces. Table 1 shows sample characteristics distribution. It was found that the mean sample weight for 'normoweight' (normal weight), 'mild to moderate malnutrition', and 'severe malnutrition' was 10.2 kg ($SD = 2.80$), 9.4 kg ($SD = 2.46$), and 6.9 kg ($SD = 2.33$), respectively. Mean sample stature was 80.6 cm ($SD = 12.38$) for the normoweight group, 82.6 cm ($SD = 15.00$) for the mild to moderate malnutrition group, and 79.0 cm ($SD = 12.58$) for the severe malnutrition group.

The results of the serum zinc levels were obtained two weeks after blood processing, while serum albumin level were obtained one day after blood processing. Based on the Kruskal-Wallis test, there was a statistically significant relationship between nutritional status and serum zinc levels in this study ($p = 0.026$). Children with the worst nutritional status had lower serum zinc levels (Table 2).

Table 3 shows the association between nutritional status and mean serum albumin level. Based on the statistical analysis, there was a significant relationship between nutritional status and mean serum albumin level ($p = 0.007$). Children with better nutritional status had a higher serum albumin level.

The correlation between serum albumin and serum zinc level was also statistically analysed by using the Spearman test. The results showed that there was a significant positive correlation between mean serum albumin and mean serum zinc level (r = 0.371; $p = 0.007$).

4 DISCUSSION

Malnutrition is still a common health problem globally, but is mainly found in developing countries. Malnutrition in children will affect a population because it disturbs children's growth and development, cognitive function later in life, and hampers the economic development of a country. Besides this, malnutrition in children will also increase morbidity and mortality from several diseases after the children reach adulthood (Nolla, 2014; Marasinghe, 2015).

The number of samples studied was 51 children, which were divided into three groups based on nutritional status. Their nutritional status was determined using a weight to height percentage ratio. Samples in this study were aged between six months and five years old and were from an urban area.

In this study, a statistically significant relationship between malnutrition and serum zinc levels was found. Statistical analysis showed that children with the worst nutrition status had lower serum zinc levels. This result is confirmed by several other studies. A research study in 2016 looked at 56 children with malnutrition in the teaching hospital of Hanyang University, South Korea; the children were aged 1 to 15 years old and had their serum and hair zinc levels evaluated. There was a statistically significant association between hair zinc levels and malnutrition, where 55% of children with malnutrition also had zinc deficiency (Han et al., 2016).

Several other studies show the same results of this study. A study in Cameroon in 2014, reported no association between serum zinc level and nutritional status (Nolla, 2014). Another study from Bangladesh in 2009 reported the same result; an association between malnutrition, serum vitamin D level and haemoglobin was found, but not with serum zinc levels (Marasinghe, 2015). A study in South Africa in 2015 also confirmed the results above and stated that there was no association between serum zinc levels and malnutrition; it was thought that a helminth infestation was a confounder (Amara, 2012).

In this research study, a statistical analysis to determine the correlation between serum albumin and serum zinc levels was conducted. The results show that there was a significant correlation between serum albumin and serum zinc levels ($r = 0.371$; $p = 0.007$). These results are supported by a 2013 study in the United States, where a significant correlation between serum albumin and serum zinc levels amongst 691 children aged between six and eleven years old was found. However, the correlation was weak, and the researchers decided that serum albumin levels were not a sensitive predictor of zinc deficiency in children with malnutrition (Bui, 2013). A study from South Korea in 2016 also reported that there was no significant correlation between serum zinc and albumin levels (Han, 2016).

Despite the results above, this study still has several weaknesses. First, the confounders for serum zinc and albumin levels, such as infection, diet pattern and knowledge about nutrition, had not been investigated in each sample, and that caused bias in the results of this study. Infection was the main confounder because samples in this study were hospitalised patients and thus were susceptible to infection. Infection can trigger inflammation and lower serum albumin levels, as well as malnutrition itself. A study from Japan in 2014 showed that serum albumin levels decreased in concomitant with increased C-reactive protein levels (the latter is a marker of inflammation) (Ishida et al., 2014). Inflammation will also affect serum zinc levels because zinc plays the role of a cofactor for enzymes in the immune system. The presence of infection and inflammation will therefore, increase zinc utilisation. It should be noted that zinc is not deposited in the human body and must be obtained from food intake (Walker & Black, 2004).

5 CONCLUSIONS

This study shows that there is a statistically significant association between malnutrition, and serum zinc and albumin levels. There is also a significant correlation between serum zinc and albumin levels.

REFERENCES

Amare, B., Moges, B., et al. (2012). Micronutrient levels and nutritional status of school children living in north west Ethiopia. *Nutrition Journal*, *11*, 1–8.
Bui, Q., Marcinkevage, J., et al. (2014). Associations among dietary zinc intakes and biomarkers of zinc status before and after a zinc supplementation program in Guatemalan school children. *Food and Nutrition Bulletin*, *32*, 143–50.
Gattoo, I., Harish, R., et al. (2015). Correlation of serum zinc level with simple febrile seizure: A hospital-based prospective case-control study. *International Journal of Pediatrics*, 509–15.
Han, H., Lee, J. & Kim, Y. (2016). Hair zinc level analysis and correlative micronutrient in children presenting with malnutrition and poor growth. *Pediatric Gastroenterology, Hepatology & Nutrition*, 259–68.
Ishida, S., Hashimoto, I., Seike, T., Nayaka, Y. & Nakanishi, H. (2014). Serum albumin levels correlate with inflammation rather than nutrition supply in burns patient: A retrospective study., *61*, 361–8.
Khubchandani, A., Sanghani, H., et al. (2003). Serum copper and zinc levels in preschool children with protein energy malnutrition. *International Journal of Research in Medical Sciences*, *2*, 7–10.
Marasinghe, E., Chackrewarthy, S., et al. (2015). Micronutrient status and its relationship with nutritional status in preschool children in urban Sri Lanka. *Asia Pacific Journal of Clinical Nutrition*, 1–16.
Nolla, N., Sop, M., et al. (2014). Assessment of nutritional status of preschool children in the Bangang rural community. *International Journal of Biotechnology and Food Science*, *2*, 44–52.
Riset, K.D. (2013). *Badan penelitian dan pengembangan kesehatan kementerian kesehatan RI.*
Walker, F. & Black, E. (2004). Zinc and the risk for infectious disease. *Annual Review of Nutrition*, 255–75.
World Health Organization. (2007). *Community-based management of severe acute malnutrition* (pp. 1–7).

Stem Cell Oncology – Adella (Ed.)
© 2018 Taylor & Francis Group, London, ISBN 978-0-8153-9272-9

Association between education, length of exposure and economic level with depression

F. Gurning
Resident of the Department of Psychiatry, Faculty of Medicine, Universitas, Sumatera Utara, Medan, North Sumatera, Indonesia

V. Camellia & H.T. Parinduri
Lecturers of the Department of Psychiatry, Faculty of Medicine, Universitas, Sumatera Utara, Medan, North Sumatera, Indonesia

ABSTRACT: Domestic violence is a social problem associated with an increased risk of mental illness in women. This study investigated the association between education level, length of exposure and economic level with the level of depression amongst woman experiencing domestic violence. This study was an observational study with a cross-sectional approach. Participants were women (82 in total) who were experiencing domestic violence, and were seeking support from PPT Bhayangkara Hospital and the psychiatry clinic of Pirngadi Hospital, Medan, Indonesia. An association was found between education level and level of depression ($p = 0.01$), length of exposure and level of depression ($p = 0.01$), and economic level and level of depression ($p = 0.01$). Factors significantly associated with a higher level of depression amongst women experiencing domestic violence were low educational level ($OR = 3,754$, $p = 0.022$), economic level ($OR = 4,436$, $p = 0.01$) and length of exposure ($OR = 4,939$, $p = 0.018$). Awareness needs to be raised through the mental health services and the government in the prevention of depression through psychosocial interventions for women experiencing domestic violence.

Keywords: domestic violence, depression, economic level, education level, length of exposure

1 INTRODUCTION

Women being abused over a long period may result in significant mental distress (Wong et al., 2012). In studies examining violence, women who report abuse have higher rates of depression (Lawrence et al., 2004). Domestic violence is associated with depression, including depressive symptoms, depressive disorders and suicide. Risk factors associated with depression in female survivors of domestic violence include age, education level, socio-economic status, and a long experience of violence (Ferrari et al., 2014).

Wong et al.'s (2012) study in Hong Kong amongst 200 women experiencing violence from their intimate partner in the Chinese community, used a Chinese version of the Beck Depression Inventory-Version II (C-BDI-II). They reported levels of depressive symptoms of: 'minimal level' (9%, $n = 18$); 'mild level' (9.5%, n = 19); 'moderate level' (7%, $n = 14$); and 'severe level' (74.5%, $n = 149$) (Wong et al., 2011).

A study by Hegarty et al. (2004) in Australia amongst abused women, reported 18% (218/1213) as currently 'probably depressed' and 24.1% (277/1147) had experienced some form of abuse in an adult intimate relationship (Hegarty & Gunn, 2004).

Abused women that experience depression are more likely to have experienced severe combined abuse and violence, greater poverty, differing social rules and sex discrimination, more negative life events abuse as a child and a poor education. They are also likely to be not married, on a low income, unemployed or receiving a pension or pregnant.

The Beck Depression Inventory-II (BDI-II) is one of the most frequently used measures of the severity of depression in adolescents and adults, by both researchers and clinicians. BDI-II consists of 21 items that assess the symptoms of depression experienced over the previous two weeks. Each item contains four statements that reflect on the varying degrees of symptom severity. Respondents are instructed to circle the number (ranging from zero to three, indicating increasing severity) that corresponds with the statement that best describes their mental state. Rating is summed to calculate a total BDI-II score, which can range from 0 to 63. BDI scores of 0–13 indicate a 'minimal level of depression', scores 14–19 indicate 'mild depression', scores 20–28 indicate 'moderate level' and scores 29–63 indicate 'severe depression' (Grothe et al., 2006).

2 METHOD

This study is an observational study with an analytic comparative design and uses a cross-sectional approach. Participants were 82 women seeking help from the Domestic Violence and Abuse Service in Medan, North Sumatera, Indonesia.

Eligible participants were women who were experiencing domestic violence or abuse which led them to seek support from Pusat Pelayanan Terpadu Bhayangkara Hospital and the psychiatry clinic of Pirngadi Hospital, Medan, between August 2015 and March 2016. The participants were women who had experienced domestic violence or abuse (emotional, physical, sexual or neglect) from adult family members, were aged between 18 and 60 years old, and were able to communicate in the language of Bahasa Indonesia. Women who suffered with other mental illnesses, had a history of medical illness, drug or alcohol problems, were currently receiving counselling, cognitive behavioural therapy or other psychological treatments, and were currently taking antidepressants or other psychopharmacologies, were excluded from this study (Ferrari et al., 2014).

Depression was assessed using the BDI-II rating scale. The results of the BDI-II was interpreted when all the data collection was complete. A bivariate analyses was used to examine the association between education level (high school and higher), length of abuse exposure greater, less than or for one year) and economic level (mild, moderate and high), with level of depression (mild, moderate and severe). Multivariate logistic regression was used to investigate the association between the independent variables and depression. The study was approved by the Medical Faculty of the Universitas Sumatera Utara Health Research Ethical Committee. Statistical tests were performed using SPSS software.

3 RESULTS AND DISCUSSION

A total of 82 women experiencing domestic violence and abuse were enrolled onto the study. The majority (93.9%) were married and aged between 31 and 40 years old (37%). Of this sample, 50% of them were in paid employment. The study revealed that 74.4% (61/82) had been experiencing abuse for more than one year, 9.8% (8/82) were experiencing physical abuse, and 8.5% (7/82) were experiencing emotional abuse. It was also found that 19.5% (16/82) were suffering a combination of physical and emotional abuse, 40.2% (33/82) neglect and emotional abuse, 18.3% (15/82) neglect, physical and emotional abuse, and 3.7% (3/82) neglect, physical, emotional and sexual abuse.

Out of 54 participants, 34 (63%) with a high school education suffered with severe depression, and for participants with education higher than high school, 25% (7/28) suffered with severe depression. Chi-square analysis showed there was significant association between education level and level of depression ($p = 0.01$). It was also found that 61 participants had been experiencing abuse for more than one year, and 37 of them (37/61, 60.7%) suffered with severe depression.

Table 1. Sample characteristics.

Variables	n	%
Age (years)		
18–30	21	25,6
31–40	37	45,1
41–50	17	20,7
>50	7	8,5
Marital Status		
Married	77	93,9
Single or separated	5	6,1
Employment status		
Paid employment	41	50
Not employed	41	50
Education		
≤Grade 12	54	65,9
>Grade 12	28	34,1
Economic level		
Low	28	34,1
Middle	34	41,5
High	20	24,4
Length of exposure		
≤1 year	21	25,6
>1 year	61	74,4

Table 2. Level of depression amongst women experiencing domestic violence.

Level of depression	BDI-II score	n	%
Mild	14–19	17	20,7
Moderate	20–28	24	29,3
Severe	29–63	41	50
Total		82	100

Table 3. Analysis of multivariate risk factors for depression in women experiencing domestic violence.

	p	OR	95% IK
Education level	0,022	3,754	1,205–11,692
Economic level	0,01	4,436	1,428–13,784
Length of exposure	0,018	4,939	1,309–18,632

Of participants who were experiencing less than one year of abuse, 19% (4/21) suffered with severe depression. It was found that the length of exposure has a significant association with level of depression ($p = 0.001$).

Analysis of the results also revealed that 28 participants had a low economic level, 34 participants had a middle economic level and 20 participants had a high economic level. Amongst low economic level participants, 71.4% (20/28) suffered with severe depression whereas amongst middle economic level participants, 50% (17/34) suffered with severe depression, and amongst the high economic level participants, 20% (4/20) suffered with severe depression. Therefore, economic level has a significant association with level of depression ($p = 0.001$).

Using structured multiphase logistic regression with the enter method, it was found that all of the independent variables had a significant association with the level of depression ($p < 0.05$). Education level ($p = 0.022$, $OR = 3,754$, 95% $CI = 1,205–11,692$), economic level

($p = 0.01$, $OR = 4{,}436$, 95% $CI = 1{,}428\text{--}13{,}784$) and length of exposure ($p = 0.018$, $OR = 4{,}939$, 95% $CI = 1{,}309\text{--}18{,}632$).

4 CONCLUSION

The main finding of this study is that there is a significant association between education level, length of exposure and economic level, with the level of depression suffered amongst women experiencing domestic violence. Awareness needs to be raised through the mental health services and the government, in the prevention of depression through psychosocial interventions for women experiencing domestic violence.

REFERENCES

Ferrari, G., Agnew-Davies, R., Bailey, J., Howard, L., Howarth, E. & Peters, T.J. (2014). Intimate partner violence and mental health domestic violence and mental health: A cross-sectional survey of women seeking help from domestic violence support services. *Global Health Action, 7*, 25519.

Grothe, K.B., Dutton, G.R, Bondelos, J., Ancona, M., Jones, G.N. & Brantley, P.J. (2006). Validation of the Beck Depression Inventory-II in a low-income African American sample of medical outpatients. *American Psychological Association, 17*(1), 110–114.

Hegarty, K., Gunn, J., Chondros, P. & Small, R. (2004). Association between depression and abuse by partners of women attending general practice: Descriptive, cross-sectional survey. *British Medical Journal*, (328).

Lawrence, S., Chau, M. & Lennon, M.C. (2004). *Depression, substance abuse, and domestic violence*. The National Center for Children in Poverty.

Warshaw, C. & Barnes, H. (2003). Domestic violence, mental health & trauma research highlights (pp. 1–4). The Chicago Community Trust.

Wong, J.Y.H., Fong, D.Y.T. & Tiwari, A. (2012). Depression in women experiencing intimate partner violence. *Essential Notes in Psychiatry*, 188–195.

Wong, J.Y.H., Tiwari, A. & Fong, D.Y.T. (2011). Depression among women experiencing intimate partner violence in Chinese community. *Nursing Research, 60*(1), 58–65.

Stem Cell Oncology – Adella (Ed.)
© *2018 Taylor & Francis Group, London, ISBN 978-0-8153-9272-9*

Correlation of irritant exposure with nasal mucociliary transportation time for gas station workers in Medan

J. Tobing, A.Y.M. Rambe, F. Sofyan & T. Ashar
Department of Otorhinolaryngology Head and Neck Surgery, Faculty of Medicine,
Universitas Sumatera Utara, Medan, North Sumatera, Indonesia

ABSTRACT: The exposure of irritant substances, such as benzene, toluene, xylene, and ethylbenzene in the air can cause a disruption in transportation time of nasal mucociliary. The aim of this study was to find out the correlation between exposure to irritant substances and their effect on nasal mucociliary transportation time for workers at a gas station in Medan city, Indonesia. The type of research was analytical with a cross-sectional study design. There are 42 samples of subjects according to the inclusion and exclusion criteria where 31 subjects went through a deceleration of nasal mucociliary transport time. The location of exposure has a significant correlation between the nasal mucociliary transport time disorder that is as many as 31 people (100%) on direct exposure. The nasal mucociliary transport time was found to slow in the gas station workers who were exposed to a direct irritant.

Keywords: benzene, general nasal mucociliary, general refuelling station, toluene, xylene

1 INTRODUCTION

Exposure to recurrent air pollution in the environment will lead to many disruptions to the human body, such as heart and lung function disorders, brain disorders, cognitive and behavioural disorders and airway problems. One source of air pollution is fuel oil which is the world's largest volume of fuel that has a complex content, with varying composition, depending on the source of its basic material (crude oil), the filtration process and other factors (Grebic et al., 2007). The aim of this study was to determine the correlation between exposure of irritant substance and disruption to transportation time of nasal mucociliary for gas station workers in Medan city.

2 METHOD

This research was analytic with a cross-sectional approach. The sample studied within this research was the gas station officer who fulfilled the inclusion criteria. The sampling formula of proportion produced at least 34 samples. This study obtained 42 samples/people.

3 RESULTS

3.1 *The characteristics of the subject's demography research*

The results of the nasal mucociliary transport examination towards the officers showed that there were 31 subjects (73.8%) who had nasal mucociliary transport disruption (nasal mucociliary transport time greater than 17 minutes). The number of subjects directly exposed to fuel at the gas station was 31 people (73.8%) while 11 people (26.2%) were not directly exposed.

3.2 Statistical analysis results

3.2.1 The correlation between location exposure with transportation time of nasal mucociliary

Table 1. The correlation between location of exposure with transportation time of nasal mucociliary.

Location of exposure	Transportation time of nasal mucociliary		p-value
	>17 minutes	≤17 minutes	
Direct	31 (100)	0	<0.001
Indirect	0	11 (100)	

3.2.2 The correlation between age and transportation time of nasal mucociliary

In the direct exposure group, significant correlation between age and transportation time of nasal mucociliary ($p = 0.001$), within the correlation value of $r = 0.560$, was found. The correlation value indicated that there was moderate correlation with the positive value, which means that increasing age of the officer would be followed by an increasing transportation time of nose mucociliary. Meanwhile, for the group of officers who were not directly exposed, there was also a positive correlation between age and transportation time of nasal mucociliary, with a strong correlation value of $r = 0.771$.

3.2.3 The correlation between sex and transportation time of nasal mucociliary

Transportation time of nasal mucociliary for the male officers in both groups was found to be longer in comparison to the female officers. In the direct exposure group, transportation time of nasal mucociliary for male officers was 22 minutes ($SD = 1.97$ minutes), while for female officers it was 19.33 minutes ($SD = 1.54$ minutes). The analysis used the Mann-Whitney test. It showed that there was a significant correlation ($p < 0.001$) between the sexes and transportation time of nasal mucociliary for the group of officers which were exposed directly. In contrast, for the group of officers who were not directly exposed, no significant correlation was found ($p = 0.104$) after being analysed by the independent t-test, even though the transportation time of nasal mucociliary in male officers was longer than the transportation time for female officers.

3.2.4 The correlation between the length of work and transportation time of nasal mucociliary

Analysis using the Spearman correlation test showed there was no significant relationship between duration of work and transportation time of nasal mucociliary ($p = 0.084$), in all research subjects.

3.2.5 The correlation between length of work and transportation time of nasal mucociliary on exposed subjects

Analysis by using the Spearman correlation test on exposed subjects in gas stations concluded that there was a significant correlation between the length of work and transportation time of nasal mucociliary ($p < 0.001$), with a correlation value of $r = 0.717$. The correlation value indicates that there was a strong and positive correlation between the length of work with the transportation time of nasal mucociliary; this means that the longer subjects are exposed (to fuel working in gas stations), the greater the transportation time of nasal mucociliary.

3.2.6 The correlation between smoking habits with transportation time of nasal mucociliary

The average transportation time of nasal mucociliary in officers who were exposed directly and smoked was 22.13 minutes ($SD = 1.96$ minutes), while the non-smoking officers had a

160

lower average of 19.38 minutes ($SD = 1.5$ minutes). The analysis by using the Mann-Whitney test showed that there was a significant correlation ($p < 0.001$) between smoking and transportation time of nasal mucociliary in officers exposed directly. The officers that were not directly exposed and who smoked, had a longer transportation time of nasal mucociliary with an average of 15.6 minutes ($SD = 1.52$ minutes) compared to non-smokers who had an average transportation time of 14 minutes ($SD = 1.41$ minutes). However, analysis by using the independent t-test, showed that there was no significant correlation between smoking habits and transportation time of nasal mucociliary in the workers that were not directly exposed ($p = 0.104$).

4 DISCUSSION

From the 31 subjects which were directly exposed, all had undergone the disruption of transportation time of nasal mucociliary, whereas from 11 subjects who were not exposed directly did not disruption of nasal mucociliary transport. Analysis by using the Fisher's Exact test showed that there was a significant correlation between the exposure location and transportation time of nasal mucociliary disruption ($p < 0.001$). This result was similar to previous research on the correlation between silver dust exposure with transportation time of nasal mucociliary conducted by Suherman (2013) in Kota Gede, Yogyakarta, Indonesia. The results showed a positive and very strong correlation between workers exposed directly to silver dust with those who were not exposed directly to silver dust; where workers were directly exposed, transportation time of nasal mucociliary any longer.

In the direct exposure group, significant correlation was found between age and transportation time of nasal mucociliary ($p = 0.001$), with a correlation value of $r = 0.560$. The correlation value indicates that there is a moderate correlation with the positive value, which means that the increasing age of the officer will be followed by increasing transportation time of nasal mucociliary. The results of this study supported a theory that states that one of the factors that affect transportation time of nasal mucociliary is age. The transportation time of nasal mucociliary increased with the increase of age, and transportation time of nasal mucociliary slowed with the degradation of age. The slowing of transportation time of nasal mucociliary was very significant for persons over the age of 60 (Valia, 2007).

The transportation time of nasal mucociliary in male officers in both groups was longer in comparison to female officers. This finding was not compatible with the study by Yadaf et al. (2011) which stated that there was no statistically significant correlation between males and females with regards to the disruption of transportation time of mucociliary ($p = 0.005$).

Analysis by using the Spearman correlation test showed that there was a strong correlation and positive value between the length of work with transportation time of nasal mucociliary. This means that the longer the subjects are exposed to fuel (working in gas stations), the greater the transportation time of nasal mucociliary. The research of Yudhanto (2015) found that there was a correlation between the length of work with the transportation time of mucociliary. There was a significant correlation between smoking habits in officers who were exposed directly, and the disruption to transportation time of nasal mucociliary, with a value of $p < 0.001$ (using the Mann-Whitney test). This was in accordance with other studies that suggested that smoking may lead to the disruption of the transportation time of nasal mucociliary. Philanthropists (2010) reported that there was a significant difference between transportation time of nasal mucociliary of smokers and those of non-smokers.

5 CONCLUSION

There was significant correlation between the exposure location and transportation time of nasal mucociliary disruption (using the Fisher's exact test with a score $p < 0.001$).

SUGGESTION

It is necessary to control the exposure of irritant substances towards the officers in each gas station, by advising officers to use personal protective equipment such as masks, especially for those exposed directly to the irritant substances. This is to minimise the slowing of the transportation time of nasal mucociliary.

It is necessary to do further research to determine the specific types of irritant substances that can disrupt the transportation time of nasal mucociliary for gas station officers.

REFERENCES

Dermawan, R. (2010). *Transport time difference mucociliar nose in smokers and non smokers.* Medan, Indonesia: University of North Sumatra.

Grebic, D.H., Jakovac, I. & Sutic, M. (2007). Short-term exposure of mice to gasoline vapor increases the metallothionein expression in the brain, lungs and kidney. *Histology and Histopathology, 22*(6), 593–601.

Suherman. (2007). Short-term exposure of mice to gasoline vapor increases the metallothionein expression in the brain, lungs, and kidney. *Histology and Histopathology, 22*(6), 593–601.

Valia. (2007). Saccharine test for the study of mucociliary clearance. *The Journal of Bronconeumology, 10*, 540–5.

Yadaf, J., Ranga, R.K. & Singh, J. (2011). Effect of aging on nasal mucociliary clearance. *Clinical Rhinology.*

Yudhanto, D. (2015). *Correlation of length of work with transportation time of mucociliar of general fuel station workers (gas station).* Yogyakarta, Indonesia: Gadjah Mada University.

Stem Cell Oncology – Adella (Ed.)
© 2018 Taylor & Francis Group, London, ISBN 978-0-8153-9272-9

Collection of stem cells in (autologous) donors by apheresis

H. Vrielink
Sanquin Blood Supply, Amsterdam, The Netherlands

ABSTRACT: Leukapheresis procedures are performed to collect Hematopoietic Progenitor Cells (HPCs) from autologous and allogeneic donors for stem cell therapies. To collect sufficient HPCs, the cells must be mobilized from the bone marrow into the peripheral circulation with G-CSF, chemotherapy, and or plerixafor. Transfusion of the specific number of HPCs is needed to guarantee sufficiently fast and reliable recovery of the bone marrow function after the myelosuppressive or myeloablative treatment in the patient. To assure safety for the donor as well as patient in this kind of therapy, solid quality in the complete chain is needed. Therefore, in many countries, by law, JACIE/FACT accreditation is required.

Keywords: stem cells, autologous, HPCs

1 INTRODUCTION

White blood cells (WBCs) can be collected with apheresis techniques. This is named leukapheresis or leukocytapheresis. Apheresis is a method of obtaining one or more blood components by machine processing of whole blood in which the residual components are returned to the donor or patient during or at the end of the process. The majority of the leukapheresis procedures are performed to collect cells for cellular therapies, of which the collections of autologous or allogeneic hematopoietic stem/progenitor cells (HPCs) are most frequent performed. HPCs are found in the bone marrow and are identified by the presence of the CD34 antigen on their surface, and therefore these cells are often named CD34 positive cells. HPCs are multipotent stem cells that can develop into all the blood cell types constituting from the myeloid (monocytes and macrophages, neutrophils, basophils, eosinophils, erythrocytes, megakaryocytes/platelets, dendritic cells), and lymphoid lineages (T-cells, B-cells, NK-cells).

In patients with haemato-oncologic malignancies such as non-Hodgkin lymphoma (NHL), multiple myeloma (MM) and Hodgkin lymphoma (HL), high-dose chemotherapy, with or without total body irradiation, is used as treatment. Because of the myelosuppressive or even myeloablative character of these treatments, subsequent stem cell transplant, in fact, administration of HPCs collected from previous cryopreserved autologous HPCs or an HLA compatible donor, is essential. Only this will guarantee sufficiently fast and reliable recovery of the bone marrow function.

2 COLLECTION STEM CELL

As said HPCs are found in the bone marrow. The cells are fixed to stroma cells. In recent history, the "bone marrow" was aspirated under general anesthesia. With the availability of hematopoietic growth factors as mobilizing agents, the connecting receptor between stroma cells and stem cells will be disrupted, the migration of HPCs into the circulating can be enhanced and therefore collected by leukapheresis techniques. In general two important drugs are in use. Subcutaneous administration of recombinant "granulocyte-colony-stimulating factor" (G-CSF) or plerixafor, in autologous situations usually in conjunction with chemotherapy, is used in this respect. Subsequent harvesting of these growth factor-mobilized

HPCs by leukapheresis techniques has almost replaced the use of bone marrow aspirate. Collection of HPCs by apheresis has some advantages over bone marrow harvesting, e.g., it is less invasive than harvesting bone marrow under general anesthesia with overnight hospitalization. Moreover, the number of HPCs that can be collected is far better than that can be obtained with marrow aspiration under anesthesia. Secondly, mobilized hematopoietic stem cell transplants usually induce a more rapidly hematological recovery due to the reinfusion of the higher number of HPCs. This, together with the so-called non-myeloablative conditioning made hematopoietic stem cell transplant (HSCT) also available for the elderly patient. In these HSCTs, the G-CSF method is the one to be used. Mobilization and one or more apheresis procedures are usually well tolerated and are performed in an outpatient setting. Side effects of G-CSF and plerixafor are usually relatively mild and consist of pain from muscles and bones, and headache. Rare complications such as splenic rupture, allergic reactions, reactivation of autoimmune disorders and vascular thrombosis, however, have been reported.

As discussed, in the bone cavity, HPCs are bound to stromal cells and various extracellular proteins. Administration of G-CSF leads to the release of a variety of serine proteases from granulocytes. This takes days. These proteases disrupt the binding between stromal cells and stem cells and with it the release of the HPCs in the peripheral circulation. Unfortunately, G-CSF mobilization has a 5–30% failure rate among healthy donors and patients. Risk factors for a sub-optimal HPC mobilization are ages above 60 years, disease status, duration of the previous chemo- and radiotherapy. Mobilization in patients is preferably achieved with chemotherapy followed with G-CSF ("chemo mobilization"). Usually, a higher number of stem cells are available in the peripheral blood stream for harvesting than after G-CSF only. Since some years, plerixafor became available for autologous HPC mobilization. Plerixafor leads direct antibody mediated interference with the CXCR4 receptor binding leading to peak levels of CD34-positive cells in the peripheral circulation 6–9 hours after administration. Plerixafor is used in combination with G-CSF when G-CSF mobilization shows to be insufficient.

Administration of G-CSF in healthy donors is typically started four days before the scheduled apheresis procedure and continues until the day of the last apheresis. On the 5th day of treatment, usually the number of circulating CD34-positive cells is maximized, and subsequent harvesting of these growth factor-mobilized HPCs by leukapheresis techniques begins. G-CSF mobilization schemes in patients are usually in conjunction with chemotherapy. In general, the leukapheresis procedure is started when the concentration of circulating CD34-positive cells is above approximately 15–20/μl. The use of G-CSF or plerixafor, together with the pre-apheresis concentration of CD34-positive cells in the de peripheral blood of the patient/donor enables prediction of the number of HPCs that can be obtained with one or two apheresis procedures. The number of CD34-positive cells to be collected in the apheresis procedure is amongst others depending on the type of transplant and the weight of the recipient. The accepted minimum dose of CD34-positive cells for hematological recovery is 2 or more $\times 10^6$ CD34-positive cells/kg of patients' body weight. Re-infusion of a higher number of CD34-positive cells such as 4–5 $\times 10^6$/kg leads primarily to a faster recovery of platelets and granulocytes. A higher number of CD34-positive cells then 4–5 $\times 10^6$/kg has almost no additive effects.

In donor apheresis programs, usually, all standardized processes are according to guidelines and specification to assure that a process has been proven to yield safe, potent and pure products with optimal safety for the recipient, but also to assure safe processes for the donor. In a stem cell transplant program, clinic, collection facility, and processing facility are working together, and we should be aware that quality is the responsibility of all those involved in the processes. To assure quality and therefore safety for donor and patient, in many countries, governments decree that all units (clinic, collection facility, and processing facility) working in one stem cell transplant program are working together in one quality program. The Joint accreditation committee of ICST and EBMT (JACIE) and the Foundation for the Accreditation of Cellular Therapy (FACT) composed together international standards for cellular therapy product collection, processing, and administration accreditation [1]. More and more governments do require a JACIE/FACT accreditation or an intention to work according to these standards with an accreditation before a specific date. Otherwise, by law, no permission is given to work in this specific field of interest.

JACIE/FACT standards are designed to provide minimum guidelines for programs, facilities and individuals performing cell transplantation and therapy or providing support services for such procedures. Therefore, JACIE/FACT standards contain standards concerning hematopoietic cellular therapy applying to quality in the clinic (part B with standards for pre- and post-transplants), the collection facility (part C) and in the processing facility (part D). Audits according to JACIE/FACT are also pointed at the interaction between the three different units. Accreditation according to the JACIE/FACT standards can solely be achieved for the complete hematopoietic cellular therapy program.

REFERENCES

Foundation for the Accreditation of Cellular Therapy (FACT). FACT-JACIE international standards for cellular therapy product collection, processing, and administration. 5th ed. Omaha, NE: FACT, 2015. (Available at: http://www.factweb.org/forms/store/CommercePlusFormPublic/ search?action=Publications [accessed March 6, 2015], and http://jacie.org) → standards of the 6th edition will be implemented worldwide in 2018.

Stem Cell Oncology – Adella (Ed.)
© *2018 Taylor & Francis Group, London, ISBN 978-0-8153-9272-9*

Transfusion of blood components in a stem cell transplant programme

H. Vrielink
Sanquin Blood Supply, Amsterdam, The Netherlands

ABSTRACT: Heavily treated oncology patients need transfusions of cellular blood components on a regular basis. Platelets, as well as units of erythrocytes, need to be ABO blood system compatible to the recipient. In platelet transfusions, rhesus D (RhD) compatibility needs to be discussed. It is preferred that all cellular blood components are leukoreduced, and for patients in a stem cell transplant programmes, gamma irradiated to prevent transfusion associated graft versus host disease.

Keywords: stem cell, platelets, gamma irradiated

1 INTRODUCTION

Patients with malignancies are usually heavily treated with cytotoxic drugs, and in some cases, also with total body irradiation. Because of this treatment, besides the malignant cells, normal cells are also damaged in many cases leading to temporary suppression, or in other situations, the complete destruction of the haemopoietic progenitor cells giving rise to severe thrombocytopenia and possibly anaemia. Usually the transfusion of a number of units of donor platelets, and in some cases units of red blood cells as well, are needed when an haemopoietic stem cell transplant programme is started. What is important is the right choice of ABO and rhesus D (RhD) blood type, and if needed, further preparations of the cellular blood component. This method is discussed further in this paper by the use of a theoretical/real-life?

2 PLATELET TRANSFUSIONS

A newly diagnosed male patient of 70 years old with multiple myeloma is being treated. During the first cycle of treatments, the platelet count decreases to 4.000 cells/µL. Since he is typed as AB RhD negative, and the number of available AB RhD negative donors is very low, discussions concerning the choice of the blood type of the component is needed. Although platelets do not express RhD antigens, RhD immunisation is possible due to erythrocytes presenting as contamination in the platelet units. It is suggested that a presence of 0.03 mL (approximately 1×10^{10} red blood cells/mL) of erythrocytes are capable of causing primary RhD immunisation (Cid & Lozano, 2005; Mollison et al., 1997). If the platelet suspension is pink in colour, it contains more than 0.3 mL of erythrocytes. The risk of RhD immunisation in leukopenic patients who are immune suppressed is between 0 and 19% (Atoyebi et al., 2000; Goldfinger & McGinniss, 1971; Lozano & Cid, 2007). In many guidelines for avoiding RhD antibody problems during pregnancy, it is recommended that platelet transfusions to female RhD negative patients of child bearing age (under 45 years old) should preferably be RhD compatible. Going back to the multiple myeloma patient case study, there is no direct need to use RhD negative donor platelets since the development of anti-D is not of any direct clinical relevance (Valsami et al., 2015).

As the patient in the case study was typed as having an AB blood group, it has been demonstrated that the transfusion of ABO blood system compatible platelets has a higher profit in the patient and are therefore of first choice. In the case of major ABO incompatibility, the patient's anti-A and/or anti-B antibodies have negative effects on the survival of the donor platelets with an impaired haemostasis of ABO compatible platelets compared to incompatible (Blumberg et al., 2012). Major ABO incompatibility in platelet transfusions can also possibly lead to a higher refractoriness. Following minor ABO incompatible platelet transfusions, a positive direct antiglobulin test can be the result of a transfusion of incompatible plasma. This is usually associated with slight haemolysis and rarely severe—even fatal—haemolysis and renal failure. Usually, an anti-A and/or anti-B titre lower than 128 is not a problem and is recommended for patients who receive multiple transfusions (Lozano & Cid, 2003; Valsami et al., 2015). Taking all this into account, the choices shown in Table 1 can be followed.

Another issue to be considered in the patient case study, is the possibility of transfusion associated graft versus host disease (TA-GvHD), caused by the presence of immunocompetent lymphocytes in the donor blood system of immune-compromised patients. This can be prevented by gamma irradiation (25 Gy) of the cellular blood component. Gamma irradiation damages the blood cells that are capable of cell division (monocytes and lymphocytes) to such an extent that they can no longer multiply, and as a result, the mixed lymphocyte culture response disappears. Although it is not known how many immunocompetent lymphocytes are required to elicit TA-GvHD, it has been shown that transfusion of leukocyte reduced components decreases the incidence, but does not protect against TA-GvHD. Therefore, irradiation of cellular blood components are (amongst others):

- acquired immunodeficiency, as is the case with allogeneic stem cell transplantation (for at least six months after transplantation), if total body irradiation formed part of the conditioning;
- autologous stem cell transplantation (for at least three months after reinfusion), after use of donor lymphocyte infusion or infusion of cytotoxic T lymphocytes for one year after transfusion;
- transfusion between first and up to, and including, third degree relatives of cell-containing blood components;
- leukaemia treatments, where this is required in the protocol (see other considerations);
- peripheral blood stem cell apheresis from mobilisation until after collection;
- bone marrow collection from six weeks prior to collection and until after collection;
- HLA compatible platelet concentrates;
- use of purine/pyrimidine antagonists and related medication (e.g. Fludarabine, Pentostatin and Cladribine) for a year after cessation of the therapy;
- in the case of anti-T cell treatment (ATG, anti-CD52 and other T cell monoclonals) for aplastic anaemia or leukaemia from the start of administration through to half a year after completion of the treatment;
- Hodgkin's lymphoma—some advocate for all stages, others only for stages 3 and 4;
- non-Hodgkin's lymphoma.

As described, the results of a transfusion of a unit of platelets can vary based on compatibility issues between donor and patient. Therefore, the effects of a platelet transfusion need to be monitored. The easiest way to do this is a patient platelet count 1 and 24 hours after the transfusion, taking into account the number of platelets in the product and the body surface

Table 1. ABO blood type of choice of donor platelets based on blood type of the recipient.

| Recipient | ABO Type for donor platelets | | | |
	1st choice	2nd choice	3rd choice	4th choice
O	O	B or A		
A	A	O		
B	B	O		
AB	AB	A	B	O

Table 2. ABO blood type of choice of donor erythrocytes based on blood type of the recipient.

Recipient	ABO type for donor erythrocytes							
	1st choice	2nd choice	3rd choice	4th choice	5th choice	6th choice	7th choice	8th choice
O pos	O pos	O neg						
O neg	O neg							
A pos	A pos	A neg	O pos	O neg				
A neg	A neg	O neg						
B pos	B pos	B neg	O pos	O neg				
B neg	B neg	O neg						
AB pos	AB pos	AB neg	A pos	A neg	B pos	B neg	O pos	O neg
AB neg	AB neg	A neg	B neg	O neg				

area of the patient (corrected count index (CCI)). One important issue in refractoriness is the HLA antibodies of the patient. The one-hour CCI will be very low, in other words, there is no increment in the platelet count of the patient. Platelets derived from an HLA compatible donor (taken from a database of HLA typed donors or first and second-degree relatives) can bring a solution. Gamma irradiation of these platelets prior to the transfusion is a requirement.

3 ERYTHROCYTE TRANSFUSIONS

Looking back at the case study within this paper, besides the thrombocytopenia, the patient also has anaemia, with a haemoglobin level of 4.0 g/dL. It is known that in an adult patient, one unit of erythrocytes results in an increase in haemoglobin of 0.8 to 1.0 g/dL therefore, three units of red blood cells are required. The choice of ABO RhD donor type for the AB RhD negative patient is more difficult. The risk of anti-RhD formation in patients who have received RhD incompatible transfusions is rather high and therefore, a blood donor that is RhD negative should be chosen. Minor ABO incompatibility is in the buffy coat, and plasma removed units of erythrocytes are not a major issue since only 15–20 mL of plasma is left in the unit, and antibody titres are usually lowered due to dilution by erythrocyte storage solutions for the unit of red blood cells. Taking these considerations into account, the preferential choice when selecting ABO RhD compatible units is shown in Table 2.

Of course, for the units of red blood cells, it should be decided whether gamma irradiation for the patient is needed or not.

A different issue to consider is whether leukoreduction is an option, or not. With leukoreduction, the white blood cell count will be below one million cells per unit of platelets and erythrocytes. Leukoreduction decreases the likelihood of FNHTR and potentially subsequent antibody (e.g. anti-HLA) formation. Leukoreduction cannot be achieved by washing the component.

REFERENCES

Atoyebi, W., Mundi, N. & Croxton, T. (2000). Is it necessary to administer anti-Rh-D to prevent Rh-D immunization after transfusion of D+ platelet concentrates. *British Journal of Haematology,, 111,* 980–983.
Blumberg, N., Heal, J.M., Philips, G.L. & Philips, R.P. (2012). Platelets – to transfuse or not to transfuse. *Lancet, 9850,* 1287–1289.
Cid, J. & Lozano, M. (1971). Risk of anti-D alloimmunization after transfusion of platelets from D+ donors to D-negative recipients. *Transfusion, 45,* 453–454.
Goldfinger, D. & McGinniss, M.H. (1971). Rh incompatible platelet transfusions—risks and consequences of sensitising immunosuppressed patients. *The New England Journal of Medicine, 284,* 942.

Lozano, M. & Cid, J. (2003). The clinical implications of platelet transfusions associated with ABO or Rh(D) incompatibility. *Transfusion Medicine Reviews, 17*, 57–68.

Lozano, M. & Cid, J. (2007). Consensus and controversies in platelet transfusion: Trigger for indication, and platelet dose. *Transfusion Clinique Et Biologique, 14*, 504–508.

Mollison, P.L., Engelfriet, C.P. & Contreras, M. (1997). *Blood transfusion in clinical medicine*. Blackwell Science Ltd.

Valsami, S., Dimitroulis, D., Gialeraki, A., Chimonidou, M. & Politou, M. (2015). Current trends in platelet transfusions practice: The role of ABO-RhD and human leukocyte antigen incompatibility. *Asian Journal of Transfusion Science, 9*, 117–123.

Stem Cell Oncology – Adella (Ed.)
© 2018 Taylor & Francis Group, London, ISBN 978-0-8153-9272-9

The effect of intranasal corticosteroids on nasal polyps as assessed by expression of Tumour Necrosis Factor Alpha (TNFα)

J.K. Siow
Clinical Associate Professor in Otorhinolaryngology, Yong Loo Lin School of Medicine, Nanyang Technological University, Singapore

A.Y.M. Rambe, E.M. Surbakti & D. Munir
Department of Otorhinolaryngology Head and Neck Surgery, Medical School, Faculty of Medicine, Universitas Sumatera Utara, Medan, North Sumatera, Indonesia

L.I. Laksmi
Department of Anatomical Pathology, Medical School, Faculty of Medicine, Universitas Sumatera Utara, Medan, North Sumatera, Indonesia

P. Eyanoer
EPI-TREAT Unit, Universitas Sumatera Utara, Medan, North Sumatera, Indonesia

ABSTRACT: Tumour Necrosis Factor Alpha (TNFα) is one of the pro-inflammatory cytokines that play an important role in the pathogenesis of nasal polyps. Fluticasone furoate is the most potent inhibitor of NF-kB activation and TNF release. The aim of this study was to determine the effect of nasal spray fluticasone furoate on TNFα expression of nasal polyps. This study was analytic with an experimental quasi-study design, performed on 16 cases of nasal polyps obtained with non-probability consecutive sampling. 16 samples, TNFα expression in nasal polyps before treatment with fluticasone furoate was mostly overexpression (87.5%) while post-treatment was found to be negative (81.3%). Data analysis showed a significant decrease in TNFα expression after therapy ($p = 0.001$). There was no significant correlation between nasal polyp decline and decreased expression of TNFα in nasal polyps after fluticasone furoate therapy ($p = 0.136$). Fluticasone furoate has been shown to decrease TNFα expression in nasal polyps and significantly reduce polyp stages.

Keywords: nasal polyps, fluticasone furoate, TNFα expression

1 INTRODUCTION

Nasal polyps are chronic inflammatory diseases of the nasal mucosa characterised by oedematous masses stemming from the inflamed mucosa (Kirtsreesakul, 2005). Tumour Necrosis Factor Alpha (TNFα) is a pro-inflammatory cytokine produced by several cell types, including epithelial cells and macrophages, which induce chronic inflammation. They play a role in the eosinophil recruitment process by increasing the adhesion of eosinophils to nasal polyps. In a study conducted by Otto and Wenzel (2008), it was found that TNFα mRNA increased significantly in nasal polyps compared to the inferior concha. TNFα has an important role in the pathogenesis of nasal polyps. This pro-inflammatory cytokine plays a role in the inflammatory process of nasal polyps by promoting the synthesis of immunoglobulin. Synthesised inflammatory mediators in fibroblasts such as metalloproteinase-1, COX-2 and IL-6 matrix are also stimulated by TNFα (Shun et al., 2005).

Nasal polyps are a manifestation of the inflammatory process, so corticosteroids are an effective therapy (Ferguson & Orlandi, 2006). Corticosteroids have extensive anti-inflammatory effects. Apoptosis is an important process in reducing the number of inflammatory cells. Corticosteroids induce the process of apoptosis of inflammatory cells in nasal polyps (Assanasen & Naclerio, 2001). Intranasal or systemic corticosteroids work by reducing the concentration of inflammatory mediators and inflammatory cells by inhibiting cell proliferation and inducing apoptosis (Jankowski et al., 2002).

Intranasal steroids have non-specific anti-inflammatory properties that can improve symptoms of nasal obstruction and drainage (Aouad & Chiu, 2011). Intranasal corticosteroids are lipophilic and can easily enter the target cell cytoplasm, binding to the glucocorticoid receptors which are common in the airway mucosa. Fluticasone furoate significantly inhibits translocation of NF-kB in fibroblasts and suppresses pro-inflammatory TNFα cytokine activity. In contrast to methylprednisolone which reduces eosinophil inflammation and albumin retention so that the size of the polyp is reduced (Sastre & Mosges, 2012).

The purpose of this study was to determine the effect of fluticasone furoate on the TNFα expression of nasal polyps.

2   METHOD

This study was analytic with an experimental quasi-study design, conducted at the ENT department of H. Adam Malik Medan Hospital, from December 2015 until July 2016. The sampling technique involved non-probability consecutive sampling. Sampling tissue obtained from the biopsy which performed in patients with suspected nasal polyps who came to the outpatient clinic ENT department of H. Adam Malik Medan Hospital. An immune-histochemical examination was conducted in the Anatomy Pathology Laboratory of FK USU to assess TNFα expression in the nasal polyps.

The sample in this study is a portion of the population that met the inclusion and exclusion criteria. The inclusion criteria included patients diagnosed with nasal polyps, males and females ($\geq$ 18 years), who were willing to be included in the study by signing informed consent and willing to use fluticasone furoate nasal spray every morning for four weeks. Exclusion criteria included histopathological examination results of malignancy, pregnancy and lactation, people with diabetes mellitus, patients with liver function disorder, patients with kidney function disorder and patients with a history of nasal surgery.

3   RESULTS

Based on TNFα expression it appears that pre-therapy the majority of the sample, as many as 14 people (87.5%), had a positive expression. Post-therapy, the number of samples with a positive expression decreased to three people (18.7%). The results of the analysis using the McNemar test showed significant differences in TNFα expression between pre- and post-therapy ($p = 0.001$).

The results of the study showed that of 13 samples with decreased expression of TNFα, there were 11 samples (84.6%) which showed reduced polyp stages. Meanwhile, of three samples with a TNFα expression that persisted, only one sample (33.3%) demonstrated decreased polyp stages. The results of the analysis using Fisher's exact test showed no significant relationship between TNFα expression and polyp stages ($p = 0.136$).

4   DISCUSSION

In this study, of 16 samples, before fluticasone furoate therapy, the highest group was obtained by overexpression of TNFα on nasal polyps, 14 samples (87.5%) while negative expression of two samples (12.5%). From the result of the bivariate data analysis, shown in Table 1, the difference table of TNFα expression on nasal polyps before and after receiving fluticasone furoate therapy, with McNemar test obtained a p value = 0.001, which showed a

Table 1. Differences in TNFα expression of nasal polyps before and after treatment with fluticasone furoate.

| | TNFα expression | | | | | | |
| | Positive | | Negative | | Total | | |
	n	%	n	%	n	%	p value*
Pre-therapy	14	87.5	2	12.5	16	100	0.001
Post-therapy	3	18.7	13	81.3	16	100	

*McNemar test.

Table 2. Changes in TNFα expression and stage in each sample before and after treatment with fluticasone furoate.

| | Nasal polyp stage | | | | | | |
| | Declining | | Fixed | | Total | | |
TNFα expression	n	%	n	%	n	%	p value*
Declining	11	84.6	2	15.4	13	100	0.136
Fixed	1	33.3	2	66.7	3	100	
Total	12	75	4	25	16	100	

*Fisher's exact test.

significant decrease of TNFα expression on nasal polyps, after administration of intranasal fluticasone furoate.

Corticosteroids induce apoptotic processes, which are important in reducing the number of inflammatory cells. The work of nasal spray corticosteroids or systemic corticosteroids is to reduce the concentration of inflammatory cells and inflammatory mediators by inhibiting cell proliferation, inducing apoptosis and inhibiting cell proliferation. The anti-inflammatory effect of corticosteroids not only affects inflammatory cells such as lymphocytes, eosinophils, neutrophils and plasma cells, but also epithelial cells and fibroblasts. Corticosteroids inhibit the release of vasoactive mediators thereby reducing fluid extravasation, vasodilation and deposit mediators. Corticosteroids also play a role in reducing the binding of inflammatory cells and inhibit the proliferation of fibroblasts and the synthesis of the extracellular protein matrix so that the inflammatory reactions that occur can be reduced. This will lead to reduced cytokines and inflammatory cells. TNFα which is one of the pro-inflammatory cytokines also decreases its expression with the role of corticosteroids, which is illustrated by the results of this study. Fluticasone furoate, in small doses, is effective in inhibiting pro-inflammatory cytokines, specifically TNFα and IL-5 (Zhang et al., 2014; Tan & Putti, 2005; Yariktas et al., 2005).

Relation of TNFα expression on nasal polyps with decreased nasal polyp stage, showing from 13 samples with decreased expression of TNFα, found 11 samples (84.6%) indicating polyp stages also decreased (Table 2). While from three samples with the TNFα expression that settled only one sample (33.3%) whose polyps stage also decreased. The result of analysis using Fisher's exact test obtained a p value = 0.136 which shows that there is no significant relationship between a decreased expression of TNFα and a decrease of polyp stage. It has been suggested that eosinophils are the dominant population of inflammatory cells found in nasal polyps and are thought to be the central effector cells responsible for the occurrence and survival of inflammatory processes in nasal polyps. The mechanisms underlying the activation, recruitment and survival of eosinophils involve complex interactions of some pro-inflammatory cells and some pathways. The increased synthesis and expression of the widely encountered cytokines (IL-1, IL-3, IL-5, IL-6, IFN-γ) and chemokines (IL-8, eotoxin and RANTES) play an important role in the activation and survival of eosinophils, which mediates the occurrence of inflammatory processes in nasal polyps. There are many studies that focus on cytokines that are responsible for the function of eosinophils, such as IL-1, IL-3, IL-4, IL-5, IL-10, GM-CSF, TNFα, although each involves different mechanisms. The ones with the greatest role are IL-3, IL-5 and GM-CSF which induce the effector function and survival of eosinophils and also stimulate eosinophils in expressing various receptors for cytokines (Anolik, 2010; Rui et al., 2002; Duda, 2015).

REFERENCES

Anolik, R. (2010). Fluticasone furoate nasal spray: Profile of an enhanced-affinity corticosteroid in treatment of seasonal allergic rhinitis. *Journal of Asthma and Allergy, 3*, 87–99.

Aouad, R.K. & Chiu, A.G. (2011). State of the art treatment of nasal polyposis. *American Journal of Rhinology and Allergy, 25*, 291–298.

Assanasen, P. & Naclerio, R.M. (2001). Medical and nasal surgical management of nasal polyps. In *Current opinion in otolaryngology and head and neck surgery* (pp. 27–36). Lippincott William and Wilkins Inc.

Duda, R. (2015). The role of inflammatory mediators in the pathogenesis of nasal polyposis: The literature review. *Romanian Journal of Rhinology, 5*(18), 81–85.

Ferguson, B.J. & Orlandi, R.R. (2006). Chronic hypertrophic rhinosinusitis and nasal polyposis. In *Head and neck surgery-otolaryngology* (4th ed, vol. 1, pp. 1–25). Lippincott Williams & Wilkins.

Jankowski, R., Bouchon, F., Coffinet, L. & Vignaud, J.M. (2002). Clinical factor influencing the eosinophil infiltration of nasal polyps. *American Journal of Rhinology, 40*, 173–178.

Kirtsreesakul, V. (2005). Update on nasal polyps: Etiopathogenesis. *Journal of the Medical Association of Thailand*, 1966–1972.

Otto, B.A. & Wenzel, S.E. (2008). The role of cytokines in chronic rhinosinusitis with nasal polyps. *Current Opinion in Otolaryngology & Head and Neck Surgery, 16*, 270–274.

Rui, X., Li, Y., Xie, M. & Wang, S. (2002). Concentration, distribution and expression of interleukin-5 in human nasal polyp tissue. *Chinese Medical Journal, 115*(9), 1386–1389.

Shun, C.T., Lin, S.K., Hong, C.Y., Kok, S.H., Juan, Y.H. & Wang, C.C. (2005). C-C Chemokine Ligand 2 gene expression in nasal polyp fibroblast: Possible implication in the pathogenesis of nasal polyposis. *The Annals of Otology, Rhinology and Laryngology, 114*(11), 879–885.

Tan, K.B. & Putti, T.C. (2005). Cyclooxigenase 2 expression in nasopharyngeal carcinoma: Immunohistochemical finding and potential implications. *Journal of Clinical Pathology, 58*, 535–538. doi: 10.1136/jcp.2004.021923.

Yariktas, M., Doner, F., Sutcu, R., Demirci, M., Dogru, H. & Yasan, H. (2005). The effect of topical corticosteroid on basic fibroblast growth factor in nasal polyp tissue. *American Journal of Rhinology, 3*, 248–250.

Zhang, N., Crombruggen, K.V., Holtappels, G., Lan, F., Katotomichelakis, M., Zhang, L., Hoffer, P. & Bachert, C. (2014). Suppression of cytokine release by fluticasone furoate vs mometasone furoate in human nasal tissue ex-vivo. *PLOS One, 9*(4), 1–8.

Stem Cell Oncology – Adella (Ed.)
© 2018 Taylor & Francis Group, London, ISBN 978-0-8153-9272-9

Immuno-expression of the p53 mutant protein in sinonasal squamous cell carcinoma

A. Yudhistira, R.A. Asnir, Farhat & D. Indriani
Department of Otorhinolaryngology, Faculty of Medicine, Universitas Sumatera Utara, Medan, North Sumatera, Indonesia

H.M.N.D. Lubis
Department of Anatomy Pathology, Faculty of Medicine, Universitas Sumatera Utara, Medan, North Sumatera, Indonesia

ABSTRACT: Sinonasal squamous cell carcinomas are malignant tumours occurring in the nasal cavity and paranasal sinuses. The p53 protein is a tumour suppressor gene, functioning in processes of cellular apoptosis, differentiation, ageing and angiogenesis. The purpose of this study was to observe the expression of the p53 mutant protein in sinonasal squamous cell carcinoma. This was an observational study in Haji Adam Malik General Hospital where we performed the immunohistochemical examination on paraffin blocks from 30 patients with sinonasal carcinoma who had undergone surgery. Out of 30 samples of sinonasal carcinoma blocks, we found 16 samples with an overexpression of the p53 mutant protein (53.3%).

Keywords: p53 mutant protein, sinonasal squamous cell carcinoma

1 INTRODUCTION

Sinonasal squamous cell carcinomas are malignant tumours occurring in the nasal cavity and paranasal sinuses (Thompson, 2006). They occur in 3% of head and neck tumours and 1% of tumours in general. They can be hard to evaluate in the early stages due to misleading symptoms which are very similar to rhinitis or sinusitis. Diagnosis of this disease can be acquired from careful history taking and physical examination including endoscopic findings. Radiologic examination is most helpful for gathering information about conditions inside the sinus cavities, while in some cases pre-operative histopathologic examination is possible where a tissue sample can be acquired nasally or via sinuscopy; in such cases diagnosis is absolute. However, many practitioners believe that radiologic imaging is enough to diagnose malignancy in the paranasal sinuses. Maxillary sinuses are the most common site of occurrence (60%–80%), followed by the nasal cavity (20%–30%) and ethmoid sinuses (around 15%). Male patients are more common than females (2:1). Therapy for sinonasal carcinoma includes surgery, chemotherapy, radiotherapy or a combination of the three regimes (Roezin, 2007; Carlson et al., 2012).

The mechanism of malignancy formation is multifactorial. However, theories are revolving around cell cycle disturbance and their system regulation (Handayani et al., 2011). The p53 protein is a tumour suppressor gene, functioning in processes of cellular apoptosis, differentiation, ageing and angiogenesis (Shahib, 2012). The p53 gene is known to be the most mutated gene in malignancies (>50% of cancer cases). Wild-type p53 is an unstable protein with unstructured regions. Their half-life is less than 30 minutes. The p53 mutant, however, has a longer half-life and can be detected with immunohistochemical examination (McDonald et al., 2004; Irish, 2003).

The aim of this study was to observe the expression of the p53 mutant in cases of sinonasal squamous cell carcinoma.

2 METHOD

This study was an observational study conducted in Haji Adam Malik General Hospital where we performed the immunohistochemical examination on paraffin blocks processed from tumours from patients with sinonasal squamous cell carcinoma who had undergone surgery. Paraffin blocks were smeared with eematoksilin eosin and damaged blocks were excluded. We acquired 30 blocks for the study.

3 RESULTS

Table 1 shows that sinonasal squamous cell carcinoma patients were mostly male (19 patients/63.3%). Age distribution peaked in the 41–60 years old group (63.3%) with one case occurring in the under 20 years of age group. Out of 30 samples, 21 were determined as non-keratinising squamous cell type (70%), and nine were keratinising squamous cell type (30%). Most patients attended at the stage IV tumour stage (11 cases/36.7%).

Table 1. Distribution of age, gender, histopathology type and tumour stage of patients with sinonasal squamous cell carcinoma.

Sinonasal carcinoma	n	%
Gender		
Male	19	63.3
Female	11	36.7
Age		
<20	1	3.3
21–40	2	6.7
41–60	19	63.3
>60	8	26.7
Histopathology type		
Keratinising squamous cell carcinoma	9	30
Non-keratinising squamous cell carcinoma	21	70
Tumour stage		
Stage I	7	23.3
Stage II	5	16.7
Stage III	7	23.3
Stage IV	11	36.7

Table 2. Distribution of area score, intensity score and the immunoreactive score of p53 mutant expression in sinonasal squamous cell carcinoma.

Scores	n	%
Area score		
0	0	0
1	12	40.0
2	10	33.3
3	8	26.7
Intensity score		
0	0	0
1	12	40.0
2	10	33.3
3	8	26.7
Immunoreactive score		
Negative	14	46.7
Overexpression	16	53.3

Table 3. Distribution of p53 mutant expression based on histopathology type and tumour stage.

Sinonasal squamous cell carcinoma	p53 mutant expression				
	Overexpression		Negative		
	n	%	n	%	Total
Keratising squamous cell carcinoma	6	37.5	3	21.4	9
Non-keratising squamous cell carcinoma	10	62.5	11	78.6	21
Tumour stage					
Stage I	2	28.6	5	71.4	7
Stage II	2	40.0	3	60.0	5
Stage III	3	42.9	4	57.1	7
Stage IV	9	81.8	2	18.2	11

Table 2 shows the immunoreactive score of the p53 mutant (area score times intensity score). In total, 16 samples exhibit overexpression (53.3%) and 14 samples exhibit negative expression (46.7%).

Table 3 shows that sinonasal carcinoma of the non-keratinising type had the most overexpression of the p53 mutant (10 samples/62.5%) while the keratinising type had six samples with p53 overexpression (37.5%). Stage IV tumours had the most overexpression of p53 mutant (9 samples/81.8%).

4 DISCUSSION

Our study showed that the occurrence of sinonasal carcinoma is more frequent in male patients (19 patients) than their female counterparts (11 patients). This is similar to a study by Roezin (2007) at Cipto Mangunkusumo General Hospital, Jakarta where they reported a ratio of sinonasal carcinoma in males:females of 2:1.

Distribution by age showed that most cases occurred in the 41–60 years age group (19 cases). This again shows similarity to a study by Thompson (2006) in the US where they reported the average age for sinonasal carcinoma as being in the 55–65 years age group.

The histopathology findings in our study showed that most cases were non-keratinising squamous cell type (21 samples). Results of histopathologic examination are varied in many studies. Salim (2010), also in Medan, reported that most cases of sinonasal carcinoma were of the keratinising squamous cell type (56.9%).

Tumour stage distribution shows us just how poorly our patients understand their ailments. Eleven patients (36.7%) came seeking treatment at stage IV. This is in tune with a report from Salim (2010) of 56.9% of cases in their study being at stage IV. A report from Turkey by Cengiz (2013) shows different results, where most cases (15 out of 36) attended at stage III.

Our study showed overexpression of the p53 mutant protein in 16 samples out of 30. Holmila (2010), from Finland, also reported a high rate of overexpression of the p53 protein (77%). Oncel (2011), from India, reported that three out of nine cases of sinonasal carcinoma showed an overexpression of the p53 protein.

5 CONCLUSION

In our study, 16 out of 30 samples of sinonasal carcinoma showed an overexpression of the p53 mutant protein (53.3%).

REFERENCES

Carlson, D.L., Barnes, L., Chan, J., Ellis, G., Harrison, L.B., et al. (2012). *Protocol for the examination if specimens from patients with carcinomas of the basal cavity and paranasal sinuses*. College of American Pathologisis. 7th edition. pp. 1–21.

Cengiz, A.B., Uyar, M., Comert, E., Dursun, E. & Erylmaz, A. (2013). Sinonasal tract malignancies: Prognostic factors and surgery outcomes. *Iranian Red Crescent Medical Journal, 15*(12), e14118.

Dhingra, P.L. (2010). Anatomy of nose. In *Disease of ear, nose, and throat* (5th ed., pp. 149–154). India: Elsevier.

Handayani et al., (2011). Ekspresi P53 Mutan dan Ki-67 pada Berbagai Varian Limfoma Sel B Jenis Sel Besar Difus dalam. *Majalah Kedokteran Indonesia, 61*(2).

Holmila, R., Bornholdt J., Heikkila, P., Sultana, T., Fevotte, J., et al. (2010). Mutation in Tp53 tumor suppressor gene in wood dust-related sinonasal cancer. *International Journal of Cancer, 127*, 578–588.

Irish, J.C., Reid, K.S., Gullane, P.J., Charoenrat, O.P. & Montgomery, P.Q. (2003). Molecular biology. In P.H. Evans, P.Q. Montgomery & P.J. Gullane (Eds.), *Principles and practice of head and neck oncology* (pp. 22–50). London: Taylor & Francis Group.

Macdonald, F., Ford, C.H.J. & Casson, A.G. (2004). *Molecular biology of cancer* (2nd ed., pp. 31–60). Ontario: Garland Science/BIOS Scientific Publishers.

Oncel, S., Cosgul. T. & Call, A. (2011). Evaluation of p53, p63, p21, p27, ki-67 in paranasal sinus squamous cell carcinoma and inverted papilloma. *Indian Journal of Otolaryngology and Head & Neck Surgery*, 63(2), 172–177.

Roezin, A. (2007). Tumor Telinga nasal dan sinonasal, dalam *Tumor Telinga Nasal Tenggorok* (pp. 178–81). Balai penerbit FK UI, Jakarta.

Salim, A. (2010). *Profil Penderita Tumor Ganas Sinonasal di RSUP H. Adam Malik Medan tahun 2005–2009*. Tesis.

Shahib, N.M. (2012). Kanker. Dalam Biologi Molekuler Medik. Edisi 1 (pp. 341–392). Penerbit PT. Alumni Bandung.

Thompson, L.D.R. (2006). *Sinonasal carcinomas in current diagnostic pathology* (pp. 40–53). USA. 12.

Stem Cell Oncology – Adella (Ed.)
© *2018 Taylor & Francis Group, London, ISBN 978-0-8153-9272-9*

The association between physical activity, sedentary behaviour and body mass index in students

U.H. Surbakti
Medical Education Study Programme, Faculty of Medicine, Universitas Sumatera Utara, Medan, North Sumatera, Indonesia

M.I. Sari
Department of Biochemistry, Faculty of Medicine, Universitas Sumatera Utara, Medan, North Sumatera, Indonesia

D.D. Wijaya
Department of Anaesthesiology and Intensive Care, Faculty of Medicine, Universitas Sumatera Utara, Medan, North Sumatera, Indonesia

ABSTRACT: Physical activity and sedentary behaviour play an important role in preventing the progression of obesity in adolescence to adulthood. This study was conducted to determine the association between physical activity, sitting time (sedentary behaviour) and Body Mass Index (BMI) in students at the Faculty of Medicine, University of Sumatera Utara. One hundred and thirty students were respondents in this study, selected based on inclusion and exclusion criteria and completion of the International Physical Activity Questionnaire (IPAQ). BMI was determined using a digital weighing scales and microtoise. All data were analysed using SPSS. Based on one-way ANOVA test analysis revealed that there was a significant association ($p = 0.007$) of physical activity toward the mean of BMI but no relationship the sedentary behaviour with BMI ($p = 0.546$). The results suggest that BMI is related to physical activity but not to sedentary behaviour.

1 INTRODUCTION

Technological developments and advancements in this modern age have positive and negative impacts on (human) life. Many activities can be done easily and quickly if they are viewed from their positive impact; however, from their negative impact, they tend to make people reluctant to move. For example, the use of an escalator can make people reluctant to climb the stairs (Booth et al., 2012).

Physical activity constitutes every movement produced by the skeletal muscles which requires energy above the acceptable resting threshold. Physical activity in daily life can be categorised as involving sport, cycling, walking, recreational activities, housework, gardening and other activities (Booth et al., 2012).

Physical inactivity occurs when body movements are minimal and can also be referred to as sedentary behaviour (behaviour that is bound to one place). Included in sedentary behaviour is watching television, reading, working in front of a computer or talking to friends on the phone or learning. Physical inactivity is counted as sitting time. Lack of physical activity and the duration of time spent in sedentary behaviour can be a risk factor for obesity (Heinonen et al., 2013; Brodersen et al., 2007). According to research Jayamani et al. (2013) comparison of women with moderate physical activity who are overweight/obese as much as 3,87 times than women with high physical activity. Previous research has shown that sedentary behaviours such as watching television and videos, using computers and playing video games are linked to obesity (Stamatakis et al., 2008).

In 2014, 11% of men and 15% of women worldwide were obese. Thus, over half a billion adults worldwide are classified as obese. This data also showed that about 3.4 million people die each year as a result of being overweight or obese. According to the Centers for Disease Control and Prevention (CDC), in 2012 the incidence of obesity reached more than 72 million people and included 20.5% of the adolescent population (World Health Organization, 2014). Adolescence is a period that is susceptible to the development of obesity as it is characterised by slowing growth and a decline in the value of physical activity. There is a risk a teenager with obesity or being overweight would be an obese or overweight adult compared to a person of normal weight (Ogden et al., 2012).

Obesity can be determined by anthropometric measurements. Anthropometric measurements exist in many forms, with one of the most widely used in nutrition surveys being the measurement of body mass index (BMI). BMI is the ratio of body weight (in kilograms) to squares of height (in metres). BMI is associated with body fat (Alaska Division of Public Health, 2011).

One group that demonstrate low physical activity are medical students (Resende et al., 2010). The age range of students can be classified as adolescence. Based on the above description, this study aimed to determine the association between physical activity, sitting time (sedentary behaviour) and BMI among students in the Faculty of Medicine, University of Sumatera Utara.

2 MATERIALS AND METHODS

This study was conducted after getting permission from the ethical committee of the Faculty of Medicine of the University of Sumatera Utara. The subjects who agreed to participate in the study were asked to fill out and sign informed consent after being given an explanation about the purpose and benefits of the research. This research involved an analytical study with a cross sectional design which searched for the relationship between the independent variables (physical activity and sedentary behaviour) and the dependent variable (BMI). It was conducted at the Faculty of Medicine, University of Sumatera Utara from March until November, 2016.

Inclusion criteria for this research included being students of the Faculty of Medicine, University of Sumatera Utara, aged between 16 to 23 years old. Exclusion criteria for this research included being students who smoked and suffered from chronic disease. An unpaired categorical analytical formula was used to determine the assumption of the number of samples. Primary data were gathered directly from the research subjects (questionnaires and BMI). Body height and weight were measured using a digital scale with a maximum capacity of 150 kg, a microtoise with a maximum length of 200 cm and an accuracy of 0.1 cm. The BMI was calculated by dividing weight and square of height. The data for physical activity and sedentary behaviour were obtained from the International Physical Activity Questionnaire (IPAQ) which had been completed by the respondents (Hagstromer et al., 2005).

Respondents' data were included and analysed using SPSS (Statistical Product and Service Solution). A one-way ANOVA was used to determine the mean value of BMI in groups categories physical activities and sedentary behaviour (sitting time).

3 RESULTS

There were 130 students who participated in this research. Table 1 shows the characteristics of the participants. The mean value for age was 20.21 ± 1.65. It was found that there were more female respondents (74 respondents or 56.9%), while there were 56 male respondents (43.1%). The mean value of body height, body weight, BMI, physical activity and sedentary behaviour were: 162.20 ± 9.10; 68.93 ± 18.90; 26.25 ± 5.83; $2.020 \pm 1.665.3$ and 6.6 ± 3.03, respectively.

Table 1. Characteristics of study population.

Variables	N (Mean, SD)	Min, Max
Age (year)	20.21 ± 1.65	16.00, 23.00
Sex		
Male n (%)	56 (43.10)	
Female n (%)	74 (56.90)	
Anthropometry		
Body height (cm)	162.20 ± 9.10	186.50, 146.50
Body weight (kg)	68.93 ± 18.90	133.00, 40.00
BMI (kg/m^2)	26.25 ± 5.83	44.27, 16.21
Physical activity (MET-minute/week)	2.020 ± 1.665.3	126.00, 6102
Sedentary behaviour (hours/day)	6.6 ± 3.03	1.30, 15.00

Table 2. Physical activity categories in relation to BMI.

	Low activity (N = 45)	Moderate activity (N = 39)	High activity (N = 48)	p*
MET (MET-minute/week)	423	1546	6468	0.007
BMI±SD (kg/m^2)	27.68 ± 6.1	26.47 ± 5.5	24.05 ± 5.3	

*One-way ANOVA test.

Table 3. Multiple comparison analysis of physical activity and BMI.

Variable	Physical activity		p*
BMI	Low activity	Moderate activity	0.99
		High activity	0.006
	Moderate activity	High activity	0.127

*Post hoc Bonferroni test.

The categories of physical activity of subjects is shown in Table 2. The respondents were divided into three physical activity categories: low activity, moderate activity and high activity. Based on MET-minute/week, the mean value of low physical activity was 423 MET-minute/week, the mean value of moderate physical activity was 1546 MET-minute/week and the mean value of high physical activity was 6.468 MET-minute/week. There were 45 respondents (34%) involved in low activity, 34 respondents (30%) involved in moderate activity and 48 respondents (36%) involved in high activity. It was found that the mean BMI for low activity was 27.69 kg/m^2, for moderate activity was 26.47 kg/m^2 and for high activity was 24.05 kg/m^2.

The result of the one-way ANOVA test showed that there was a significant difference ($p = 0.007$) in physical activity with BMI. As Table 3 shows, after multiple comparative analysis using the post hoc Bonferroni test, it was found that there was a significant difference ($p = 0.006$) in the mean BMI between respondents involved in low activity and respondents involved in high activity, but a significant difference was not found ($p = 0.99$) in the respondents involved in low activity and in the respondents involved in high activity. There was also no significant difference ($p = 0.127$) in the mean BMI between the respondents involved in moderate activity and the respondents involved in high activity.

It was also found that for the sitting time (sedentary behaviour) divided in three categories (shown in Table 4). The mean value of the sedentary behaviour in less than four hours was 2.7 hours/day, the sedentary behaviour four to eight hours was 5.5 hours/day, and sedentary behaviour more than eight hours was10.3 hours/day. The mean value of BMI in sedentary

Table 4. Sedentary behaviour categories in relation to BMI.

	Less than 4 Hours (N = 19)	4 to 8 Hours (N = 67)	More than 8 Hours (N = 44)	$p*$
Sedentary behaviour (hours/day)	2.7	5.5	10.3	0.546
BMI±SD (kg/m²)	25.12 ± 6.5	25.5 ± 6.5	26.18 ± 5.4	

*One-way ANOVA test.

behaviour less than four hours was 25.12 kg/m²; the mean value of BMI in sedentary behaviour four to eight hours was 25.50 kg/m²; and the mean value of BMI in sedentary behaviour more than eight hours was 26.18 kg/m².

4 DISCUSSION

In this research, the mean value of the respondents' BMI was 26.25 kg/m². This high mean value of BMI was caused by the large number of obese students who participated in this research. The rate of one of the respondents' weight even reached 133 kg. Students tend to lack a healthy lifestyle, such as not sleeping until late at night and a lack of exercise. Students do not have time to exercise or undertake recommended physical activity. This was because their study schedule was from 8.00 a.m. to 5.00 p.m. The curriculum and examination pattern of the students at the Faculty of Medicine was tight so that they had less time to concentrate on extracurricular activities. They only had spare time in the evening (Wattanapisit et al., 2016). These are risk factors for obesity (World Health Organization, 2014).

In this research categories physical activity of the students: the mean value of low physical activity was 423 MET-minute/week, the mean value of moderate physical activity was 1546 MET-minute/week and the mean value of high physical activity was 6.468 MET-minute/week. The result of a one-way ANOVA test showed that there was a significant difference ($p = 0.007$) in the mean BMI of the respondents involved in low activity (27.68 ± 6.1), moderate activity (26.47 ± 5.5) and high activity (24.05 ± 5.3), respectively.

Research conducted by Labban (2014) revealed that there was a correlation between physical activity and weight, height and obesity status. This indicates that physical activity plays an important role in body metabolism through fatty acid oxidation, gluconeogenesis processes and burning calories to hamper fatty adiposity (Sugondo, 2014). A previous study in the Faculty of Medicine, University of Sumatera Utara shows the effect of nutrients cause obesity (Sari & Sari, 2017).

Based on the research conducted by Kaplan, it was found that a person with higher IMT group was inclined to have a risk of being affected by diabetes, hypertension and cardiovascular disease. A high mortality rate occurred in IMT ≥ 25 kg/m² and ≥ 30 kg/m² (Kaplan et al., 2014).

Adolescents with good physical activity will mostly not be affected by obesity, compared with inactive adolescents. An adolescent with obesity or who is overweight will be an obese adult, compared with an adolescent of normal weight (Rauner et al., 2013).

Physical inactivity occurs when body movements are minimal and can also be referred to as sedentary behaviour (behaviour that is bound to one place). Sedentary behaviour is assessed by measuring sitting time using the IPAQ (Resende et al., 2010). Most of the respondents tended to engage in sedentary behaviour from four to eight hours with the mean value being 6.6 hours/day. This may happen because most of the students of the Faculty of Medicine had to follow the curriculum of the Faculty of Medicine such as courses of lectures, practical work, laboratory skills and tutorials, which enabled them to sit down in the same position for a prolonged period of time.

The research conducted by Krishnakumar et al. (2013) found similar results to those of the present study. In that research, it was found that the average sitting time for students of the Faculty of Medicine in Bangalore, India, reached six to seven hours per day. Students of the Faculty of Medicine in Casablanca, Morocco, also had a similar average sitting time of six hours per day (Otmani, 2016).

The results of this research showed that there was no difference in the mean value of sedentary behaviour between BMI. Different results from Labban, (2014) suggest that longer sitting times will result in higher BMI values. The existence of a trend that refers to the decrease in physical activity due to work activities that cause more sitting and transportation activities.

5 CONCLUSION

There was a significant difference in the mean value of BMI between low, moderate and high physical activity levels in students at the Faculty of Medicine, University of Sumatera Utara, but no difference in the mean value of BMI between sedentary behaviour. These findings indicate that physical activity modulates obesity in students at the Faculty of Medicine, University of Sumatera Utara because most of the students had to follow the curriculum including courses of lectures, practical work, laboratory skills and tutorials which involved prolonged periods of sitting.

ACKNOWLEDGEMENTS

The writer gratefully acknowledges that this research was supported by the Ministry of Research and Technology and the Higher Education Republic of Indonesia. The support was under the research grant DIPA USU of 2016. Also, thanks to the Dean of the Faculty of Medicine, University of Sumatera Utara, who provided the facility for carrying out this research.

REFERENCES

Alaska Division of Public Health. (2011). *State of Alaska measuring height/weight and calculating guidelines for schools.*

Booth, F., Roberts, C. & Laye, M. (2012). Lack of exercise is a major cause of chronic diseases. *Comprehensive Physiology, 2*(2), 1143–1211.

Brodersen, N.H., Steptoe A., Boniface D.R. & Wardle J. (2007). Trends in physical activity and sedentary behavior in adolescence: Ethnic and socioeconomic differences. *British Journal of Sports Medicine, 41*(3),140–144.

Hagstromer, M., Oja, P. & Sjostrom, M. (2005). The International Physical Activity Questionnaire (IPAQ): A study of concurrent and construct validity. *Public Health Nutrition, 9*(6), 755–762.

Heinonen, I., Helajärvi, H., Pahkala, K., Heinonen, O.J., Hirvensalo, M., Pälve, K., et al. (2013). Sedentary behaviours and obesity in adults: The cardiovascular risk in young Finns study. *BMJ Open, 3*(6), pii: e002901. doi: 10.1136/bmjopen-2013–002901.

Jayamani, V., Gopichandran, V., Lee, P., Alexander, G., Christopher, S. & Prasad, J.H. (2013). Diet and physical activity among women in urban and rural areas in South India: A community based comparative survey. *Journal of Family Medicine and Primary Care, 2*, 334–338.

Kaplan, R.C., Aviles-Santa, M.L., Parrinello, C.M., Hanna, D.B., Jung, M., Castaneda S.F., et al. (2014). Body mass index, sex, cardiovascular disease risk factors among Hispanic/Latino adults: Hispanic community health study/study of Latinos. *Journal of the American Heart Association, 3*, e000923. doi:10.1161/JAHA.114.000923.

Krishnakumar, P., Khrisna, P. & Rasu, T. (2013). Prevalence and pattern of physical activity among medical students in Bangalore, India. *Electron Physician, 5*(1), 606–610.doi: 10.14661/2013.606–610.

Labban, L. (2014). The association between physical activity, overweight and obesity among Syrian university students. *Saudi Journal of Sports Medicine, 14*(5), 121–127.

Ogden, C.L., Carrol, M.D., Kit, B.K. & Flegal, KM. (2012). Prevalence of obesity and trends in body mass index among US children and adolescents, 1999–2000. *JAMA, 307*(5), 483–490.

Otmani, N., Serhier, Z. & Housbane, S. (2016). Physical activity among medical students in Casablanca, Morocco. *Imperial Journal Interdisciplinary Research, 2*(2), 566–576.

Rauner, A., Mess, F. & Woll, A. (2013). The relationship between physical activity, physical fitness and overweight in adolescents: A systematic review of studies published in or after 2000. *BMC Pediatrics, 13*, 19.

Resende, M.A., Resende, R.B.V., Tavares, R.S., Santos, C.R.R.. & Barreto-Filho, J.A.S. (2010). Comparative study of the pro-atherosclerotic profile of students of medicine and physical education. *Arquivos Brasileiros de Cardiologia, 95*(1), 21–29.

Sari, M.I. & Sari, D.I. (2017). Nutrient intake, apolipoprotein A5–1131T > C polymorphism and its relationship with obesity. *Materials Science and Engineering, 180*. 012094 doi:10.1088/1757–899X/180/1/0120941011001.

Stamatakis, E., Hirani, V. & Rennie, K. (2009). Moderate-to-vigorous physical activity and sedentary behaviours in relation to body mass index-defined and waist circumference-defined obesity. *British Journal of Nutrition, 101*(5), 765–773.

Sugondo, S. (2014). Obesitas. In S.Setiadi., I. Alwi, A.W. Sudoyo, M. Simadibrata, B. Setiyohadi, & A.F. Syam (Eds.), *Buku Ajar IlmupenyakitDalam. Edisi VI*: 2559–2569. Jakarta: Interna Publishing.

Wattanapisit, A., Fungthongcharoen, K., Saengow, U. & Vijitpongjinda, S. (2016). Physical activity among medical students in Southern Thailand: A mixed methods study. *BMJ Open, 6*, e013479. doi:10.1136/ bmjopen-2016.

World Health Organization. 2014. *Global status report on noncommunicable diseases*. Geneva.

Stem Cell Oncology – Adella (Ed.)
© *2018 Taylor & Francis Group, London, ISBN 978-0-8153-9272-9*

The role of a Simplified Selvester Score as a predictor of successful fibrinolytics in STEMI

Syaifullah, I.N. Kaoy, Z. Mukhtar, H. Hasan, N.Z. Akbar & H.A.P. Lubis
Department of Cardiology and Vascular Medicine, Universitas Sumatera Utara, Adam Malik Hospital, Medan, Indonesia

ABSTRACT: Fibrinolytics are one of the modalities of treatment for STEMI patients. Successful fibrinolytics have been associated with better clinical outcomes. We sought to explore whether the Simplified Selvester Score could predict successful fibrinolytic therapy electrocardiographically. Fifty-three STEMI patients who received fibrinolytic therapy with streptokinase were enrolled in this retrospective study. The Simplified Selvester Score was estimated on the first admission by ECG. STEMI patients were divided into two categories: successful or failed fibrinolytic therapy, based on ECG. The optimal cut-off Simplified Selvester Score was analysed. Patients with successful fibrinolytics have a lower Simplified Selvester Score (2.3 ± 1.6 vs 5.1 ± 1.7; $p = 0.001$). In multivariate analysis, a Simplified Selvester Score ≤ 3.5 remained significantly associated with successful fibrinolytic therapy and appeared to be a strong predictor for successful fibrinolytic therapy ($p = 0.004$: OR = 6.8; 95% CI [1.55, 37.05]). A Simplified Selvester Score ≤ 3.5 can be used as a predictor of successful fibrinolytic therapy in STEMI patients.

Keywords: fibrinolytics, Selvester Score, STEMI

1 INTRODUCTION

STEMI is a leading cause of cardiovascular disease worldwide. The immediate therapeutic goal of reperfusion therapy is to restore full antegrade flow in the infarct-related epicardial coronary artery, as well as to achieve adequate myocardial perfusion at the tissue level. Fibrinolytic therapy is one reperfusion modality. It is well established that early and complete resolution of ST segment elevation is a powerfull predictor of successful fibrinolytic therapy. Successful ST segment resolution as an electrocardiographic sign of restored myocardial perfusion may vary according to how far the infarction process has progressed (Al-Daydamony, 2014; Ghaffari, 2013; Gusto Investigators, 1993; Steg, 2012).

During the evolution of acute STEMI, pathologic Q waves evolve and R-wave regression develops. Measurements of these ECG parameters at presentation may reflect the progression of the infarct process and predict the extent of myocardial salvage to be gained from successful fibrinolytic therapy (Granger, 1992; Grines, 2003).

The Simplified Selvester Score was initially developed to estimate electrocardiogaphically the size of myocardial infarction and scars. It has been validated with high sensitivity and specificity and high intra and inter-observer agreement (Selvester, 1985). We choose to study the ability of the Simplified Selvester Score as a pre-fibrinolytic predictor of successful management of STEMI because the electrocardiogram (ECG) remains a simple yet powerful tool and is easily available in the assessment of reperfusion efficacy.

2 METHODS

This was a single centre study in which a total of 53 STEMI patients received fibrinolytic therapy in the form of streptokinase by intravenous infusion, at a dose of 1,500,000 U over 30–60 minutes from January 2015 until December 2016. Standard anti-ischaemic medications were allowed and remained unchanged during the study period. All patients underwent resting high-quality 12-lead ECG recordings, from which the following was estimated:

1. QRS score calculated according to the simplified form of the Selvester scoring system based on 37 criteria capable of generating 29 points.
2. ST segment elevation measured 20 ms after the J point. The height (in mm) of ST segment elevations was measured in leads I, aVL and V1 through V6 for anterior infarctions, and in leads II, III, aVF, V5 and V6 for inferior infarctions.

The ST segment was measured in the single lead with the highest elevations. The resting ECG was analysed for all patients 90 minutes following the initiation of fibrinolytic therapy, the sum of ST segment resolution was measured, classified into two groups: successful fibrinolytic therapy with a sum of ST segment resolution ≥ 50%, and failed thrombolytic therapy if a sum of ST segment resolution < 50%.

All statistical analyses were performed using statistical software, and a p value < 0.05 was considered significant. A receiver operating characteristic curve analysis was used to determine the optimum cut-off values of the Simplified Selvester Score to predict successful fibrinolytic therapy. Clinical, laboratory and procedural data were compared with the use of Student's t-test or Mann-Whitney U test for continuous variables and the Chi-square or Fisher's exact test for categorical variables (expressed as counts and percentages). The correlation of the Simplified Selvester Score and troponin T was analysed by a correlation test. Continuous variables were analysed for normal distribution using the Kolmogorov–Smirnov test. To address concerns over confounding variables affecting successful fibrinolytics, we also performed a multivariate logistic regression analysis which significant variables in bivariate analysis before were included. The study protocol was reviewed and approved by our local institutional human research committee.

3 RESULTS

From a total of 53 STEMI patients, 33 patients (62%) had successful fibrinolytic therapy and 20 patients (38%) had failed fibrinolytic therapy. The mean age of our study population was 52 ± 7.8 years, and the mean Simplified Selvester Score was 3.5 ± 2.6. The baseline characteristics of the overall cohort, as well as the two individual study groups, are shown in Table 1. The median time from symptom onset to reperfusion was four hours. Compared to the successful fibrinolytic group, patients in the failed fibrinolytic group had a longer onset to reperfusion 4.5(1–10) vs 3(0.5–8) hours respectively, $p < 0.05$, were more likely to be diabetic [10 (50%) vs 7 (21.2%) respectively, $p < 0.05$], with a higher troponin level [0.25 (0–2.39) vs 0.03 (0–7.8) µg/l respectively, $p < 0.05$]. The Simplified Selvester Score was higher in the failed than the successful fibrinolytic group [5.1 ± 2.1 vs 2.3 ± 1.6 respectively, $p < 0.05$].

There was a good significant positive correlation between the Simplified Selvester Score and troponin level with a correlation coefficient $r = 0.53$.

The receiver operating characteristic (ROC) curve identified a cut-off value of ≤ 3.5 as the optimal cut-off value of the Simplified Selvester Score, with a sensitivity of 75% and specificity of 64%.

On bivariate analysis, some variables are significant: Diabetes mellitus (odds ratio [OR] 0.27; $p = 0.019$); Dislipidaemia (odds ratio [OR] 2.8; $p = 0.082$); chest pain onset ≤ three hours (odds ratio [OR] 4.8; $p = 0.013$); Diastolic BP ≥ 70 mmHg (odds ratio [OR] 3.0; $p = 0.092$); Troponin level ≤ 0.11 (odds ratio [OR] 6; $p = 0.03$) and the Simplified Selvester Score ≤ 3.5 (odds ratio [OR] 5.3; $p = 0.006$. From the multivariate analysis, a Simplified Selvester Score of ≤ 3.5 was an independent predictor for successful fibrinolytic therapy in STEMI patients who received fibrinolytic treatment ($p = 0.004$: $OR = 6.8$; 95% CI [1.51, 37.06]) (Table 2).

Table 1. Baseline characteristics.

Characteristics	Successful fibrinolytics (n = 33)	Failed fibrinolytics (n = 20)	Sig (p)
Age (year)	53 ± 7.6	51 ± 8.3	0.78
Male (%)	32 (97%)	19 (95%)	0.67
Smoking	28 (84.8%)	18 (90%)	0.59
Hypertension	12 (36.4%)	7 (35.0%)	0.92
Dyslipidaemia	18 (54.5%)	6 (30.0%)	0.08
Diabetes mellitus	7 (21.2%)	10 (50%)	**0.03**
Chest pain onset (hour)	3 (0.5–8)	4.5 (1–10)	**0.016**
Systolic BP (mmHg)	129 ± 23.7	126 ± 26.1	0.62
Diastolic BP (mmHg)	84 ± 12.5	80 ± 17.5	0.35
Hear rate (times/i)	7 (20–107)	62 (46–94)	0.30
Killip II–IV	4 (12.1%)	0 (0%)	0.14
Location of infarct			
– Anterior	18 (54.5%)	8 (40%)	0.31
– Non-anterior	15 (45.5%)	12 (60%)	
Hb (g/dL)	14.7 ± 1.2	14.8 ± 1.9	0.09
Ht	42 ± 4	43 ± 4	0.44
Leucocyte (/µL)	12530 ± 3184	12291 ± 3480	0.99
Thrombocyte	247000 (162000–415000)	273000 (175000–544000)	0.53
Troponin (µg/l)	0.03 (0–7.8)	0.25 (0–2.39)	**0.012**
Simplified Selvester Score	2.3 ± 1.6	5.1 ± 2.1	**0.001**

Table 2. Multivariate model analysis of independent factors of successful fibrinolytic therapy.

Variable	p	OR	95% CI for OR	
			Lower	Upper
Selvester Score	0.004	6.842	1.511	37.065
Diastolic BP	0.031	4.245	1.594	40.186

4 DISCUSSION

The present study demonstrated that a Simplified Selvester Score of ≤ 3.5 was independently associated with successful fibrinolytic therapy in STEMI patients.

It seems appealing to identify those who are more likely to benefit from fibrinolysis in this patient category. Evaluation of the Simplified Selvester Score on admission ECG recordings would simply and readily offer the chance for this stratification. In this way, one would avoid giving fibrinolytic therapy (with its notorious risk of bleeding) to patients who are less likely to get its benefit and restrict it only to those who are more likely to improve (Schroder, 1995; Selvester, 1985).

The extent of myocardial damage in STEMI patients suggested a worse prognosis. Troponin T prone to describe this. Our study showed a good correlation with troponin level and also the Simplified Selvester Score. An advantage of the QRS scoring system is that it requires only an adequately obtained 12-lead ECG, which is universally available, inexpensive, safe and noninvasive.

In our study, the optimum cut-off point of the Simplified Selvester Score of ≤ 3.5 predicted successful fibrinolytic therapy with high sensitivity and specificity. Ghaffari et al. (2013) also found a cut-off point of ≥ 3.5 in failed fibrinolytic therapy. In bivariate and multivariate analysis, the Simplified Selvester Score is associated with predicting successful fibrinolytic therapy, but this finding must be tested in a larger sample involving multicentres.

The main practical result of our study is that the Simplified Selvester Score can be used to predict incomplete ST segment resolution in those patients presenting with a high calculated Simplified Selvester Score and avoid administrating fibrinolytic therapy in a subset of these patients who arrive late to the emergency department with some ongoing chest discomfort, where the benefit of fibrinolytic therapy might be negligible or those deemed to be at high risk of thrombolytic (TLT)-related complications (e.g. elderly). It can also help in more accurate selection of STEMI patients for primary PCI in those centres with PCI facilities available.

This study has some limitations. First, our study was a single centre study. Second, using the complete version of the scoring system (54 criteria for a total of 32 points) might have changed the results. The simplified version may underestimate infarct size because it excludes posterior extension of inferior infarcts. Third, we studied patients with their first STEMI, where this scoring system performs best, so the results are not applicable to patients with previous MI. We also excluded patients with left bundle branch block, left anterior or posterior fascicular block, left ventricular hypertrophy or right ventricular hypertrophy. Fourth, we used only SK for TLT which has a lower reperfusion, patency and TIMI-3 flow rate than the newer generation of thrombolytics (e.g. alteplase, reteplase or TNK-t-PA).

5 CONCLUSION

The Simplified Selvester Score can reliably predict the occurrence of adequate successful fibrinolytics in patients with first acute STEMI receiving fibrinolytic therapy. Using the cut-off value of ≤ 3.5, the Simplified Selvester Score can predict adequate ST segment resolution with a high sensitivity and specificity.

REFERENCES

Al-Daydamony, M.M. & Kandeel, N.T. (2014). Value of modified Selvester Score in prediction of successful reperfusion in patients with acute myocardial infarction. *The Egyptian Heart Journal, 66*, 28.

Ghaffari, S., Kazemi, B., Saeidi, G., et al. (2013). The value of the simplified QRS scoring system in predicting st-segment resolution after thrombolysis in patients with acute myocardial infarction. *European Journal of Cardiovascular Medicine, III*(1), 268–275.

Granger, C.B., Califf, R.M. & Topol, E.J. (1992). Thrombolytic therapy for acute myocardial infarction. *Drugs, 44*, 293–325.

Grines, C.L., Serruys, P. & O'Neill, W.W. (2003). Fibrinolytic therapy. Is it a treatment of the past? *Circulation, 107*, 2538–2542.

Gusto Investigators. (1993). An international randomized trial comparing four thrombolytic strategies for acute myocardial infarction. *The New England Journal of Medicine, 329*(1993), 673–682.

Schroder, R., Wegscheider, K., Schroder, K. & Dissmann, R. (1995). Extent of early ST segment elevation resolution: A strong predictor of outcome in patients with acute myocardial infarction and a sensitive measure to compare thrombolytic regimens. A substudy of the International Joint Efficacy Comparison of Thrombolytics trial. *Journal of the American College of Cardiology, 26*, 1657–1667.

Selvester, R.H., Wagner, G.S. & Hindman, N.B. (1985). The Selvester QRS scoring system for estimating myocardial infarct size. The development and application of the system. *Archives of Internal Medicine, 145*, 1877–1881.

Six, A.J., Louwerenburg, J.H. & Kingma, J.H. (1991). Predictive value of ventricular arrhythmias for patency of the infarct-related coronary artery after thrombolytic therapy. *British Heart Journal, 66*(2), 143–146.

Steg, P.G., James, S.K., Atar, D, et al. (2012). ESC guidelines for the management of acute myocardial infarction in patients presenting with ST-segment elevation. *European Heart Journal, 33*, 2569–2619.

Stem Cell Oncology – Adella (Ed.)
© 2018 Taylor & Francis Group, London, ISBN 978-0-8153-9272-9

Cryptosporidium sp. findings in AIDS patients: A case report

D.M. Darlan
Parasitology Department, Faculty of Medicine, Universitas Sumatera Utara, Medan, North Sumatera, Indonesia

M.F. Rozi
Faculty of Medicine, Universitas Sumatera Utara, Medan, North Sumatera, Indonesia

R.H. Saragih
Tropical and Infectious Disease Division, Internal Medicine Department, Universitas Sumatera Utara, Medan, North Sumatera, Indonesia

ABSTRACT: *Cryptosporidium sp.* is a common intestinal parasite infecting immunocompromised patients. This organism causes chronic diarrhoea. Infection is related to the ingestion of oocyst-contaminated drinking water or food. For immunocompromised individuals, this infection could have a higher mortality and vary in clinical manifestation. We report on three patients, aged 33–40 years, suffering from chronic diarrhoea caused by *Cryptosporidium sp.* These patients were diagnosed with AIDS and a very low CD4 count (< 5%). The inadequacy of antiretroviral cause progressively decrease CD4 count according to host factors, it explains *Cryptosporidium sp.* is still a burden for AIDS patient, especially with very low CD4 count. There was no medication given to these patients including paromomycin or nitazoxanide, continuing antiretroviral therapy was the only medication given to patients. Diarrhoea frequency decreased after 8–10 days adminstration to hospital and discharge was done to these patients.

Keywords: cryptosporidium, AIDS, HIV, diarrhoea

1 INTRODUCTION

Cryptosporidium is an apicomplexan protozoa causing infections in the gastrointestinal tract and lungs (Leitch & He, 2011). There are two species associated with human infection, *Cryptosporidium parvum* and *Cryptosporidium hominis* (Widerstrom et al., 2014). In the early 1980s, several cases were confirmed as related to HIV infection. In the 1990s, cryptosporidium was also linked to waterborne outbreaks of diarrhoea, with approximately 403,000 people being infected by this organism in Wisconsin (White, 2015; MacKenzie et al., 1994).

Although this organism is a protozoa, it has a complex life cycle, with infection occurring when a fully sporulated oocyst is ingested by a human through contaminated water or food (Levinson, 2014). Excystation occurs in the upper part of the small intestine and penetration by the enterocyte will ensue, producing watery diarrhoea. Unfortunately, oocysts of this organism are thick-walled, which explains their resistance to chlorination or other disinfecting agents (Fritsche & Pritt, 2017).

Most studies have shown that self-limiting diarrhoea is the main clinical manifestation in immunocompetent hosts worldwide, but chronic diarrhoea will ensue if the host is immunocompromised. The focus of treatment for this infection is supportive care, especially fluid replacement therapy (Flynn, 2016). Comparison studies using nitazoxanide and a placebo showed no difference, particularly in the HIV-infected population (Agnamey, 2010).

2 CASE REPORT

The first patient, a 40-year old female was admitted to Adam Malik General Hospital for diarrhoea lasting for more than three days. She tested positive for HIV infection five years previously and underwent antiretroviral therapy. Unfortunately, her CD4 count progressively decreased, until now her absolute CD4 count was 17 cell/µL. This woman did not have any special condition or family history of systemic disease. She was negative for the Hepatitis B virus and Hepatitis C virus antibodies. For prophylaxis of *Pneumocystis carinii* pneumonia, co-trimoxazole was given to this patient.

The second patient, a 33-year old woman with chronic diarrhoea lasting for more than seven days was admitted to the same hospital. She was diagnosed with HIV eight years previously. This woman presented to hospital with fever and profuse watery diarrhoea. She also reported abdominal cramp. She also received co-trimoxazole as prophylactic medication. Her absolute CD4 count was just 2 cell/µL.

The third patient, a 35-year old man became debilitated with watery diarrhoea and fatigue. He experienced that for more than five days, and first line antiretroviral therapy was given to this patient. This man was a stage IV HIV-infected individual with pulmonary tuberculosis. This patient was also positive for HIV infection for eight years. Because of the high-burden of infection, this patient was also malnourished. The medication history of this patient included first category for pulmonary tuberculosis (isoniazid, pyrazinamide, rifampicin and ethambutol), antiretroviral therapy and co-trimoxazole. His absolute CD4 count was 8 cell/µL.

All patients underwent further examination, especially microbiological and parasitological examination. Nevertheless, faecal smear under microscope examination revealed only *Cryptosporidium sp.* in all samples. We do not use any anti-parasitic medication for cryptosporidiasis due to opportunistic infection in immunocompromised patients, especially those with AIDS. Using anti-parasitic medication is only considered for the paediatric population, not the HIV-infected population. Maintaining the fluid and nutritional status were the goals of therapy for this infection. Thus, continuing antiretroviral treatment was the only option here. After 8–10 days hospitalisation, diarrhoea frequency had decreased and resolved several days afterward.

3 DISCUSSION

Cryptosporidiidae are named based on the host they infect and approximately five common cryptosporidium species usually infect humans. However, more than 90% of human infections are caused by *Cryptosporidium parvum* (*C. parvum*) and *Cryptosporidium hominis* (*C. hominis*) (Rossle & Latif, 2013). Sporulated oocysts are an infective stage for this organism and have been found in 87% of water samples sourced from the United States and Canada (Yoder & Beach, 2010). Hardy, chlorine-resistant oocysts can spread by direct person-to-

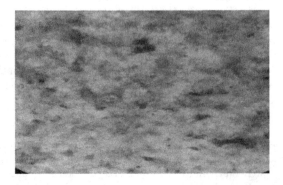

Figure 1. *Cryptosporidium sp.* under microscopic examination. (1000x magnification field).

person contact and survive for up to 12 months in cold water (Chalmers & Katzer, 2013). After oocyst ingestion, excystation in the upper small bowel will occur, with each oocyst consisting of four sporozoites and the sporozoites penetrate the enterocyte. Sporozoites will develop into their mature form in the enterocyte (Xiao & Griffiths, 2013).

Diarrhoea caused by this organism presents in four different populations: childhood diarrhoea in developing regions; travellers' to developing regions diarrhoea; diarrhoea in immunocompromised patients; and outbreaks in developed countries (Lima & Guerrant, 2016).

Clinical manifestation similarities are found in giardiasis, isosporiasis and cyclosporiasis. After a 3–12 day incubation period, clinical manifestation will be present. Watery diarrhoea is the main symptom, which may be associated with other symptoms, such as: abdominal cramps (96% of patients); anorexia, malaise, flatulence, nausea, vomiting (65%); and mildly elevated temperature (59%) (Davies & Chalmers, 2009). Cryptosporidiosis is associated with a higher mortality rate and more severe symptoms when an immunocompromised host is infected. Moreover, the CD4 count can be a predictor for this infection. There is no effective therapy for this infection because of its resistance to many antiprotozoal drugs, particularly for immunocompromised patients. Vaccine is also unavailable, however, ongoing research is still trying to find a vaccine using microRNAs (Checkley et al., 2015).

After excystation from the oocyst, sporozoites will invade mucosal epithelium and Peyer's patch M cells. Intestinal Epithelial Cells (IECs), as a part of the innate immune system, have their own Toll-Like Receptors (TLRs) and intracellular Nod-Like Receptors (NLRs) which finally detect cryptosporidium. Presentation to CD4$^+$ will ensue using IECs via MHC-II (Leitch & He, 2011). After recognition, CD4$^+$ will be activated and play a major role in the acquired immune response (Checkley et al., 2015). Several studies have shown that two chemokines, CXCL-10 and CXCL-8, were attracting immune cells while infection developed (Rescigno, 2011). However, cell-mediated immunity is severely affected by HIV, which explains the inadequate clearance of this organism. Nevertheless, many observations have shown that the humoral immune response to cryptosporidium is quite strong in AIDS patients, even greater than those in immunocompetent patients. Unfortunately, the humoral immune response and antibody production, are not associated with clearance of this infection. IFN-Υ is still required for an effective immune response to eradicate cryptosporidium. As noted, IFN-Υ is produced by the Th1 (a subset of CD4 lymphocytes) (Santarlasci et al., 2013). IFN-Υ can accelerate the immune response, as it inhibits proliferation of cryptosporidium in cultured enterocytes and it increases transcription factor for TNFα and NF-kB, which also increases the amount of TNFα. In addition, patients with a low CD4 count will suffer from a severe form of this infection. Meanwhile, CD8$^+$ does not have several roles in cryptosporidiosis but requires further study to prove its function (Reijasse et al., 2001). In vitro studies have shown that peripheral blood mononuclear cells (PBMCs) of AIDS patients do not have normal respones to the cryptosporidium antigen (Leitch & He, 2011).

Borad and Ward summarised their studies using mice and humans, confirming that the severity of cryptosporidiosis is related to the CD4$^+$ count. Those with a CD4$^+$ of less than 50 cell/mm^3 are susceptible to a severe form of the disease, otherwise those with a CD4$^+$ count more than 180 cells/mm^3 are not susceptible to severe disease or self-limiting disease (Rossle & Latif, 2013). *Cryptosporidium sp.* can also induce inflammation without tissue invasion. Several studies tried to prove the toxin related to boost the inflammation but it remains elusive (Bouzid et al., 2013).

Nutritional support and replacement of fluid therapy are vital in immunocompromised hosts infected by this organism. Anti-motility drugs, such as loperamide or diphenoxylate/ atropine, can be used to relieve symptoms related to abdominal cramp and diarrhoea (Spark et al., 2015). Nitazoxanide has been approved by the FDA for treatment of cryptosporidium. However, clinical studies have shown that nitazoxanide has failed to eradicate this organism in the immunocompromised population and malnourished children (Checkley et al., 2015). Azithromycin, spiramycin and bovine anti-cryptosporidium immunoglobulin were considered as treatment for cryptosporidiosis, unfortunately, all were not superior to a placebo in AIDS patients (Cabada & White, 2010).

4 CONCLUSIONS

Chronic diarrhoea caused by *Cryptosporidium sp.* is a common infection in those with a very low CD4 count or AIDS patients. The use of anti-parasitic drugs is still debatable because of the lack of effectiveness. The main goals of therapy for those suffering from opportunistic infection, particularly *Cryptosporidium sp.* are fluid replacement therapy and nutritional support. Continuing antiretroviral drugs are the major mainstay for this infection to restore immune function over a period of time.

REFERENCES

Agnamey, P., Djeddi, D., Vanrenterghem, A,. et al. (2010). Childhood cryptosporidiosis: A case report. *Journal of Parasitology Research.*

Bouzid, M., Hunter, P.R., Chalmers, R.M. & Tyler, K..M. (2013). Cryptosporidium pathogenicity and virulence. *Clinical Microbiology Reviews, 26*(1), 115–134.

Cabada, M.M. & White, A.C. Jr. (2010). Treatment of cryptosporidiosis: Do we know what we think we know? *Current Opinion in Infectious Diseases, 23*(5), 49.

Chalmers, R.M. & Katzer, F. (2013). Looking for cryptosporidium: The application of advances in detection and diagnosis. *Trends in Parasitology, 29*(5), 237–248.

Checkley, W., White, A.C., Jaganath, D., et al. (2015). A review of the global burden, novel diagnostics, therapeutics, and vaccine targets for cryptosporidium. *The Lancet Infectious Diseases, 15*, 85–94.

Davies, A.P. & Chalmers, R.M. (2009). Cryptosporidiosis. *BMJ, 339*, 963–966.

Flynn, P.M. (2016). Cryptosporidium, isospora, cyclospora, and microsporidia. In *Nelson textbook of pediatrics.* New York: Elsevier.

Fritsche, T.R. & Pritt, B.S. (2017). Medical parasitology. In *Henry's clinical diagnosis and management.* New York: Elsevier.

Leitch, G.J. & He, Qing. (2011). Cryptosporidiosis-an overview. *Journal of Biomedical Research, 25*(1), 1–16.

Levinson, W. (2014). Intestinal & urogenital protozoa. In *Review of medical microbiology and immunology.* New York: McGraw-Hill.

Lima, A.A.M. & Guerrant, R.L. (2016). Cryptosporidiosis. In *Goldman-Cecil medicine.* New York: Elsevier.

MacKenzie, W.R., Hoxie, N.J., Proctor, M.E., et al. (1994). A massive outbreak of *Cryptosporidium* infection transmitted through the public water supply. *The New England Journal of Medicine, 331*, 161–167.

Reijasse D., Canioni D., de Serre, N.P.M., Canioni, D., et al. (2001). Cytotoxic T cells in AIDS colonic cryptosporidiosis. *Journal of Clinical Pathology, 54*, 298–303.

Rescigno, M. (2011). The intestinal epithelial barrier in the control of homeostasis and immunity. *Trends in Immunology, 32*(6), 256–258.

Rossle, N.F. & Latif, B. (2013). Cryptosporidiosis as threatening health problem: A review. *Asian Pacific Journal of Tropical Biomedicine, 3*(11), 916–924.

Santarlasci, V., Cosmi, L., Maggi, L., et al. (2013). IL-1 and T helper immune responses. *Frontiers in Immunology, 4*, 1–5.

Spark, H., Nair, G., Castellanos-Gonzalez, A. & White, A.C. (2015). Treatment of cryptosporidium: What we know, gaps, and the way forward. *Current Tropical Medicine Reports, 2*(3), 181–187.

White, A.C. (2015). Cryptosporidiosis (Cryptosporidium Species). In *Mandell, Douglas, and Bennett's principles and practices of infectious diseases.* USA: Elsevier.

Widerstrom, M., Schonning, C., Lilja M., et al. (2014). Large outbreak of *Cryptosporidium hominis* infection transmitted through the public water supply, Sweden. *Emerging Infectious Disease, 20*(4), 581.

Xiao, L. & Griffiths, J.K. (2013). Cryptosporidiosis. In *Hunter's tropical medicine and emerging infectious diseases* (9th edition). New York: Elsevier.

Yoder, J.S. & Beach, M.J. (2010). Cryptosporidium surveillance and risk factors in the United States. *Experimental Parasitology, 124*, 31–39.

Stem Cell Oncology – Adella (Ed.)
© 2018 Taylor & Francis Group, London, ISBN 978-0-8153-9272-9

Endoscopic approach in maxillary tumours

A.B. Zulkiflee & N. Prepageran
Department of Otorhinolaryngology, Faculty of Medicine, University of Malaya,
Kuala Lumpur, Malaysia

ABSTRACT: With the advent of dynamic and better resolution camera systems, an endoscopic approach is more popularly acceptable than conventional methods. Thus, surgical intervention in maxillary pathology has shifted into less invasive procedures with lower morbidity and better disease surveillance.

Keywords: endoscopic, maxillary tumours

1   INTRODUCTION

Maxillary tumours are traditionally excised via an open approach even at early disease stages. However, with current advanced video technology and better resolution of camera systems, the tumours can be removed endoscopically, promising better outcomes.

2   CASE PRESENTATION

A 49-year-old man presented to our centre with a persistent unilateral nose blockage with a protruding mass in the left nostril. He was then further assessed using computer tomography. The mass was noted to occupy his entire unilateral sinuses; however, there was no evidence of orbital and intracranial involvement. He was then scheduled for endoscopic excision of the tumour.

A complete excision was successfully performed with a microdebrider. He has been under clinical surveillance at our centre. To date, no recurrence has been noted. His histopathology reported inverted papilloma.

3   DISCUSSION

Tumours in the maxillary sinus originate either from the apical point or medial wall of the sinus. In some cases, they extends into the nasal cavity and with further involvement of other sinuses, such as the ethmoidal and frontal sinuses. These tumours distort the natural anatomy of the region, providing a technical challenge to head and neck surgeons.

Traditionally, the tumours are removed using an open approach in which a facial incision is made along the lower lid of the eyes and continuously parallel to the nasal area and down to the philtrum. This is called a Weber-Ferguson incision.

However, the approach has become less popular since the 1980s, when the endoscope became evolutionised with better resolution and also became more easily available on the market. Currently, endoscopic training and technique has been markedly improved with better camera systems so that early maxillary tumours can be removed endoscopically. This minimally invasive approach promises better outcomes and improved monitoring for patients.

4 CONCLUSION

Currently, an endoscopic approach for maxillary tumours is widely acceptable. However, intensive training for endoscopic surgeons and delicate instruments are required.

REFERENCES

Lawson, W., LeBenger, J., Som, P., et al. (1989). Inverted papilloma: An analysis of 87 Cases. *Laryngoscope, 99*, 1117–1124.

Pagella, F., Giourgos, G., Matti, E., Canevari, F.R. & Carena, P. (2011). Endoscopic treatment of maxillary inverted papilloma. *Rhinology, 49*, 369–374.

Phillips, P., Gustafson, R. & Facer, G. (1990). The clinical behavior of inverting papilloma of the nose and paranasal sinuses: Report of 112 cases and review of the literature. *Laryngoscope, 100*, 463–469.

Wormald, P.J., Ooi, E., van Hasselt, C.A. & Nair, S. (2003). Endoscopic removal of sinonasal inverted papilloma including endoscopic medial maxillectomy. *Laryngoscope, 113*, 867–873.

Stem Cell Oncology – Adella (Ed.)
© 2018 Taylor & Francis Group, London, ISBN 978-0-8153-9272-9

Sensitivity and specificity of the urine nitrite test and gram staining in diagnosing UTIs in children

N. Fidelia, R. Ramayanti, S. Nafianti, Rusdidjas, O.R. Ramayani,
R.S. Siregar & B. Siregar
*Department of Child Health, Faculty of Medicine, Universitas Sumatera Utara,
Medan, North Sumatera, Indonesia*

ABSTRACT: Urine culture is the gold standard in the diagnosis of a Urinary Tract Infection (UTI). More simple tests are often used instead of urine cultures. To compare the sensitivity and specificity of the urine nitrite test and gram staining with urine culture, a cross-sectional study was conducted at RSUP H Adam Malik, from February to July 2017, with participants recruited by consecutive sampling. The data collected were sample characteristics, clinical manifestations, causal organisms, nitrite test, gram staining and urine culture results. The data were analysed using Fisher's exact test with $p < 0.05$. A total of 60 samples were included. The organism encountered was *Escherichia coli*. The most frequent clinical manifestation was fever, exhibited by 37 children with UTIs. The sensitivity and specificity of the nitrate test were 64.8% and 86.9%, respectively, while the sensitivity and specificity of gram staining were 94.5% and 100%, respectively. Gram staining is a good alternative test for diagnosing UTIs, but nitrite testing still needs further research.

Keywords: nitrite test, gram staining, urine culture, urinary tract infection

1 INTRODUCTION

Early detection of urinary tract infection (UTI), such as urine dipstick test, microscopic examination and urine culture, is necessary because of the incidence of UTI misdiagnosis (Najeeb, 2015). Urinalysis was conducted in children aged over three years old who exhibited dysuria, frequency, haematuria, abdominal pain and urinate incontinence (Robinson, 2014). The urine dipstick test is a method for detecting leucocyte esterase and nitrite (White, 2011). Gram staining and the urine dipstick test are considered as useful, simple, practical and effective methods for early diagnosis of UTIs (Zorc, 2005; Whiting, 2005). Urine culture is unavailable in some health care facilities. The nitrite test is an alternative, but its accuracy compared to urine culture is controversial. Gram staining is a simple test with high accuracy (Zorc, 2005).

A meta-analysis study from the American Academy of Pediatrics (AAP) in 2011 revealed that sensitivity and specificity of gram staining were 81% and 83%, respectively, while the sensitivity and specificity of the urine nitrite test were 53% and 98%, respectively (Subcommittee, 2011). A meta-analysis study in 2010 by William et al. indicated that the sensitivity of the urine nitrite test was 49%, while gram staining was 91% (Cantey, 2015). A study in Indonesia noted that the sensitivity and specificity of gram staining were 88% and 100%, respectively (Putri, 2013).

All of those studies pictured a controversy of sensitivity and specificity of urine nitrite test, however, they revealed a high sensitivity and specificity for gram staining. Therefore, it is necessary to determine the sensitivity and specificity of the urine nitrite test and gram staining so that clinicians can choose the best, quickest, most accurate and reliable examination at all levels of health care facilities. Thus, the diagnosis and management of UTIs in children could be well performed, leading to a satisfactory outcome.

2 METHOD

The study protocol and the informed consent process were approved by the Research Ethics Committee of the Universitas Sumatera Utara Medical School, Indonesia. This was a descriptive study with a cross-sectional approach.

The 60 participants were recruited by consecutive sampling. We enrolled children aged from 13 to 18 years old with suspected UTIs based on symptoms, urine dipstick test, gram staining and urine culture. The samples were children who could do midstream urine collection, agreed to participate and filled the informed consent form. UTI was suspected in patients who had symptoms such as dysuria, frequency, urgency, vomiting, abdominal and flank area pain, decreased appetite and costovertebral angle tenderness, including children with unexplained fever which can occur in all age groups, and children with congenital anomaly of the urinary tract (Bou, 2017; Saheed, 2016). The study was conducted from February to July 2017 in H Adam Malik General Hospital, Department of Child Health. The exclusion criteria were children who received antibiotic therapy one week before the examination, corticosteroid therapy or who used a urine catheter. All urine specimens were collected using clean-catch midstream urine collection.

The urine specimens were transported to the Microbiology Laboratory of H Adam Malik General Hospital within the hour. MacConkey agar was used for the urine culture. UTI was diagnosed with bacteriuria of $\geq 10^5$ CFU/ml. The gram staining was performed by one physician. The urine dipstick test (Verify Urinalysis) procedure was conducted.

We used SPSS version 15.0 to examine the data. The data were tabulated and presented in a frequency distribution 2×2 table. The relation between the nitrite test and the urine culture was analysed using a Chi-square test with Fisher's exact test.

3 RESULTS

Sixty children aged 3 to 18 years old were included in this study. Twenty-nine samples (48.3%) had gram-negative staining. Twenty-seven samples (45%) had a positive nitrite test. The median age of participants was ten years old, and from the Kolmogorov-Smirnov test, there

Table 1. Distribution of sample characteristics.

Characteristic	Frequency ($n = 60$)
Gender, n (%)	
Boy	30 (50)
Girl	30 (50)
Median age, year (minimum–maximum)	10 (3–18)
Gram staining, n (%)	
Gram-negative	29 (48.3)
Gram-positive	6 (10)
Bacteria absent	25 (41.7)
Nitrite, n (%)	
Positive	27 (45)
Negative	33 (55)
Urine culture, n (%)	37 (61.7)
Bacteria present	23 (38.3)
Bacteria absent	

was significant result, $p < 0.05$ (Table 1). A positive result with UTI mostly was found in girls 21 (56.8%) and boys 16 (43.2%).

There were 31 gram-negative samples (83.7%). The most common types of bacteria causing UTIs were *Escherichia coli* eight (21.6%), *Klebsiella pneumoniae* five (13.5%) and *Enterobacter faecalis* four (10.8%) (Table 2).

The clinical manifestations of UTIs in children attending the Adam Malik General Hospital are described in Table 3. The most common symptom found with a UTI in this study was fever 21 (56.8%).

The other common clinical symptoms were dysuria and abdominal pain; both had a proportion of 24.3%.

Table 4 shows the ratio of nitrite test to urine culture, with the sensitivity and specificity of the nitrite test being 64.8% and 86.9%, respectively. Table 5 shows that the sensitivity and specificity of gram staining were 94.5% and 100%, respectively.

Based on Fisher's exact text, the association between the nitrite test and the organisms resulting from the urine culture was significant, with $p = 0.014$ and PR (95% CI) 14.375 (Table 6).

Table 2.   Distribution of organisms causing UTIs.

Organism		Frequency, n (%)
Gram-negative	*Escherichia coli*	8 (21.7)
	Klebsiella pneumoniae	5 (13.5)
	Enterobacter faecalis	4 (10.8)
	Morganella morgagni	3 (8.1)
	Citrobacter freundii	2 (5.4)
	Enterobacter cloacae	2 (5.4)
	Pseudomonas aeruginosa	2 (5.4)
	Serratia fonticola	2 (5.4)
	Acinetobacter baumanii	1 (2.7)
	Bordatella ronchiseptica	1 (2.7)
	Pantoea spp	1 (2.7)
Gram-positive	*Enterococcus faecium*	1 (2.7)
	Staphylococcus sciuri	1 (2.7)
	Staphylococcus gordonii	1 (2.7)
	Streptococcus agalactiae	1 (2.7)
	Streptococcus hemolyticus	1 (2.7)
	Streptococcus mitis	1 (2.7)

Table 3.   Distribution of clinical manifestations of UTIs in children.

Clinical manifestation	Frequency, n (%)
Fever	21 (56.8)
Dysuria	9 (24.3)
Abdominal pain	9 (24.3)
Frequency	5 (13.5)
Dysfunctional voiding	4 (10.8)
Urgency	3 (8.1)
Flank pain	3 (8.1)
Decreased appetite	3 (8.1)
Vomiting	2 (5.4)
Costovertebral angle tenderness	1 (2.7)

Table 4. Comparison between the nitrite test result and urine culture.

Nitrite test	Urine culture		Sn (%)	Sp (%)	PPV (%)	NPV (%)	PLR	NLR	A (%)
	Positive	Negative							
	n (%)	n (%)							
Positive	24 (88.9)	3 (11.1)	64.8	86.9	88.8	60.6	4.9	0.4	73.3
Negative	13 (39.4)	20 (60.6)							

*Sn: sensitivity, Sp: specificity, PPV: positive predictive value, NPV: negative predictive value, PLR: positive likelihood ratio, NLR: negative likelihood ratio, A: accuracy.

Table 5. Comparison between gram staining and urine culture.

Nitrite test	Urine culture		Sn (%)	Sp (%)	PPV (%)	NPV (%)	PLR	NLR	A (%)
	Positive	Negative							
	n (%)	n (%)							
Positive	24 (88.9)	3 (11.1)	64.8	86.9	88.8	60.6	4.9	0.4	73.3
Negative	13 (39.4)	20 (60.6)							

*Sn: sensitivity, Sp: specificity, PPV: positive predictive value, NPV: negative predictive value, PLR: positive likelihood ratio, NLR: negative likelihood ratio, A: accuracy.

Table 6. Association between nitrite test and organism from urine culture.

Nitrite test	Urine culture		P*	PR (95% CI [1.452, 142.351])
	Gram-negative n (%)	Gram-positive n (%)		
Positive	23 (95.8)	1 (4.2)	0.014	14.375
Negative	8 (61.5)	5 (38.5)		

4 DISCUSSION

Acute UTIs are relatively common in children. School-aged children may have symptoms similar to adults, including dysuria, frequency or urgency. Females have a high risk of UTI infection (White, 2011).

Common uropathogens include *Escherichia coli* (accounting for approximately 85% of UTIs in children). Gram-negative bacteria are the most common (White, 2011; Bou, 2017). In this study, in accordance with the results of previous studies, the most common organism-causing encounter is *Escherichia coli* followed by *Klebsiella pneumoniae*. Furthermore, UTIs are caused by coliform and *Enterococcus spp*. This is due to their presence in high numbers on the perineum (Saheed, 2016).

UTIs are more common in girls than boys. According to the AAP, in 2011 the incidence of UTIs in girls was 8% and in boys was 2%. UTI rates are largely unchanged from 6 to 16 years of age (Chang, 2006; Trapote, 2011). In Indonesia, the risk of UTIs in prepuberty is 3%–5% in girls and 1%–2% in boys (Pardede, 2001). UTI prevalence in children ranges from 3%–73%, with a median of 20% found in some studies (Whiting, 2005). In this study, the number of a girls suffering from UTIs is 56.8% of all proven UTI samples.

Usually, in children over two years of age, midstream urine can be taken. Research in France concluded that direct urine sampling is better than through a urine catheter

(Mori, 2007). A study in New York concluded that the midstream urine sample is less likely to be contaminated with bacteria (Dayan, 2000). Research in Spain, in 2012, introduced the concept of urine collection by the midstream method (Bou, 2017). Some studies concluded a sensitivity of clean-catch midstream urine sampling of 98% to 100%, whereas a specificity of 71% to 97% was reported (Holm, 2016). Midstream urine collection has decent sensitivity and specificity besides its superiority in patient comfort, reduced trauma and ease of sampling compared to other urine sampling methods.

Urinalysis and the dipstick urine test cannot replace urine culture as the gold standard for investigating UTIs. Research in Nigeria showed a sensitivity and specificity of urine nitrite testing of 66.2% and 93.5%, respectively (Maya, 2011). A study in Iran revealed the sensitivity of the nitrite test as being 79% (Ayazi, 2007). In the present study, the sensitivity of the nitrite test was 64.8% and the specificity was 86.9%. The sensitivity of gram staining was 94.5% and the specificity was 100%.

The relationship between the nitrite test and gram of bacteria using Fisher's exact test showed $p = 0.014$, indicating a statistically significant relationship with a PR value of 14.375 (95% CI [1.452, 142.351]). The change of nitrate to nitrite in urine by gram-positive bacteria is unclear. In positive gram, the change was found in staphylococcus with a negative coagulase, with some of the nitrite yields positive (Sato, 2005). A study in Riyadh, in 2010, showed a sensitivity of urine nitrite to gram-negative organisms of 45%–60%, while for specificity the range was 85%–98%%. Overall, positive nitrite found in gram-positive ranged from 5.5% (0% to 50% and to gram-negative 49.7% (21.4% to 55.2%) (Majid, 2010).

5   CONCLUSION

This study showed that the sensitivity and specificity of gram staining are high. The nitrite test showed high specificity. The nitrite test and gram urine staining are good alternative diagnostic and screening tests for UTIs in children in areas with limited facilities and health workers.

REFERENCES

Ayazi, P. & Daneshi, M.M. (2007). Comparison of urine culture and urine dipstick analysis in diagnosis of urinary tract infection. *Acta Medica Iranica, 45*(6), 501–504.
Bou, A.S. (2017). *Comparison between bladder stimulation with midstream clean-catch urine and bladder catheterization to obtain non-contaminant urine specimens in febrile children up to 6 months of age: A cross-sectional study*. Universitat de Girona.
Cantey, J.B., Gaviria-Agudelo, C., TeKippe, E.M. & Doern, C.D. (2015). Lack of clinical utility of urine gram stain for suspected urinary tract infection in pediatric patients. *Journal of Clinical Microbiology, 53*, 1282–1285.
Chang, S.L. & Shortliffe, L.D. (2006). Pediatrics urinary tract infections. *Pediatric Clinics of North America, 53*, 379–400.
Dayan, P.S., Chamberlain, J.M., Boenning, D., Adirim, T. & Schor, J.A. (2000). A comparison of initial to the later stream urine in children catheterized to evaluate for a urinary tract infection. *Pediatric Emergency Care, 16*(2), 88–90.
Holm, A. & dan Aabenhus, R. (2016). Urine sampling techniques in symptomatic primary-care patients: A diagnostic accuracy review. *BMC Family Practice, 17*(72), 1–9.
Majid, F.A. & Buba, F. (2010). The predictive and discriminant values of urine nitrites in urinary tract infection. *Biomedical Research, 21*(3), 297–299.
Mava, Y., Ambe, J.P., Bello, M., Watila, I. & Pius, S. (2011). Evaluation of the nitrite test in screening for urinary tract infection in febrile children with sickle cell anemia in Maiduguri-Nigeria. *Nigerian Medical Journal, 52*(1), 45–48.
Mori, R., Lakhanpaul, M. & Verrier-Jones, K. (2007). Diagnosis and management of urinary tract infection in children: Summary of NICE guidance. *BMJ, 335*, 395–397.
Najeeb, S., Munir, T., Rehman, S., Hafiz, A., Gilani, M. & Latif, M. (2015). Comparison of urine dipstick test with conventional urine culture in diagnosis of urinary tract infection. *Journal of the College of Physicians and Surgeons Pakistan, 26*(2), 108–110.

Pardede, S.O., Tambunan, T., Alatas, H., Trihono, P.P. & Hidayati, E.L. (2011). Konsensus Infeksi saluran kemih pada Anak. Unit Kerja Koordinasi Nefrologi (UKK); Badan penerbit Ikatan Dokter Anak Indonesia, Jakarta, pp. 1–31.

Putri, A.U., Rina, O., Rosmayanti, Ramayanti, R. & Rusdidjas, (2013). Comparison of urine gram stain and urine culture diagnose urinary tract infection in children. *Paediatrics Indonesia*, *53*(2), 121–124.

Robinson, J.L., Finlay, J.C., Lang, M.E. & Bortolussi, R. (2014). Urinary tract infection in infants and children: Diagnosis and management. *Paediatrics and Child Health*, *9*(6), 315–319.

Saheed, A.M., Aurangzeb, S.M. & Saadia, M. (2016). A review on common bacteria causing urinary tract infection. *Pakistan Journal of Medicine and Health Sciences*, *10*(2), 513–517.

Sato, A.F., Svidzinski, A.E., Consolaro, E.L. & Boer, C.G. (2005). Urinary nitrite and urinary tract infection by gram-positive cocci. *J Bras Patol Med Lab*, *41*, 397–404.

Subcommittee on urinary tract infection, steering committee on quality improvement and management. (2011). Urinary tract infection: Clinical practice guideline for the diagnosis and management of the initial UTI in febrile infants and children 2 to 24 months. *Peds*, *128*, 595–610.

Trapote, R.C.A., Laita, J.A.C., Subías, J.E., Rodríguez, G.M.F., Díaz, A.G. & Rodríguez, S.G. (2011). Epidemiology of UTI and its complication in children. Dalam: Clinical practice guideline for urinary tract infection in children. *Ministry of Science and Research*, 45–52.

White, E. (2011). Diagnosis and treatment of urinary tract infections in children. *American Family Physician*, *83*(4), 409–415.

Whiting, P., Westwood, M., Watt, I., Cooper, J. & Kleijnen, J. (2005). Rapid tests and urine sampling techniques for the diagnosis of urinary tract infection (UTI) in children under five years: A systematic review. *BMC Pediatrics*.

Zorc, J.J., Kiddoo, D.A. & Shaw, K.N. (2005). Diagnosis and management of pediatric urinary tract infections. *Clinical Microbiology Reviews, 18*(2), 417–422.

Stem Cell Oncology – Adella (Ed.)
© *2018 Taylor & Francis Group, London, ISBN 978-0-8153-9272-9*

Ascariasis incidence in children who received single and repeated educational lectures

M.A. Boediman, M. Lubis, O.R. Ramayani & P.D.H. Simbolon
Department of Child Health, Medical School, Faculty of Medicine, Universitas Sumatera Utara, Medan, North Sumatera, Indonesia

ABSTRACT: The World Health Organization (WHO) have recommended albendazole 400 mg for the eradication ascariasis. Despite effective treatment options, reinfection following treatment alone is inevitable. A case-control study was conducted to investigate the difference in incidence of ascariasis in children who received education on sanitation and personal hygiene once with recurrent in Singkuang village, South Tapanuli, North Sumatera from April to October 2016. The subjects were elementary school children selected using a cluster sampling technique. Statistical analysis was performed by Chi-square and Fisher's exact test. One hundred and seventy elementary school children were divided into two groups, with 85 subjects in the control group. The incidence of ascariasis was found to be 24% in the control group and 3% in the case group. Children who received recurrent education tended to be 8.4 times more likely not to succumb to ascariasis. There were significant differences in the incidence in both groups ($p = 0.001$).

Keywords: ascariasis, children, educational lecture, parasitic worm

1 INTRODUCTION

The incidence of soil-transmitted helminths (STH) in developing countries remains high. The main cause of intestinal parasitic infections is *Ascaris lumbricoides* (Clarke et al., 2017; Yap et al., 2016). The groups most vulnerable to this infection are school-age children, with an intensity peaking in the 5–14 year-age group (Yap et al., 2016). Among STH, ascariasis is the most common worm infection, with an estimated worldwide incidence of 25% (0.8 to 1.22 billion people) (Bethony et al., 2006).

The World Health Organization's (WHO) policy for control of ascariasis centres on three groups, preschool-aged children (pre-SAC), school-aged children (SAC) and women of child bearing age, on the basis that heavy infection in these groups will have a detrimental impact on anaemia, child growth and development. The current WHO guidelines focus on school-aged children, both for monitoring infection and as a target for treatment, although treatment of pre-SAC and women of childbearing age is also recommended where sustainable delivery mechanisms exist, especially in areas of intense transmission. The guidelines recommend treating SAC annually where any STH prevalence falls between 20% and 50% and twice a year where it exceeds 50% (Anderson et al., 2015). At present, the control strategy for STH infection promoted by the WHO is based solely on the eradication of periodic worms or deworming in high-risk communities (Clarke et al., 2017). By treating the highest risk group, environmental contamination is reduced and consequently, infection in the wider community decreases. School-based deworming programmes have been shown to contribute towards achieving several of the Millennium Development Goals (MDG).

Despite effective treatment options for STH infections, reinfection following treatment alone is inevitable (Jia et al., 2012). One strategy that has been identified to reduce reinfection following deworming treatment is health education, focussing on teaching hygienic and sanitary behaviours. The simplest and cheapest strategy is handwashing. Previous studies have assessed the effectiveness of handwashing in reducing the prevalence of ascariasis (Mahmud et al., 2015). Regular education in schools can be a way of conveying the right method of handwashing to a child. A school-based health hygiene education intervention was effective in increasing STH knowledge and in reducing ascariasis (Gyorkos et al., 2013). Education on health, especially prevention of ascariasis disease, for both parents and children is an important factor in breaking the chain of transmission as well as the incidence rate of ascariasis disease (Schmidlin et al., 2013; Corneiro et al., 2002).

2 METHOD

This study took place in Singkuang village, Mandailing Natal, North Sumatera from April 2016 until October 2016. The subjects were elementary school children selected using a cluster sampling technique. The exclusion criteria were students who refused to take worm medicines and incomplete follow the execution. All children who fulfilled the inclusion criteria were enrolled in the study. Primary school data collection in Singkuang village, the selection of elementary school will be conducted randomly. Elementary schools that were selected were randomised for one or three-time extension interventions. Basic baseline data on parents' and children's knowledge of helminth infection and its prevention were collected based on the available questionnaires. Examination of faeces by the parasitology officer of the Faculty of Medicine, the University of North Sumatra was conducted using the Kato Katz method. All participants who suffered and did not suffer from a worm infection were given the anthelmintic medication, albendazole 400 mg, in a single dose. The participants were randomly grouped into case and control groups. Single education was performed in the control group and repeated three times in the case group. We tested the validity of the education lecture instrument by using Pearson's correlation test and obtained a result for Cronbach's alpha coefficient of 0.86. Repeat examination of faeces was conducted three months after and assessed the incidence rate of ascariasis in both new and reinfected children. Data were analysed using the Statistical Package for Social Sciences (SPSS) for Windows, version 19 (2010), with a 95% confidence interval and a p value <0.05 was considered as significant. Randomisation was used Microsoft Excel Randomisation. The analysis was performed using a Chi-square and Fisher's exact test. Ethical approval was granted by the Research Ethics Committee, Medical Faculty, University of North Sumatera.

3 RESULTS

One hundred and seventy elementary school children from Singkuang village, Mandailing Natal, North Sumatra, were enrolled and divided into two groups, with 85 subjects in the control group.

The study population characteristics showed that the mean age of children in the control group was 10.1 (SD 1.97) years and in the case group 8.8 (SD 2.04) years. Both groups were dominated by males. Based on the class, children in the control group were mostly in fifth class (23.5%), while in the case group they were mostly in first grade (28.2%). The number of siblings and the order in the family of children in each group was almost the same. Children in both groups mostly had short stature and normal nutritional status. Parents of children in both groups have incomes ranging from 500,000 to 1,000,000 Rupiah, with most occupations being either fishermen or farmers. More than 80% of children's parent's education is up to elementary school. From the total sample, 50 students suffered from ascariasis. This shows that the prevalence of ascariasis in this study was 29.4%.

This study reported that after six months follow-up, we found 96.5% (82/85 samples) and 76.5% (65/85) samples in the uninfected state, the remaining was 3.5% and 23.5% samples in reinfection state, respectively for intervention and control group. The relative risk ratio for both groups was 8.410. The findings from the six months follow-up assessment showed

Table 1. Educational relationship of sanitation and hygiene with the occurrence of ascariasis.

	Ascariasis				
Education	No	Yes	RR	95% CI	p*
Multiple	82	3	8.410	[2.394, 29.543]	0.001
Single	65	20			

Table 2. Factors related to the success of education.

Variable	Wald	p*	Constants	95% CI
Gender	1.215	0.270	3.914	[0.346, 44.311]
Age	0.843	0.359	1.669	[0.559, 4.978]
Class of school	0.023	0.880	0.791	[0.037, 16.728]
Family order	3.203	0.074	0.390	[0.139, 1.094]
Number of siblings	0.800	0.371	0.720	[0.351, 1.478]
Parental education	2.165	0.141	16.695	[0.393, 709.63]
Parental employment	3.986	0.046	184.404	[1.100, 30917.9]
Parental income	2.576	0.109	0.013	[0.000, 26.111]

that there were differences in the incidence in both groups ($p = 0.001$). Children who received recurrent education tended to be 8.4 times more likely not to succumb to ascariasis (Table 1).

This study also looked for factors related to the success of the education programme. The results of the logistic regression test on factors related to the success of education in this study showed that the parent's occupation is the only factor affecting the success of education, where the success of education will increase 184 times in children of parents with civil service employees compared with children of parents with other jobs (Table 2).

4 DISCUSSION

In Indonesia, the prevalence of ascariasis remains high, especially in children aged one to ten years. Research conducted by Rahmad in Sibolga, North Sumatra, showed a prevalence of ascariasis of 55.8% and in Karo of 18.3% (Rahmad, 2008). Meanwhile, research by Ginting (2009) in Samosir reported a higher figure of 55.8%. Another study in the area of North Sumatra, Deli Serdang by Rahma reported a prevalence of 84.4% (Rahma, 2011). The present research was conducted in the North Sumatera province, Mandailing Natal Regency. This region consists of coastal and tropical lowlands. The results showed a prevalence of ascariasis of 29.4%. This figure is lower than the prevalence in the Sibolga and Deli Serdang areas which are both coastal and lowland areas. This may be due to a lack of STH infection screening conducted in the study area.

Ascaris infection is more common in children aged 6–12 years (Mahmud et al., 2015). This is because children still have a lack of knowledge or consciousness about personal hygiene and health. The presence of Intestinal Parasitic Infections (IPIs) have a statistically significant association with the educational status of the household heads, the absence of washing facilities, home cleanness conditions and type of toilet used ($p < 0.05$) (Abbosie & Seid, 2014). The economic and educational level of parents also affects the incidence of ascariasis in children (Nematian et al., 2004). Parents with low economic levels tend to use health facilities more often associated with prevention of health or ascariasis. Low-educated parents will have less knowledge, including in the health field. One of the things they often ignore is personal hygiene and the environment. Also, poorly educated parents will find it difficult to provide good health education to their children, including the prevention of worms.

STHs are easily treated with one of four drugs: albendazole and mebendazole, and to a lesser extent, levamisole and pyrantel pamoate (Anderson et al., 2015). In line with the WHO strategy for controlling STH infections in endemic countries, a national school-based deworming programme currently provides annual delivery of albendazole to school children (Kepha, 2017). However, reinfection commonly occurs due to the inability of the human host to mount protective immunity to reinfection by intestinal helminths (Jia et al., 2012). The impacts on both prevalence and intensity of infection were significantly higher among children receiving four-monthly treatments of albendazole compared to those who received a single annual treatment (Kepha, 2017). But if treatment combined with inadequate hygiene and sanitation. Ziegelbauer et al. (2012) to restrict or eliminate re-exposure in environments continuously contaminated with the egg or larval free-living transmission stages of these parasitic worms (Gabrie et al., 2014; Seid et al., 2015; Walker et al., 2011).

The major strengths of this study include the large sample size, the randomised design, the high response and follow-up rates, appropriate statistical adjustment for clustering by schools, the matched-paired design and potential confounders. One limitation of this study is related to the open-label design. Although difficult to assess, it may be possible that students' knowledge of their exposure status (i.e. whether they received the intervention or not) may have biased their self-reported responses to the behaviour questions, leading to potential measurement error. Another limitation is that we only had one follow-up period (i.e. four months) and we cannot conclude if knowledge of STH transmission and the protective effects on the intensity of *Ascaris lumbricoides* infection can be maintained over longer time periods.

5 CONCLUSION

There is a significant difference in the incidence of ascariasis between children receiving education on sanitation and recurrent hygiene with those who only receive a once off educational lecture.

REFERENCES

Abbosie, A. & Seid, M. (2014). Assessment of the prevalence of intestinal parasitosis and associated risk factors among primary school children in Chencha town, Southern Ethiopia. *BMC Public Health*, *14*, 166–174.

Anderson, R.M., Turner, H.C., Truscott, J.E., Hollingsworth, T.D. & Brooker, S.J. (2015). Should the goal for the treatment of soil transmitted helminth (STH) infections be changed from morbidity control in children to community-wide transmission elimination? *PLOS Neglected Tropical Diseases*, 9(8), 1–8.

Bethony, J., Brooker, S., Albonico, M., Geiger, S.M., Loukas, A. & Diemert, D. (2006). Soil-transmitted helminth infections: Ascariasis, trichuriasis, and hookworm. *The Lancet*, *367*, 1521–1532.

Clarke, N.E., Clements, A.C.A., Doi, S.A., Wang, D. & Campbell, S.J. (2017). Differential effect of mass deworming and targeted deworming for soil-transmitted helminth control in children: A systematic review and meta-analysis. *The Lancet*, *389* (10066), 287–297.

Corneiro, F.F., Cifuentes, E., Tellez-Rojo, M.M. & Romieu, I. (2002). The risk of Ascaris lumbricoides infection in children as an environmental health indicator to guide preventive activities in Caparaó and Alto Caparaó, Brazil. *Bulletin of the WHO, 80*, 40–46.

Gabrie, J.A., Rueda, M.M., Canales, M., Gyorkos, T.W. & Sancezh, A.L. (2014). School hygiene and deworming are key protective factors for reduced transmission of soil-transmitted helminths among schoolchildren in Honduras. *Parasites & Vectors, 7*, 354.

Ginting A. (2009). *Faktor-Faktor yang berhubungan dengan kejadian kecacingan pada Anak Sekolah Dasar di Desa tertinggal Kecamatan Pangururan Kabupaten Samosir Tahun 2008*. Medan: Universitas Sumatera Utara.

Gyorkos, T.W., Maheu-Giroux, M., Blouin, B. & Casapia, M. (2013). Impact of health education on soil-transmitted helminth infections in schoolchildren of the Peruvian Amazon: A cluster-randomized controlled trial. *PLOS Neglected Tropical Diseases, 7*, e2397.

Jia, T.W., Melville, S., Utzinger, J., King, C.H. & Zhou, X.N. (2012). Soil-transmitted helminth reinfection after drug treatment: A systematic review and meta-analysis. *PLOS Neglected Tropical Diseases, 6*, e1621.

Khepa, S., Mwandawiro, C.S., Anderson, R.M., Pullan, R.L. & Nuwaha, F. (2017). Impact of single annual treatment and four-monthly treatment of hookworm and Ascaris lumbricoides, and factors associated with residual infection among Kenyan school children. *Infectious Diseases of Poverty, 6*, 30.

Mahmud, M.A., Spigt, M., Bezabih, A.M., Pavon, I.L., Dinant, G. & Velasco, R.B. (2015). Efficacy of handwashing with soap and nail clipping on intestinal parasitic infections in school-aged children: A factorial cluster randomized controlled trial. *PLOS Medicine, 10*, 1–16.

Nematian, J., Nematian, E., Gholamrezanezhad, A. & Asgari, A. (2004). Prevalence of intestinal parasitic infections and their relation with socio-economic factors and hygienic habits in Tehran primary school students. *Acta Tropica, 92*, 179–186.

Rahma, M.W. (2011). *Hubungan antara higiene dengan infeksi cacing Soil Transmitted Helminths pada siswa-siswi SD Negeri No. 101837 Suka Makmur, Kecamatan Sibolangit, Kabupaten Deli Serdang Tahun 2011.* Medan: Universitas Sumatera Utara.

Rahmad, Z.R. (2008). *Hubungan higiene perorangan siswa dengan infeksi kecacingan anak SD Negeri di Kecamatan Sibolga Kota Sibolga.* Medan: Universitas Sumatera Utara.

Schmidlin, T., Hurlimann, E., Silue, K.D., Yapi, R.B., Houngbedji, C. & Kouadio, B.A. (2013). Effects of hygiene and defecation behavior on helminths and intestinal protozoa infections in Taabo, Cote d'Ivoire. *PLOS One, 8*, e65722.

Seid, M., Dejeniae, T. & Tomass, Z. (2015). Prevalence of intestinal helminths and associated risk factors in rural school-children in Were-Abaye Sub District, Tigray Region, Northern Ethiopia. *Acta Parasitologica Globalis, 6*, 29–35.

Walker, M., Hall, A. & Basanez, M. (2011). Individual predisposition, household clustering and risk factors for human infection with Ascaris lumbricoides: New epidemiological insights. *PLOS Neglected Tropical Diseases, 5*, e1047–1057.

Yap, P., Utzinget, J., Hattendorf, J. & Steinmann, P. (2016). Influence of nutrition on infection and reinfection with soil-transmitted helminthes: A systematic review. *Parasites & Vectors, 229*(7), 1–14.

Ziegelbauer, K., Speich, B., Mausezahl, D., Bos, R., Keiser, J. & Utzinger, J. (2012). Effect of sanitation on soil transmitted helminth infection: Systematic review and meta-analysis. *PLOS Medicine, 9*, e1001162.

Stem Cell Oncology – Adella (Ed.)
© 2018 Taylor & Francis Group, London, ISBN 978-0-8153-9272-9

Comparative time achieved VAS ≤ 3 oxycodone and fentanyl post-operative analgesia

V. Kumar, A. Hanafie, H. Arifin & H.A. Nasution
Department of Anesthesiology and Intensive Therapy, Faculty of Medicine,
Universitas Sumatera Utara, Medan, North Sumatera, Indonesia

ABSTRACT: Fentanyl has a potency ratio 100 times stronger than morphine. Oxycodone is a receptor agonist of mu and kappa opioids, structurally similar to codeine, but pharmacodynamically similar to morphine. The aim of this study was to determine the comparison of time achievement of VAS ≤ 3 on oxycodone. This study used a double-blind, randomised clinical trial, collecting 48 samples from participants aged 21–60 years, PS ASA I-II. Oxycodone (A): fentanyl (B) (initial bolus 5 mg than continuous infusion dose of 1 mg/hour: initial bolus 5 cc of NaCl 0.9% than continuous infusion dose of 0.5 mcg/hour) with significance level 95% ($p < 0.05$). Average length of surgery fentanyl: oxycodone (218.96 ± 53.38 minutes: 191.87 ± 80.10, $p > 0.05$). Oxycodone is faster in achieving VAS ≤ 3 compared with fentanyl intravenous infusion.

Keywords: effectiveness, fentanyl, opiates, oxycodone, visual analogue score

1 INTRODUCTION

Fentanyl has a potential ratio 100 times stronger than morphine (Barash, 2013). According to the South African Anesthesiologist's Guide, the average fentanyl dose for post-operative pain is 1–5 mcg/kg/day (SASA, 2009).

Opioid drugs are most commonly used in the first 24 hours post-operatively. Patients who have frequently received previous opioid administration may become resistant to commonly used opioid doses (Fabregat, 2011).

Kloub in 2015 examined the efficacy of oxycodone for the treatment of short-term pain in post-operative patients. This study involved 263 patients undergoing various surgical procedures. It was reported that 220 patients (83.7%) had no pain and 20 patients (7.6%) reported pain with a score of five more than those concluded. Oxycodone is effective in the treatment of short-term pain in most types of surgery (Kloub, 2015).

Park in 2015 studied 74 patients undergoing elective laparoscopic hysterectomy or laparoscopic myomectomy with a random choice to obtain fentanyl or oxycodone using IV-PCA (potential ratio 1:60). Patients were also examined for post-operative pain, side effects and patient satisfaction. There was a significant difference in patient satisfaction with analgesics observed during the post-operative period. Patients in the oxycodone group showed a low intake of opioids (10.1 ± 8.5 ml vs. 16.6 ± 12.0 ml, $p = 0.013$). It was found that oxycodone and fentanyl showed similar effects (Park, 2015), differences in VAS values and adverse events after the administration of oxycodone is 1 mg/hour and fentanyl dose 0.5 mcg/kgbb/hour intravenously continuously in overcoming post-surgical pain of long bone surgery under general anaesthesia on the grounds of finding alternatives to opioid analgesic drugs that have an effect the same for post-operative pain management with general anaesthesia techniques without side effects that could harm the patient.

2 METHODS

The design of this study involved a double-blind, randomised controlled clinical trial. The aim was to determine the differences in VAS values and adverse events after oxycodone doses of 1 mg/hour and fentanyl doses of 0.5 mcg/kgbb/hr of intravenous continuous pain in post-surgical pain with general anaesthesia. This research was conducted at RSUP.H. Adam Malik. The research was conducted after ethical clearance was published until the number of samples was met.

The study population involved elective patients scheduled to undergo long bone surgery under general anaesthesia techniques using ETT. The study sample fulfilled the inclusion and exclusion criteria. Once calculated statistically, all samples were divided into:

a. Group A received an oxycodone bolus of 5 cc and continued with an intravenous continuous 1 cc/hour continuous maintenance dose.
b. Group B received fentanyl doses of 0.5 mcg kg bw continuous intravenously.

Inclusion criteria: aged 21–60 years; undergoing long bone surgery; physical status of ASA 1 and 2; with ideal body weight according to BMI; patients agreed to participate in the study. Exclusion criteria: patients who received opioid analgesics before surgery. Criteria of Disconnect Test (Drop Out): Occurred emergency heart and lung, allergic reactions occur after the use of drugs studied.

The patients received an explanation about the procedure to be followed and provided informed consent. Both groups of patients were given preloading fluid Ringer Lactate 10 ml/kg BW. Both groups were prepared for general anaesthesia. Premedication with fentanyl 2 mcg/kg, midazolam 0.05 mg/kg, awaited onset 5 minutes. Patients were induced with propofol 2 mg/kg, rocuronium muscle paralytic 1 mg/kg, after the onset of 1 min, a direct laryngoscopy was performed with a laryngoscope and the trachea was intubated with an appropriate size endotracheal tube. Surgery begins, the maintenance of sedation using Isoflurane, maintenance of analgesia with fentanyl according to hemodynamic response, and maintenance of muscle paralysis using rocuronium.

After surgery, having fulfilled the extubation criteria, the patient was extubated and the time was recorded as T0 and the VAS was assessed using the VAS drawing table, by asking the patient to indicate on the scale the point corresponding to their perception of pain experienced. This assessment was conducted directly by researchers who are not involved in the administration of drugs to these patients. The time of initiation of the study in which group A received an oxycodone bolus 5 mg was followed by intravenous 1 mg/hour continuous maintenance for 24 hours, while group B received fentanyl with the initial bolus using 0.9% NaCl 0.5 doses of 0.5 mcg/kgbw/hour intravenously for 24 hours. If, during the study, the patient was still in pain (VAS > 3) then oxycodone was increased by 1 mg per hour until VAS < 3 is reached. Fentanyl was increased by 0.5 mcg to VAS < 3.

The patient was observed in the recovery room and transferred to the ward when the Aldrette Score was 10. The VAS assessment and the side effects of the drug were performed directly by the researchers at 0 (T0), 1 (T1), 2 (T2), 3 (T3), 4 (T4), 6 (T5), 12 (T6) and 24 (T7) after surgery ends. T0 begins after the patient is extubated and fully awake. The results of observational data in both groups were statistically comparable.

3 RESULTS

No statistically significant differences in age, sex and ASA between the two study groups was demonstrated ($p > 0.05$).

Statistically, there was no significant difference in pre-operative VAS between the two study groups ($p > 0.05$).

Based on the above table, it can be seen that the average duration of group operation given fentanyl was 218.96 ± 53.38 minutes and the mean duration of group operation given

Table 1. Distribution of research subjects by age, sex and ASA.

| Characteristics | Drugs given | | Total | p value |
	Morphine	Oxycodone		
Age (year)				
19–29	11 (45.8%)	7 (29.2%)	18 (37.5%)	
30–39	3 (12.5%)	2 (8.3%)	5 (10.4%)	0.604
40–49	4 (16.7%)	6 (25.0%)	10 (20.8%)	
50–59	6 (25%)	9 (37.5%)	15 (31.3%)	
Total	24 (100%)	24 (100%)	48 (100%)	
Sex				
Male	13 (54.2%)	15 (62.5%)	28 (58.3%)	0.558
Female	11 (45.8%)	9 (37.5%)	20 (41.7%)	
Total	24 (100%)	24 (100%)	48 (100%)	
ASA				
ASA 1	10 (41.7%)	8 (33.3%)	19 (39.6%)	0.551
ASA 2	14 (58.3%)	16 (66.7%)	29 (60.4%)	
Total	24 (100%)	24 (100%)	48 (100%)	

*Fisher's exact test.

Table 2. Distribution of research subjects based on pre-operative VAS values.

| VAS Pre-Op | Drugs | | Total | p value* |
	Fentanyl	Oxycodone		
4	15 (62.5%)	11 (45.8%)	26 (54.2%)	0.247
5	9 (37.5%)	13 (54.2%)	22 (45.8%)	
Total	24 (100%)	24 (100%)	48 (100%)	

*Chi-square tests.

Table 3. The average difference in surgery duration based on the drugs given.

| Drugs given | n | Duration of operation (Minutes) | | | | | Value of p* |
		Mean	Std. Deviation	Median	Minimum	Maximum	
Fentanyl	24	218.96	53.38	217.5	50	310	0.185
Oxycodone	24	191.87	80.997	200	65	365	

*Mann-Whitney test.

Table 4. The average time difference to achieve VAS ≤ 3 based on the drugs given.

| Drugs given | n | Time to reach VAS 3 (Hours) | | | | | Value of p* |
		Mean	Std. Deviation	Median	Minimum	Maximum	
Fentanyl	24	2.58	0.50	3	2	3	0.001
Oxycodone	24	1.46	0.509	1	1	2	

*Mann-Whitney test.

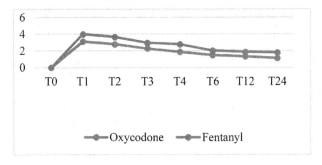

Figure 1. Average VAS score of oxycodone and fentanyl T0–T7 Groups.

oxycodone was 191.87 ± 80.10 minutes. Based on statistical tests with Mann-Whitney test showed no difference in the duration of surgery between the two study subjects ($p > 0.05$).

Based on statistical tests with Mann-Whitney test showed no time difference to achieve VAS ≤ 3 between the two study subjects ($p < 0.05$).

From the graph above, the oxycodone group has a lower average VAS value compared to the fentanyl group from T1–T7. At T0, both groups have the same VAS. This is because there are still effects of analgesic drugs used during surgery.

4   DISCUSSION

This study assessed the effectiveness of oxycodone analgesics and continuous infusion fentanyl in monitoring post-operative pain in long bones. From the sample characteristic data, it can be seen that the age between the two sample groups did not have a statistically significant difference. Thus, the samples taken were relatively homogeneous ($p > 0.05$). Similarly, sex, ASA physical status, VAS pre-op and duration of operation between the two groups of samples were not statistically significant ($p > 0.05$).

Based on the statistical test of the average dose used to achieve VAS ≤ 3 it was found that the mean dose of fentanyl group drug group was 0.4058 ± 0.054 mcg more than the group given oxycodone by as much as 1.46 ± 0.51 mg. The Mann-Whitney test showed significant differences between the two groups ($p < 0.05$).

The results of the clinical trial showed that the oxycodone group required a faster time to achieve VAS ≤ 3 with a mean time of 1.46 hours compared with the fentanyl group with an average time of 2.58 hours. The Mann-Whitney test results in this study also showed that the average dose of drugs produced in the oxycodone group had a smaller dose range of 1.46 ± 0.51 mg compared with fentanyl of 0.4058 ± 0.054 mcg.

A study conducted by Kim et al. in 2014 found that oxycodone IV-PCA was more favourable than IV-PCA fentanyl for laparoscopic hysterectomy surgery regarding oxycodone consumption accumulation, pain control and favourable effects related to price. This is in line with this study, where the use of oxycodone by continuous infusion is more effective in reducing VAS ≤ 3 compared with fentanyl use.

This study did not assess the incidence of adverse events occurring from both drugs. In further studies, an assessment of possible side effects due to the use of this drug may be possible.

REFERENCES

Choi Yoon-Ji, Park Sang-Wook, Kwon Hyun-Jung, dkk. (2015). Efficacy of early intravenous bolus *oxycodone* or fentanyl in emergence from general anaesthesia and postoperative analgesia following laparoscopic cholecystectomy: A randomised trial. *Journal of International Medical Research, 43*(6), 809–818.

Kim Nan-Seol, Kang Kyu Sik, Yoo Sin Hyeon, dkk. (2014). A comparison of oxycodone and fentanyl in intravenous patient-controlled analgesia after laparoscopic hysterectomy. *Korean Journal of Anesthesiology*, *68*(3), 261–266.

Kloub, G. (2015). Effect of oxycodone in post-operative pain management. *Journal of Pain and Relief*, *4*, 217. doi:10.4172/21670846.1000217.

Kokki, H., Kokki, M. & Sjovall, S. (2012). Oxycodone for the treatment of postoperative pain. *Expert Opinion on Pharmacotherapy*, *13*(7), 1045–1058.

Morgan, G.E., Mikhail, M.S. & Murray, M.J. (2013). Perioperative pain management & enhanched outcomes. In *Clinical anesthesiology* (5th ed., pp. 1087–105). Lange Medical Books/McGraw-Hill.

Oczak et al. (2017). Analgesic efficacy, adverse effects, and safety of oxycodone administered as continuous intravenous infusion in patients after total hip arthroplasty. *Journal of Pain Research*, *10*, 1027–1032.

Pain Assessment and Management Initiative (PAMI). *Pain management and dosing guide*. November 2016.

Park Joong-Ho, Lee Chiu, Shin Youngmin, dkk. (2015). Comparison of oxycodone and fentanyl for postoperative patient-controlled analgesia after laparoscopic gynecological surgery. *Korean Journal of Anesthesiology*, *68*(2), 153–158.

Stem Cell Oncology – Adella (Ed.)
© 2018 Taylor & Francis Group, London, ISBN 978-0-8153-9272-9

Depressive syndrome in patients with breast cancer

M.M. Amin & E. Effendy
*Department of Psychiatry, Faculty of Medicine, Universitas Sumatera Utara, Medan,
North Sumatera, Indonesia*

E.T. Pasaribu
*Department of Surgery, Faculty of Medicine, Universitas Sumatera Utara, Medan,
North Sumatera, Indonesia*

P. Pariwatcharakul
Department of Psychiatry, Faculty of Medicine, Siriraj Hospital, Mahidol University, Thailand

ABSTRACT: It is common to believe that depression can lead to more severe disease. Breast cancer is the most studied cancer in terms of its psychosocial effects and not surprisingly, many studies of the prevalence of depression in cancer are studies of women with breast cancer. Aim: To determine the level of depressive syndrome in breast cancer patients by using the BDI questionnaire. Method: The respondents amounted to 66 breast cancer patients who come to the Clinic of Surgical Oncology and General Surgery at Adam Malik Hospital, and Hospital Haji Medan. Results: It was found that moderate depressive syndrome was most prevalent in patients with breast cancer (42.4%), followed by severe (25.8%), mild (19.7%) and minimal (12.1%) depression severity.

Keywords: depression, BDI, breast cancer

1 INTRODUCTION

In psychiatry, depression points to a clinical syndrome composed of diminished mood (painful feelings and sadness), difficulty in thinking and psychomotor retardation (Campbell, 1981). A survey by the Indonesian Psychiatry Association reported that 94% of Indonesians had depressive symptoms ranging from mild to severe (Sadock et al., 2007).

The age of onset for severe depressive disorder was about 40 years, with 50% of all patients having an onset between the ages of 20 and 50 years. Severe depressive disorders could also occur in childhood or old age. Maguire reported that up to 80% of the psychological and psychiatric problems of cancer patients were under detected. The barriers identifying depression in cancer patients included the following: no reports by cancer patients; the inability of doctors to recognise depression in cancer; patients consider depression to be 'appropriate'; difficulties distinguishing depression from other psychological conditions; signs and symptoms that accompany cancer; and fear of psychiatric disorder stigma (Wah, 2004).

There were few reasons why depression and anxiety were not diagnosed in cancer patients; for example, lack of time during office visits, misinterpretation of depression and anxiety as 'normal' reactions, depression-related symptoms and anxiety-related cancer, focusing only on medical issues and therapeutic absence. Some risk factors for the occurrence of anxiety and depression in cancer patients are organic mental disorders, less controlled physical symptoms, lack of communication between staff and patients, previous history of mood disorders and lack of support from family and friends (Jones, 2011). Depressive symptoms in cancer patients may be from psychiatric comorbidity, symptoms of a medical disorder or psychological reaction. Moreover, the overlapping symptoms between depression and physical illnesses, for example vegetative symptoms, result in complexity in making a diagnosis of depression. Few approaches were used in previous epidemiological studies of depression in patients with physical illnesses, including inclusive and exclusive approaches (Gross et al., 2007).

Depression develops in those who have had cancer in relation to the medical illness itself, to factors related to management and the nature of a person. The frequency of depression is associated with the type of cancer. The severity of the disease is also a predictive factor, with metastatic disease leading to higher rates of depression than cancer detected at an early stage. The presence or absence of social support and a person's ability to overcome problems also contributed to the development of depression in cancer patients (Gross et al., 2007).

2 METHODS

This study was an analytic study with a cross-sectional design to assess whether there was a depressive syndrome in patients with breast cancer and whether the depressive syndrome in breast cancer patients was different based on age, education, marital status, tribe, occupation, income and stage of cancer.

Subjects in the study were patients diagnosed with histopathologic breast cancer, as well as all stages administered by RSUP H. Adam Malik, Medan and Haji Hospital, Medan, with the following inclusion criteria: (1) Breast cancer patients diagnosed on histopathologic examination; (2) Age $\geq$ 30 years; (3) First contact with investigator; (4) Cooperative and willing to fill out the questionnaire; (5) Never received therapy for breast cancer. Exclusion criteria included: (1) Having psychiatric disorders before taking the study; (2) Having other general medical conditions.

3 RESULTS

The respondents amounted to 66 breast cancer patients who came to the Clinic of Surgical Oncology and General Surgery at Adam Malik Hospital and Haji Hospital, Medan within the four months of the study.

Table 1 shows that the sample was dominated by the age group 40–49 years old (63.6%), elementary education (65.2%), marital status (77.3%), Batak (39.4%), monthly income <Rp 500,000.00 (75.8%) and stage IIIB (63.6%) for clinical stage of cancer disease.

Our findings show that medium depressive syndrome was most prevalent in patients with breast cancer (42.4%), followed by severe (25.8%), mild (19.7%) and minimal (12.1%) depressive syndromes.

Table 3 shows that depressive syndrome in patients with breast cancer is most common in stage IIIB (76.5%) in the form of severe depressive syndrome. There was no significant difference in depressive syndrome in patients with breast cancer based on clinical stage of breast cancer.

Table 4 shows that age risk factors for the occurrence of depressive syndrome in patients with breast cancer were aged 30–39 years (PR = 6.180; 95% IK 1.518 to 34.139).

Table 1. Characteristics of age, education, marital status, tribe, employment, revenue and clinical stage of breast cancer.

Characteristics of respondents		Total	%
Age	30–39 yr	8	12.1
	40–49 yr	23	34.8
	50–59 yr	22	33.3
	60–69 yr	11	16.7
	≥70 yr	2	3.0

(*Continued*)

Table 1. (*Continued*).

Characteristics of respondents		Total	%
Mean = 50.4 yr (*SD* = 10.1)			
Education	No education	2	3.0
	Primary	43	65.2
	Lower secondary	8	12.1
	Higher secondary	8	12.1
	University	5	7,6
Marital Status	Married	51	77.3
	Not married	15	22.7
Tribe	Batak	26	39.4
	Java	20	30.3
	Aceh	9	13.6
	Malay	6	9.1
	Etc.	5	7.6
Occupation	Employed	33	50.0
	Unemployed	33	50.0
Income/Month	<Rp 500,000	50	75.8
	Rp 500,000–1,000,000	9	13.6
	>Rp 1,000,000	7	10.6
Staging of	III A	9	13.6
breast cancer	III B	42	63.6
	III C	8	12.1
	IV	7	10.6

SD = Standard Deviation.

Table 2. Depressive syndrome in breast cancer patients.

Depressive syndrome	Total	%
Minimal	8	12.1
Mild	13	19.7
Moderate	28	42.4
Severe	17	25.8
Total	66	100.0

Table 3. Distribution of clinical stages of breast cancer with depressive syndrome.

Staging of breast cancer	Depressive syndrome								p
	Minimal		Mild		Moderate		Severe		
	n	%	n	%	n	%	n	%	
IIIA	0	0	3	23.1	4	14.3	2	11.8	
IIIB	6	75.0	6	46.2	17	60.7	13	76.5	0.647*
IIIC	2	25.0	2	15.4	3	10.7	1	5.9	
IV	0	0	2	15.4	4	14.3	1	5.9	
Total	8	100	13	100	28	100	17	100	

Table 4. Risk factor age for occurrence of depressive syndrome in breast cancer patients.

Variable	Prevalence ratio (PR)	p	95% (IK)	
			Lowest	Highest
≥60 yr	6.640	0.084		
50–59 yr	2.481	0.115	0.682	33.798
40–49 yr	3.170	0.075	0.878	15.242
30–39 yr	6.180	0.013	1.518	34.139

4   DISCUSSION

Overall, this study showed that among 66 breast cancer patients, 58 of them had depressive syndrome (87.9%). However, in previous studies on depression in breast cancer patients, Ell et al. reported that from 250 breast cancer patients, 76 of them (67%) suffered severe depressive disorders (Ell et al., 2007) and Burgess et al. (2005) reported that in 107 breast cancer sufferers, 48% suffered depression after one year from breast cancer diagnosis, while 25%, 23%, 22% and 15% of them developed depression after breast cancer diagnosis two, three, four and five years later, respectively. The differences encountered from the results of this study with those reported by Ell et al. were due to the use of different instruments, as this study used the BDI while Ell et al. used the Patient's Health Questionnaire-9. Our findings are different compared to those reported by Burgess et al. because in our study, other than using the BDI which was assessed only once, Burgess et al. used the Structured Clinical Interview for DSM and assessed it over a period of five years after breast cancer diagnosis. Another point that should be considered is the bias of the use of the BDI in this study of women, low education and parents tending to have higher BDI values (Beck, 2000).

We also found that depressive syndrome in most breast cancer patients occurs in stage IIIB (76.5%) in the form of severe depressive syndrome. There was no significant difference in depressive syndrome in patients with breast cancer based on clinical stage of breast cancer. Similar results were obtained by Burgess et al. (2005) who conducted a study of 170 breast cancer patients and reported that the number of axillary nodules present and the size and histology of the tumours were unrelated to depression and anxiety. The age risk factors for the occurrence of depressive syndrome in patients with breast cancer were 30–39 years (PR = 6.180; 95% IK 1.518 to 34.139). The results of this study are consistent with the results of the Ell et al. (2005) who found that those <50 years of age tended to be depressed and the theory that one risk factor for depression in the female population was being younger (Burgess et al., 2005).

5   CONCLUSION

Although depression as a psychiatric illness still has a stigma for those that experience it, depression can worsen the prognosis of cancer. Special attention should be made to women who have breast cancer and depressive syndrome concurrently, so that treatment for their condition can be made using a comprehensive approach by the physician.

REFERENCES

Beck, A.T. (2000). Beck Depression Inventory (BDI). In Rush, A.J. et al, (Eds.), *Handbook of psychiatric measures* (pp. 519–22). Washington, DC: American Psychiatric Association.

Burgess, C. et al. (2005). Depression and anxiety in women with early breast cancer: Five year observational cohort study. *BMJ*, *330*, 702.

Campbell, R.J. (1981). *Psychiatric dictionary* (5th Ed.). New York: Oxford University Press.

Ell, K. et al. (2005). Depression, correlates of depression, and receipt of depression care among low-income women with breast or gynecologic cancer. *Journal of Clinical Oncology*, *23*, 3052–3060.

Gross, A.F. et al. (2007). Is depression an appropriate response to having cancer? A discussion of diagnostic criteria and treatment decisions. *Primary Care Companion to the Journal of Clinical Psychiatry*, *9*(5), 382–387.

Jones, R.D. (2011). Depression and anxiety in oncology: The oncologist's perspective. *The Journal of Clinical Psychiatry*, *62*(8), 52–55.

Lederberg, M.S. (2006). Psycho-oncology. In Sadock, B.J., et al (Eds.), *Kaplan & Sadock's comprehensive textbook of psychiatry* (pp. 2201–2202, 8th Ed.). Philadelphia: Lippincott Williams & Wilkins.

Sadock, B.J. et al. (2007). *Kaplan & Sadock's synopsis of psychiatry: Behavioral sciences/clinical psychiatry* (10th Ed.), Philadelphia: Wolters Kluwer Lippincott Williams & Wilkins.

Wah, T.M. (2004). Depression in advanced cancer. *Hong Kong Society of Palliative Medicine Newsletter*, *3*, 27–30.

Stem Cell Oncology – Adella (Ed.)
© *2018 Taylor & Francis Group, London, ISBN 978-0-8153-9272-9*

Infant feeding practices and anaemia in 9-month-old infants

D.P. Amri, T. Sembiring, P. Sianturi, T. Faranita & W. Pratita
*Department of Child Health, Faculty of Medicine, Universitas Sumatera Utara, Medan,
North Sumatera, Indonesia*

ABSTRACT: The incidence of anaemia in infants is still high and nutritional deficiency is suggested as the main factor due to inappropriate feeding practices. To evaluate the relationship between feeding practices and anaemia in 9-month-old infants, a cross-sectional study was conducted in 6 *Puskesmas* in Medan from August–October 2016. Chi-square tests and multivariate analyses were used in the statistical analysis. The incidence of anaemia was 66.7%. No significant association between anaemia and exclusive breastfeeding ($P = 0.214$, 95% CI) was found. The variables associated with anaemia were: starting complementary feeding at <6 months old ($P = 0.032$, PR = 2.830, CI 95%), using steamed rice as an initial Complementary Food (CF) ($P = 0.021$, PR = 12 318, 95% CI) and CF not containing animal protein ($P = 0.013$, PR = 14 160, 95% CI). Anaemia in 9-month-old infants was associated with the infant's age when complementary feeding was first started, the type of CF first given, and the animal protein content in the CF.

Keywords: anaemia, infant feeding, 9-month-old infants

1 INTRODUCTION

Appropriate feeding practice is an important factor in ensuring optimal nutrition for infant growth and development (Luo et al., 2014). Incorrect feeding practice could cause both macro- and micro-nutrient deficiency, especially protein and iron, progressing into nutritional deficiency anaemia (Luo et al., 2014; Maguire et al., 2013). Anaemia has become a major health issue in Indonesia, as it has caused serious, irreversible impairment on infant and child growth and development (Maguire et al., 2013). When an infant reaches the age of nine months, it enters a critical phase of feeding practice, providing the nutritional requirement for rapid growth/development, while simultaneously stimulating its oral and motor skills. Therefore, the Centres for Disease Control and Prevention (CDC) recommends anaemia screening for infants aged 9–12 months by measuring blood haemoglobin (Hb) levels, with the test repeated six months later (McDonagh et al., 2015).

2 METHOD

2.1 *Study design*

This study used a cross-sectional design, conducted from August 2016 to October 2016 in 6 community health centres (*puskesmas*) and 42 integrated health service posts (*posyandu*) in Medan, North Sumatera. Infants were brought to these *puskesmas* or *posyandu* by their parents to measure their body weight or to undergo routine vaccination.

2.2 *Sample and subjects*

Sample was recruited with consecutive sampling method. The inclusion criteria were infants aged nine months, full-term born with birth weight ranged from 2.500 grammes to 4.000 grammes.

The exclusion criteria were infants who had never been given breastmilk, or infants with chronic diseases, such as heart problems and congenital heart disease. Infants who had ever been diagnosed with blood disorders, or had ever been pale since birth without any known diagnosis, or had received a blood transfusion even once in their lifetime were also excluded from this study.

2.3 Data collection

The subjects of this study were 9-month-old infants brought to *puskesmas* or *posyandu*, as mentioned above. The subjects who met the inclusion criteria were recruited using the consecutive sampling method. Parents were interviewed to obtain a socio-economic characteristic of the family along with infant feeding practices (e.g. breastfeeding exclusively, the age when complementary feeding started, when the first complementary food was given, the animal protein content, the preparation of complementary food and the frequency of giving one type of complementary food). The subjects' body weight and length were measured, and blood haemoglobin levels measured using a *HemoCue® Hb 201⁺ System* device. This research received ethical approval from the Ethical Research Committee, Faculty of Medicine, University of Sumatera Utara, and has also been approved by the local public health office, *puskesmas* and *posyandu*, in which this research took place.

2.4 Statistical analysis

The data sets were analysed using statistical software SPSS 17.0. The association between infant feeding practice and anaemia was analysed using the Chi-square test. The relationship between each variable of feeding practice and anaemia was examined using multivariate logistic regression analysis, generating a Prevalence Ratio (PR) value for each variable mentioned above.

3 RESULTS

Ninety-nine infants aged nine months were examined in this study, each of whom underwent body weight and length examinations, as well as a general physical examination and haemoglobin level measurement. Demographic characteristics were also obtained from the parents and these can be seen in Table 1. Anaemia was more prevalent in infants given complementary

Table 1. Subject characteristics.

	Anaemic	
Characteristic	No (n = 33)	Yes (n = 66)
Sex, n(%)		
Male	19 (58)	38 (58)
Female	14 (42)	28 (42)
Body weight, n(%)		
Normal	32 (97)	53 (80)
Underweight	1 (3)	11 (17)
Severely underweight	(0)	2 (3)
Body length, n(%)		
Normal	31 (94)	63 (95)
Stunting	2 (6)	2 (3)
Severe stunting	(0)	1 (2)
Nutritional status, n(%)		
Normal	31 (94)	53 (80)
Malnutrition	2 (6)	11 (17)
Severe malnutrition	(0)	2 (3)

Table 2. Association between anaemia and exclusive breastfeeding, starting age of complementary feeding, and type of first complementary food in 9-month-old infants.

Characteristic	Anaemic		
	No (n = 33)	Yes (n = 66)	P-value
Exclusive breastfeeding, n(%)			
Yes	11(46)	13(54)	0.214
No	22(29)	53(71)	
Complementary feeding started at, n(%)			
6 months old	21(46)	25(54)	0.027*
6 months old	12(23)	41(77)	
First complementary food is given, n(%)			
Milk or fine porridge	32(39)	51(61)	0.026*

Table 3. Factors associated with anaemia in 9-month-old infants.

Variable	P-value	PR	CI 95%
Complementary feeding started at <6 months old	0.032*	2.830	1.093 to 7.324
Steamed rice as the first complementary food	0.021*	12.318	1.472 to 103.068
Complementary food not containing animal protein	0.013*	14.160	1.749 to 114.614

feeding at age < 6 months, and in infants given steamed rice as their first complementary food and there was no association between exclusive breastfeeding and anaemia in the infants. These results are displayed in Table 2.

This study also examined indicators of good infant feeding practice as recommended by WHO *Global Strategy for Feeding Infant and Young Children* 2003 and is displayed in Table 3. Multivariate regression logistic analysis showed that the lack of animal protein content in complementary food was the strongest factor related to anaemia in 9-month-old infants (Table 3).

Table 3 association between anaemia and animal protein content in complementary food, preparation of complementary food and introduction of complementary food in 9-month-old infants.

4 DISCUSSION

This study showed that anaemia prevalence in 9-month-old infants in Medan city was still high (67%). The main factors related to anaemia in Indonesia are feeding practices, using low-iron-content foods and a high prevalence of parasitic infections. The most common type of anaemia in the first 1000 days of life is nutritional deficiency anaemia, caused by iron deficiency (Lozoff et al., 2016).

In this study, the exclusive breastfeeding rate was still low (23%). Although not statistically significant, the prevalence of anaemia was lower in infants given exclusive breastfeeding compared to those who were not. This result is similar to studies conducted in other countries, such as Brazil and China, which showed that infants given exclusive breastfeeding had a lower anaemia prevalence at the age of 6–12 months, albeit this was not statistically significant (Assis, 2004). A longitudinal study in Peru found that maternal Hb level and iron status while breastfeeding correlated with infant Hb level and iron status (Finkelstrein, 2013). A study in Cambodia examining 928 infants aged 3–24 months also revealed similar results, namely, 6- to 12-month-old infants who were exclusively breastfed by anaemic mothers were 1.77 times more likely to develop anaemia (Reinbott, 2016). Low maternal Hb level and iron status could be the reason why anaemia was more prevalent in exclusively breastfed infants. However, this study did not measure maternal nutritional status nor Hb level.

An inappropriate feeding practice when starting complementary food could be another reason why exclusively breastfed infants may develop anaemia because complementary feeding practices greatly affected iron storage in the infant's body (Assis, 2004).

This study has found that infants who were started on complementary feeding at <6 months old were more likely to develop anaemia than infants who were started at 6 months old (PR = 2.83). This result is similar to a randomised controlled trial examining the iron level and growth pattern in 119 full-term infants in Iceland. It was found that infants given complementary feeding at 6 months old had a higher serum ferritin level compared to infants given this at 4 months old (Jonsdottir, 2013).

It was also found that infants who were given steamed rice or coarse porridge had a 12.318 times higher risk of developing anaemia than infants who were given fine porridge or milk porridge as their first complementary food ($P = 0.026$). A similar result was also found in a study conducted in China, whereby, infants given coarse steamed rice as their first solid food had a higher risk of developing anaemia than infants who were given fine porridge or milk porridge (Luo et al., 2014).

Animal protein has the highest iron content and thus can be considered as the best source of iron; it includes red meat, duck meat, lamb meat, and liver (Grote et al., 2015). In this study, complementary food containing animal protein could prevent anaemia if given daily to the infant ($P = 0.006$). Infants who were given complementary food without any animal protein content had a 14.160 times higher risk of developing anaemia.

This research had several limitations. Firstly, it was a cross-sectional study which could not evaluate a cause-effect mechanism between the variables of infant feeding practice and anaemia. Additionally, data about infant feeding practice was collected through interview, which could be influenced by recall-bias from the parents.

In conclusion, there was no association between exclusive breastfeeding and anaemia in 9-month-old infants. Factors associated with anaemia in 9-month-old infants were the infant's age when complementary feeding was first started, the type of complementary food first given, and the animal protein content in the complementary food.

REFERENCES

Clark, K.M., Li, M., Zhu, B., Liang, F., Shao, J., Zhang, Y., ... Lozoff, B. (2016). Breastfeeding, mixed, or formula feeding at nine months of age and the prevalence of iron deficiency and iron deficiency anemia in two cohorts of infants in China. *The Journal of Pediatrics, 104*, 1–10.

Grote, V., Verduci, E., Scaglioni, S., Vecchi, F., Contarini, G., Giovanni, M., ... Agostoni, C. (2015). Breast milk composition and infant nutrient intakes during the first 12 months of life. *European Journal of Clinical Nutrition*, 1–7.

Jonsdottir, O.H., Thorsdottir, I., Hibberd, P.L., Fewtrell, M.S., Wells, J.C., Palsson, G.I., ... Kleinman, R.E. (2013). The timing of the introduction of complementary foods in infancy: A randomized controlled trial. *American Academy of Pediatrics, (130)*, 1038–45.

Lozoff, B., Jiang, Y., Li, X., Zhou, M., Richard, B., Xu, G., ... Li, M. (2016). Low-dose iron supplementation in infancy modestly increases infant iron status at nine months without decreasing growth or increasing illness in a randomized clinical trial in rural China. *Community and International Nutrition*, 1–10.

Luo, R., Shi, Y., Zhou, H., Yue, A., Zhang, L., Sylvia, S., ... Rozelle, S. (2014). Anemia and feeding practices among infants in rural Shaanxi province in China. *Nutrients, (6)*, 5975–91.

Maguire, J.L., Salehi, L., Birken, C.S., Carsley, S., Mamdani, M., Thorpe, K.E., ... Parkin, P.C. (2013) Association between total duration breastfeeding and iron deficiency. *American Academy of Pediatrics, 131(5)*, e1531–38.

McDonagh, M., Blazina, I., Dana, T., Cantor, A., Bougatsos, C. (2015). Routine iron supplementation and screening for iron deficiency anemia in children ages 6 to 24 months: A systemic review to update US preventive services task force recommendation. *Evidence synthesis no. 122*. Rockville, MD: Agency for Healthcare Research and Quality.

Vendt, N., Grünberg, H., Leedo, S., Tillmann, V., Talvik, T. (2007). Prevalence and causes of iron deficiency anemias in infants aged 9 to 12 months in Estonia. *Medicina, 43(12)*, 947–52.

Stem Cell Oncology – Adella (Ed.)
© 2018 Taylor & Francis Group, London, ISBN 978-0-8153-9272-9

Low survival rate in high-grade osteosarcoma: A retrospective study at a single institution in Indonesia

Andriandi
Department of Orthopaedics, Faculty of Medicine, Universitas Sumatera Utara, Medan, North Sumatera, Indonesia

ABSTRACT: Osteosarcoma is a very rare malignant bone tumour, it is an aggressive bone neoplasm. Combination of surgical removal and systemic multidrug chemotherapy is the current treatment strategy. This study aims to evaluate the prognostic factors influencing the survival rate in our centre. A retrospective cohort study of patients diagnosed with osteosarcoma between January 2012 and December 2014 was carried out. A total of 58 osteosarcoma patients were included in this study, including 36 men (62%) and 22 women (38%), with a mean age at diagnosis of 15 years. The median survival of this group was 12 months. Patients with no pulmonary metastases after treatment had better survival rates of 18 and 90% at two years. The overall survival of osteosarcoma patients in this study is low. Patients who did not comply with treatment had a worse survival rate. Patients with pulmonary metastases have a significantly increased risk of death.

Keywords: amputation, osteosarcoma, prognosis, survival analysis

1 INTRODUCTION

Osteosarcoma is a very rare malignant bone tumour. It is an aggressive bone neoplasm arising from primitive transformed cells of mesenchymal origin (Ayerza et al., 2010). It is such a fatal disease that "months to metastasis", rather than actual survival time, was used to measure the outcomes of treatment in studies of early stage. The combination of surgical removal of the tumour and systemic multidrug chemotherapy is the current treatment strategy for conventional osteosarcoma. Primary chemotherapy, surgery, and adjuvant chemotherapy are the most frequent approaches in osteosarcoma (Bacci et al., 2005; Bacci et al., 2006; Bielack et al., 2002).

It is now generally accepted that surgical amputation is adopted for high malignancy osteosarcoma (Bispo et al., 2009). Some surgeons hold the view that immediate and aggressive removal of the tumour will prevent the progression of the fracture-induced disease and, consequently, amputation is considered to be a better option for osteosarcoma patients with a pathologic fracture. Survival after amputation is no different from that after Limb Salvage Surgery (LSS) with neoadjuvant therapy in patients with osteosarcoma (Ayerza et al., 2010). The question of whether LSS correlates with higher local rates of recurrence remains a controversial topic. Recent literature suggests that local recurrence has only a small influence on overall survival in patients with high-grade osteosarcoma. The other crucial factor determining the risk of local recurrence is the resection margins of a primary tumour. With LSS, the surgical margin obtained will always be narrower than with amputation (Bramwell et al., 1992; Chang et al., 2002; Cho et al., 2011).

Before the advent of neoadjuvant chemotherapy for osteosarcoma, there was a 5-year overall survival (OS) rate of only 10–20%. In the 1950s, there was no optional therapy that could significantly increase the survival rate, with a 5-year survival rate of 22%. However, with the aid of effective chemotherapeutic drugs, the survival rate of osteosarcoma has been significantly improved since the late 1970s. The 5-year survival rate using a multidisciplinary approach varies from 60 to 70% (Enneking et al., 1980; Huvos et al., 1977; Kager et al., 2003).

The drugs currently used in the neoadjuvant treatment of osteosarcoma are doxorubicin (or adriamycin, ADM), cisplatin (CDDP), methotrexate (MTX), ifosfamide (IFO) and etoposide (ETO).

We conducted a retrospective study to assess the efficacy of four drug regimens with methotrexate, cisplatin, adriamycin, and ifosfamide (MTX-CDDP-ADM-IFO) chemotherapy for high-grade osteosarcoma patients who underwent a limb amputation. We analysed the response and survival of the patients in a series of patients based on 2-survival rates.

2 METHOD

This was a retrospective cohort study of all patients diagnosed as having osteosarcoma between January 2012 and December 2014 within our centre, the Haji Adam Malik General Hospital. The patients with osteosarcoma were identified through a search of the computerised databases. As a part of the staging process, routine haematological and biochemical investigations were performed using radiology. The final diagnosis was determined by pathologists after performing the biopsy. The patients were staged according to Enneking's Staging System (1980) for musculoskeletal sarcoma.

The survival parameters were described using frequencies and percentages and the survival rate at two years was calculated. Differences in the survival functions between levels in predictors were tested using the log-rank test. We plotted the Kaplan–Meier survival curves to depict the survival function over time between levels of the predictor (Kaplan et al., 1958).

To identify the significant prognostic factors for the multivariable analysis, we used the Cox proportional hazard regression. The proportional hazard assumption was checked in Stata. In all of our analyses, P-values (two-sided) of less than 0.05 were deemed statistically significant.

3 RESULTS

A total of 58 osteosarcoma patients were included in this study, including 36 men (62%) and 22 women (38%), with a mean age at diagnosis of 15 years (3–43 years). Five (9%) patients had hand, proximal humerus, shoulder, and pelvic osteosarcoma. Thirty-three (57%) patients were diagnosed with osteosarcoma in the distal femur, 13 (39%) in the right thigh and 18 (55%) in the left thigh. Eighteen (31%) patients were diagnosed with osteosarcoma in the proximal tibia: 15 (83%) in the right cruris and 3 (16%) in the left cruris. The median follow-up was 32 months (ranging from 36 to 48 months).

The overall survival and disease-free survival analysis for all subjects are depicted in Table 1. The survival parameters for both groups are also shown in the table. The results from this study were variable. We found that 21 (36%) who didn't undergo any chemotherapy protocol and 11 (52%) patients among are alive in 2 years survival rate, 2 (18%) of them survive non-chemotherapy group didn't undergo limb salvage or amputation, and 10 (47%) patients die under 1 years after diagnosed, 3 (30%) of them survive with chemotherapy group didn't underwent limb salvage or amputation. Thirty-seven (64%) patients who diagnosed as osteosarcoma and underwent chemotherapy protocol, which 10 (27%) patients were alive in 2 years survival rate and 27 (73%) patients died under one year after treatment, all of the patients in this group had undergone amputation.

For the 58 osteosarcoma patients in this study, 36 (62%) patients had been diagnosed with pulmonary metastases at presentation, 1 (3%) of whom survived after undergoing the chemotherapy protocol and amputation. Twenty-two (38%) patients had no pulmonary metastases at presentation, and at the end of treatment, 20 (91%) patients survived with 18 (90%) of these having undergone chemotherapy and amputation, and 2 (10%) not receiving any treatment at all. Pulmonary metastases at the time of diagnosis were associated with poor survival rates of 1 and 3% at two years. Patients with no pulmonary metastases after treatment had better survival rates of 18 and 90% at two years. Of the 21 (36%) patients who survived, 19 (90%) completed treatment and had a 90% survival rate for 2 years, and none

Table 1.   Detailed prognostic parameters and survival outcomes.

Survival parameter	Total cases = 58			Univariate analysis (log-rank)
	Case number	<2 year survival	>2 year survival	
Survival overall	58	39	19	
Complete treatment				
No	21	18	3	
Yes	37	21	16	
Gender				
Male	36	25	11	p = 0.52
Female	22	14	8	
Age group				
<12 years	11	5	6	p = 0.41
≥12 years	47	34	13	
Age group				
0–10	7	2	5	
10–20	36	23	11	
20–30	11	8	3	p = 0.10
30–40	2	2	–	
>40	2	2	–	
Surgery (amputation)				
No	6	6	–	
Yes	52	33	19	p = 0.00
Lung Metastasis				
Yes	22	15	12	
No	36	24	7	p = 0.83
Survival overall	37	21	16	
Complete treatment				
No	–	–	–	
Yes	37	21	16	
Gender				
Male	20	12	8	p = 0.50
Female	17	9	8	
Age group				
<12 years	9	4	5	p = 0.62
≥12 years	28	17	11	
Age group				
0–10	6	2	4	
10–20	26	17	9	
20–30	3	1	2	p = 0.75
30–40	1	1	0	
>40	1	1	0	
Surgery (amputation)				
No	–	–	–	
Yes	37	21	16	p = 0.00
Lung Metastasis				
Yes	11	5	6	
No	26	16	10	p = 0.59

Table 2. Survival predictor in patients with high-grade osteosarcoma—multivariate analysis.

Predictor	Hazard ratio	Standard error	95% CI	P-value
Female	1.00	0.26	0.4–1.5	0.57
Male	0.85			
Complied Surgery + Chemotherapy	1.00			

Not Complied
  Surgery without chemotherapy
  No surgery + No chemotherapy
	3.31	1.7	1.6–6.6	0.00

At or above 12 years old	0.90	0.33	0.4–1.8	
Less than 12 years old	1.00	0.21	0.3–1.2	
Had Lung Metastasis	0.70			0.78
No Lung Metastasis	1.00			0.23

had a local recurrence, irrespective of the methods of surgical treatment and chemotherapy, and 2 and 10% survival rate at 2 years and none had a local recurrence, irrespective of the methods of surgical treatment and chemotherapy.

4   DISCUSSION

This study included all 58 consecutive patients managed in our institution over a period of 3 years. This analysis will provide an additional perspective to discuss with patients, particularly as the acceptance of treatment is still low in developing countries. The overall survival for all subjects in this study was slightly lower than in other studies (Chang et al., 2002; Ogihara et al., 1991; Yip et al., 1996). The overall survival of patients who for all the patients was 33% above two years, whereas it was 43% above two years for the group of the patient that performed completed treatment (amputation and complete chemotherapy). The group of patients who did not comply with the treatment had poor survival, with a 14.3% survival rate at above two years.

In our study, we included patients who did not complete, or refused, treatment even as their disease progressed. These patients were either from a lower socioeconomic group or had a poor educational status. However, with the addition of chemotherapy, the survival rate had no significant improvement. The combination of chemotherapy and surgery should be the standard choice of treatment, including pre- and post-operative chemotherapy. Ablation was the only treatment in this study, while limb-sparing surgery couldn't be applied due to the staging and condition of patients where the presentation was large and extensive systemic metastases (Bacci et al., 2005; Bacci et al., 2006; Lewis et al., 2007; Li et al., 2011).

Local recurrence was not found in this study, as compared to other studies. Amputation conferred only a marginal benefit against local recurrence; however, it was the treatment of choice for large tumours and patients with a worse perceived prognosis (Ayerza et al., 2010). This study showed that patients had a poor survival rate and this had been confirmed by other studies. Microscopic pulmonary metastasis spread was present in 62% of osteosarcoma patients at the time of diagnosis. Pulmonary metastasis at initial diagnosis and multiple nodules were associated with poor prognosis (Kager et al., 2003; Pakos et al., 2009). From the patients who complied, this study found that in patients with pulmonary metastasis, the survival rate above two years was 38% compared to the patient with no pulmonary metastasis with a survival rate of 55% at two years.

This study also showed that the survival rate is still low because most of the patients came with pulmonary metastasis. The patients with pulmonary metastasis who did not comply had a survival rate above two years of almost 20% which is less than the group of patients who complied.

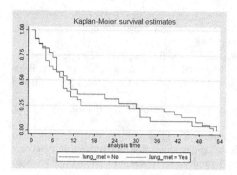

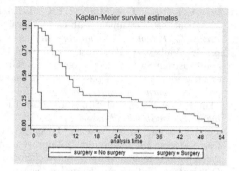

Figure 1. Kaplan–Meier graph showing the survival rate in patients who completed treatment and amputation of the primary tumour and that of those who did not complete treatment.
– had metastasis; - - - - no metastasis.

Figure 2. Kaplan–Meier graph showing the survival rate in patients who underwent limb amputation.
– complied; - - - - not complied.

5 CONCLUSIONS

The overall survival of osteosarcoma patients in this study is low. Amputation is preferred and this study conferred only a marginal benefit against local recurrence and treatment of choice for those with large tumours and a worse perceived prognosis. Patients who do not comply with treatment have a worse survival rate. Within our centre, of those with osteosarcoma, older patients and patients with pulmonary metastases have a significantly increased risk of death.

REFERENCES

Ayerza, M.A., Farfalli, G.L., Aponte-Tinao, L, & Muscolo, D.L. (2010). Does increased rate of limb-sparing surgery affect survival in osteosarcoma? *Clinical Orthopaedics and Related Research*, *468*(11), 2854–9.

Bacci, G., Longhi, A., Versari, M., Mercuri, M., Briccoli, A., & Picci, P. (2006). Prognostic factors for osteosarcoma of the extremity treated with neoadjuvant chemotherapy: 15-year experience in 789 patients treated at a single institution. *Cancer, 106*(5), 1154–61.

Bacci, G., Mercuri, M., Longhi, A., Ferrari, S., Bertoni, F., Versari, M., & Picci, P. (2005). Grade of chemotherapy-induced necrosis as a predictor of local and systemic control in 881 patients with non-metastatic osteosarcoma of the extremities treated with neoadjuvant chemotherapy in a single institution. *European Journal of Cancer, 41*(14), 2079–85.

Bielack, S.S., Kempf-Bielack, B., Delling, G., Exner, G.U., Flege, S., Helmke, K., ... Winkler, K. (2002) Prognostic factors in high-grade osteosarcoma of the extremities or trunk: An analysis of 1,702 patients treated on neoadjuvant Cooperative Osteosarcoma Study Group protocols. *Journal of Clinical Oncology, 20*(3), 776–90.

Bispo, R.Z. & de Camargo, O.P. (2009). Prognostic factors in the survival of patients diagnosed with primary non-metastatic osteosarcoma with a poor response to neoadjuvant chemotherapy. *Clinics, 64*(12), 1177–86.

Bramwell, V.H., Burgers, M., Sneath, R., Souhami, R., van Oosterom, A.T., Voûte, P.A., ... Somers, R. (1992). A comparison of two short intensive chemotherapy regimens in osteosarcoma of limbs in children and young adults: The study of the European Osteosarcoma Intergroup. *Journal of Clinical Oncology 10*(10), 1579–91.

Chang, H.C., Pho, R.W.H., Kumar, V.P., Kour, A. & Satku, K. (2002). Extremity osteosarcoma—a Southeast Asian Experience. *Annals of the Academy of Medicine, Singapore, 31*(5), 598–606.

Cho, Y., Jung, G.H., Chung, S.H., Kim, J.Y., Choi, Y. & Kim, J.D. (2011). Long-term survivals of stage IIb osteosarcoma: A 20-year experience in a single institution. *Clinics in Orthopedic Surgery, 3*(1), 48–54.

Enneking, W.F., Spanier, S.S. & Goodman, M.A. (1980). A system for the surgical staging of musculoskeletal sarcoma. *Clinical Orthopaedics and Related Research, 153*, 106–20.

Huvos, A.G., Rosen, G. & Marcove, R.C. (1977). Primary osteogenic sarcoma: Pathological aspects in 20 patients after treatment with chemotherapy enbloc resection and prosthetic bone replacement. *Archives of Pathology & Laboratory Medicines, 101*(1), 14–18.

Kager, L., Zoubek, A., Pötschger, U., Kastner, U., Flege, S., Kempf-Bielack, B., ... Cooperative German-Austrian-Swiss Osteosarcoma Study Group. (2003). Primary metastatic osteosarcoma: Presentation and outcome of patients treated on neoadjuvant Cooperative Osteosarcoma Study Group protocols. *Journal of Clinical Oncology, 21*(10), 2011–18.

Kaplan, E.L. & Meier, P. (1958). Non-parametric estimation from incomplete observations. *Journal of the American Statistical Association, 53*(282), 457–81.

Lewis, I.J., Nooij, M.A., Whelan, J., Sydes, M.R., Grimer, R., Hogendoorn, P.C., ... European Osteosarcoma Intergroup (2007). Improvement in histologic response but not survival in osteosarcoma patients treated with intensified chemotherapy: A randomized phase III trial of the European Osteosarcoma Intergroup. *Journal of the National Cancer Institute, 99*(2), 112–28.

Li, X., Ashana, A.O., Moretti, V.M. & Lackman, R.D. (2011). The relation of tumour necrosis and survival in patients with osteosarcoma. *International Orthopaedics, 35*(12), 1847–53.

Ogihara, Y., Sudo, A., Fujinami, S., Sato, K. & Miura, T. (1991). Current management, local management and survival statistics of high-grade osteosarcoma. Experience in Japan. *Clinical Orthopaedics and Related Research, 270*, 72–8.

Pakos, E.E., Nearchou, A.D., Grimer, R.J., Koumoullis, H.D., Abudu, A., Bramer, A.J., ... Ioannidis, J.P. (2009). Prognostic factors and outcomes for osteosarcoma: An international collaboration. *European Journal of Cancer, 45*(13), 2367–75.

Souhami, R.L., Craft, A.W., van der Eijken, J.W., Nooij, M., Spooner, D., Bramwell, V.H., ... Machin, D. (1997). Randomised trial of two regimens of chemotherapy in operable osteosarcoma: A study of the European Osteosarcoma Intergroup. *The Lancet, 350*(9082), 911–17.

Yip, K.M., Leung, P.C. & Kumta, S.M. (1996). Osteosarcoma in Hong Kong. *Clinical Orthopaedics and Related Research, 323*, 49–59.

Stem Cell Oncology – Adella (Ed.)
© *2018 Taylor & Francis Group, London, ISBN 978-0-8153-9272-9*

Relationship of depressive syndrome level with duration of detention and type of crime

M. Affandi, H.T. Parinduri & M.S. Husada
Department of Psychiatry, Faculty of Medicine, Universitas Sumatera Utara, Medan,
North Sumatera, Indonesia

ABSTRACT: In the course of reform of the criminal justice system in Indonesia, detention is one problem that has not received serious attention. Loss of freedom for a person can cause a decrease in dignity and self-esteem allowing stress to manifest. Further, the changes that occur in the life of a prisoner who is full of pressure and loss can increase the likelihood of depression.

Keywords: Beck Depression Inventory-II (BDI-II), Detention, Depression

1 INTRODUCTION

People in detention are more likely to experience psychiatric disorders that may not be treated. Studies conducted in Australia noted that among prisoners treated in hospitals for 12 months, the primary cause of hospitalisation were depressive disorders at a rate of 15.4% among women and 7.8% among men (Hughes, 2012). Roy Walmsley in the World Prison Population List (2010) stated that in Indonesia there are 117,863 detainees with an estimated total population of 232.5 million so, the average proportion of detainees per 100,000 of population is 51 (Walmsley, 2008).

The detention of a suspect is essentially a loss of liberty. In the Indonesian context, detention of a person has long been regarded as at the discretion of an official who has the authority to detain without having to justify the validity of his/her unilateral decision. Therefore, for such a long period in state detention houses and without an adequate process of detention testing becomes one of the factors deteriorating the situation and conditions in places of detention in Indonesia (Eddyono, 2009).

In Indonesia, pre-trial detention is commonly termed as the arrest. However, such detention is a detention before the criminal justice process has begun. In other words, detention is carried out within the framework of investigation and the prosecution conducted by investigators and prosecutors. For the purpose of this research, the term used shall be 'pre-trial detention' (Semendawai et al., 2009).

Pre-trial detainees may lose their jobs, be forced to abandon their education and be displaced from their homes. They are exposed to illness and suffer from physical and mental disorders that last long after their term of detention ends. Their families also suffer from loss of income and educational opportunities, including a multi-generational impact where children of detainees experience decreased educational attainment and reduced income for the rest of their lives (Berry, 2010).

Among the mental disorders that occur in custody, the most common is depression. Several studies have reported a significant association between the symptoms of depression and antisocial behaviour. Although depression is associated with antisocial and criminal behaviour, there is also evidence to suggest that, once a person is arrested for criminal behaviour, he/she can suffer from depression due to social, economic, and family factors, as well as the punishment experienced. Galvan, Romero, Rodríguez, Durand, Colmenares & Saldivar reported that there was a relationship between the frequency of visits in prison and the symptoms of depression, especially in women. For example, women who had not had a visit for about a month or more displayed levels of depression. The most common type of crime committed by both men and women is persecution, then abduction and robbery in women as well as murder and immorality (rape) in men (Lanz & Díaz, 2013).

The history of previous psychiatric disorders and the presence of physical illness is a risk factor for the occurrence of depression while in custody. In young adult arrestees, economic/occupational factors and length of stay in detention are risk factors for neurotic disorders. However, in respect of detention of elderly prisoners, Fazel et al. (2001) stated that there is no relationship between depression and work and length of stay in detention.

2 METHOD

2.1 Study design

This study is an analytical study with a cross-sectional study approach to prisoners in Medan Police prison in March 2015. Inclusion criteria are Medan Police prisoners, aged between 18–60 years old, with a minimum junior high school education and willing to take part in the study. Exclusion criteria are having a history of previous psychiatric disorders such as anxiety, depression, etc., not drug prisoner resistance and poor general medical conditions. The psychometric test used in this research is the Beck Depression Inventory-II (BDI-II), with the data analysed using the Chi-Square statistical technique.

2.2 Setting and sample

This study required 80 prisoners in Medan Police prison in March 2015 with Inclusion criteria are Medan Police prisoners, aged between 18–60 years old, minimum junior high school and willing to take part in the study. Exclusion criteria are having a history of previous psychiatric disorders such as anxiety, depression, etc., not drug prisoner resistance and poor general medical conditions. The instrument used in this research is Beck Depression Inventory-II (BDI-II), then the data is analysed by using the Chi-Square statistical technique.

2.3 Ethical consideration

This research will be conducted after obtaining approval from the Research Ethics Committee at the Faculty of Medicine, Universitas Sumatera Utara. Subjects meeting the inclusion-exclusion criteria, will be interviewed with Mini International Neuropsychiatric Interview (MINI) techniques, version ICD-10 (A1). If the subjects who meet the criteria have a tendency towards depression they will then be asked to complete an informed consent form. After obtaining a detailed and clear explanation on participation in this research, the subjects were asked to give information regarding their identity and demographic characteristics. The research subjects were then asked to complete the Beck Depression Inventory-II (BDI-II) questionnaire consisting of 21 questions. After completion, all the questionnaires were collected and the data analysis performed.

2.4 Data analysis

The processing and statistical analysis of the data obtained was computerised using the Statistical Package for Social Sciences (SPSS) programme.

3 RESULTS

Table 1 shows that most of the participants are aged 31–40 years (38.75%), male (68.75%), unmarried (56.25%), in work (68.75%), have a high school education level (51.25%), a duration of detention <3 months (61.25%) and committed the crime of murder/persecution (43.75%).

Table 2 shows that the highest level of depressive syndrome is mild (43.75%), with moderate at 31.25% and severe at 25.0%.

Table 3 shows that the level of severe depressive syndrome was highest in a duration of detention <3 months (24.5%), moderate in a duration of detention >3 months (35.5%) and mild in a duration of detention <3 months (46.9%). There was no significant difference between depressive syndrome level and the duration of detention (p = 0.742).

Table 4 shows that the level of severe depressive syndrome is highest in the immorality type of crime (29.2%), moderate also in the immorality type of crime (37.5%) and mild in the

Table 1. Participants' characteristics.

Variable	Amount (n = 80)	%
Age (years)		
18–30	20	25.0
31–40	31	38.75
41–50	19	23.75
51–60	10	12.5
Gender		
Male	55	68.75
Female	25	31.25
Marital status		
Unmarried	45	56.25
Married	35	43.75
Job status		
Work	55	68.8
No work	25	31.3
Education		
Junior High School	21	26.3
Senior High School	41	51.3
College	18	22.5
Duration of detention		
<3 months	49	61.25
>3 months	31	38.75
Type of crime		
Murder/Persecution	35	43.75
Robbery/Theft	21	26.25
Immorality	24	30.0

Table 2. Depressive syndrome level in Medan Police prisoners.

Depressive syndrome level	n	%
Mild	35	43.75
Moderate	25	31.25
Severe	20	25.0
Total	80	100

229

Table 3. Relationship of depressive syndrome level with duration of detention.

| Duration of detention | Depressive syndrome level | | | p |
	Mild n(%)	Moderate n(%)	Severe n(%)	
<3 months	23(46.9)	14(28.6)	12(24.5)	0.742
>3 months	12(38.7)	11(35.5)	8(25.8)	
Total	35(43.75)	25(31.25)	20(25.0)	

Table 4. Relationship of depressive syndrome level with the type of crime.

| Type of crime | Depressive syndrome level | | | p |
	Mild n(%)	Moderate n(%)	Severe n(%)	
Murder/Persecution	17(48.6)	10(28.5)	8(22.9)	0.822
Robbery/Theft	10(47.6)	6(28.6)	5(23.8)	
Immorality	8(33.3)	9(37.5)	7(29.2)	
Total	35(43.75)	25(31.25)	20(25.0)	

murder/persecution type of crime (48.6%). There was no significant difference between the level of depressive syndrome and the type of crime (p = 0.822).

REFERENCES

Berry, D. (2010). Dampak social Ekonomi dari penahanan pra-persidangan. New York: Open Society Justice Initiative.

Eddyono, SW. (2009). Penahanan Pra Persidangan Dalam Rancangan KUHAP. Jakarta Selatan: Institute for Criminal Justice Reform.

Fazel, S., Hope, T., O'Donnell, I. & Jacoby, R. (2001). Hidden psychiatric morbidity in elderly prisoners. The British Journal of Psychiatry, 179, 535–9.

Hughes, L.D. (2012). Psychosocial treatments for depression in UK criminal justice—A review of the evidence. Scottish Universities Medical Journal, 1–13.

Lanz, P.M. & Díaz, M.J. (2013). Domestic violence, alcohol consumption and depression in criminal population. Scientific Research, 4(3), 153–158.

Semendawai, A.H., Sriyana, Wiryawan S.M., Eddyono S.W., Wahyudi, Wagiman, W. (2009). Pemetaan awal situasi penahanan dan pra peradilan di Indonesia. Jakarta Selatan: Institute for Criminal Justice Reform.

Walmsley, R. (2008). World Prison Population List. (9th ed). London: International Centre for Prison Studies.

Stem Cell Oncology – Adella (Ed.)
© *2018 Taylor & Francis Group, London, ISBN 978-0-8153-9272-9*

Correlation of BDNF and cognitive function in smoking Batak male schizophrenic patients

E. Effendy, M.M. Amin, N. Utami & F.H. Sitepu
Department of Psychiatry, Faculty of Medicine, Universitas Sumatera Utara, Medan, North Sumatera, Indonesia

ABSTRACT: Schizophrenia is a complex neurodevelopmental disorder with impaired cognitive function as a major element. BDNF may be a marker of abnormal neuronal development and neurotransmission in schizophrenia. Cognitive function often correlates significantly with awareness of pain, social skills and the presence of a delayed return to normal life. The purpose of this study was to look at the association of serum levels of BDNF and cognitive function in Batak male, schizophrenic patients who smoke and have a history of using risperidone treatment. This study was a cross-sectional, correlative numerical study in order to assess cognitive function using the Montreal Assessment Cognitive Instrument Indonesia (MoCA-Ina) version. BDNF serum levels were analysed using the quantitative sandwich enzyme, immunoassay. There was a significant correlation between the MoCA-Ina score and BDNF serum levels with a correlation value of 0.441 showing a positive correlation with moderate correlation strength (r = 0.4 – <0.6).

Keywords: Schizophrenia, BDNF, Cognitive

1   INTRODUCTION

Schizophrenia is a complex neurodevelopmental disorder with impairment of cognitive function as a central feature. This confirmed by a number of studies performed on patients who suffer from schizophrenia where clinical symptoms and social functioning of patients are consequences of neurocognitive deficits. The cognitive deficit is a core aspect of the schizophrenic condition (Fisekovic et al., 2012).

Over two decades of research has highlighted the relationship of cognitive performance with the neurotrophins system. Neurotrophins are a unique family of polypeptide growth factors with similar structures that are involved in the process of brain development, differentiation and survival of neurons, synaptic plasticity, and connectivity. The neurotrophins comprise of nerve growth factor (NGF), brain-derived neurotrophic factor (BDNF), neurotrophin-3 (NT-3), and neurotrophin-4 (NT-4) (Bath et al., 2006). BDNF, a member of the neurotrophic family, is common in the mammalian brain and plays an important role in the development, regeneration, survival, maintenance, and function of the neuron (Zhang et al., 2015; Niitsu et al., 2011). BDNF is a protein highly involved in the development of the nervous system of all mammals, and in the regulation of synaptic transmission. During the period of development, BDNF has been involved in the survival of stem cells, neurogenesis, and neuronal differentiation along with polarisation and neuronal guidance. BNDF also regulates the plasticity aspect of the brain and is thus involved in cognitive function (Rowbotham et al., 2015).

The smoking rate in schizophrenics is estimated between 40–90%, higher than among the general population or individuals with severe mental illness. The reasons for smoking in schizophrenics are not well understood, but these patients may be trying to reduce the side effects of treatment and the negative symptoms and/or cognitive deficits associated with schizophrenia, suggesting that they are smoking tobacco or nicotine as self-medication (Zhang et al., 2010).

A study conducted by Kim et al. found that serum levels of BDNF in smokers, as compared to non-smokers, supports the idea of a possible relationship between BDNF and smoking. They found that the smoking group had significantly lower levels of BDNF in baseline while the BDNF serum level after two months of quitting was significantly higher. A study by Zhang et al. found that the BDNF level was significantly higher in smokers (7.8 ± 3.2 ng/ml) than non-smokers (6.4 ± 2.1 ng/ml). Furthermore, higher BDNF levels are associated with a large number of smoked cigarettes (Zhang et al., 2010).

2 METHOD

2.1 Study design

This study design is a cross-sectional study that assessed differences in serum levels of BDNF and cognitive function in smoking Batak male, schizophrenia patients.

2.2 Setting and sample

Participants were recruited from the inpatient ward in a psychiatry facility in Professor. Muhammad Ildrem Mental Hospital, Medan, Indonesia with the following inclusion criteria: (a) those who had been diagnosed with schizophrenia in a stable phase by a psychiatrist, (b) from the Batak clan, (c) smoker, (d) aged between 20–40 years old who understood the purpose of this study and agreed to participate with written consent, (e) and with their last education being in junior high school. Exclusion criteria: (a) suffering from other mental illness, (b) suffering from other neurologic disease.

This study required 22 participants and each participant who was suitable, with respect to the inclusion and exclusion criteria, had their body mass index (BMI) ratio measured (weight to height ratio). Blood samples were then taken to check the levels of BDNF. The serum level of BDNF was analysed using the quantitative sandwich enzyme, immunoassay. After the serum level of BDNF results had been accepted, the cognitive function was calculated using the Montreal Cognitive Assessment Indonesia version (MoCA-Ina).

2.3 Ethical consideration

The present study was conducted after receiving approval from the institutional review board at the Faculty of Medicine of the University of Sumatera Utara. The recruitment of research participants was conducted through individual interviews with schizophrenia inpatients that met the selection criteria. When the potential participants agreed to take part in the study, we asked them to sign the consent form. The purpose and the procedures of the study were explained, including voluntary participation and withdrawal.

2.4 Data analysis

The results were analysed using the statistical software package SPSS for Windows.

3 RESULTS

From the 22 participants took part in the study, the majority of participants were 31–40 years old (86.4%), married participants (12, 54.5%), and the duration of illness number of participants was the same for 2–3 years and >3 years. Participants' characteristics are presented in Table 1.

Table 1. Participants' characteristics.

Variable	n	%
Age		
20–30 years	3	13.6
31–40 years	19	86.4
Marital status		
Unmarried	10	45.5
Married	12	54.5
Duration of illness		
2–3 years	11	50
>3 years	11	50

Table 2. Mean of MoCA-Ina score.

Variable	Mean	SD	p
MoCA-Ina	20.64	6.02	0.362*

*Shapiro-Wilk test.

Table 3. Mean of serum level of BDNF.

Variable	Mean	SD	p
BDNF	26651	6084	0.715*

*Shapiro-Wilk test.

Table 4. Correlation score of MoCA-Ina and serum level of BDNF.

	Serum level of BDNF
MoCA-Ina score	r = 0.441
	p = 0.4
	n = 22

The mean of MoCA-Ina score was found to be 20.64 ± 6.02. From the results, using the Shapiro-Wilk test, $p = 0.362$ ($p > 0.05$), so the data was normally distributed.

The mean of serum level of BDNF was found to be 26651 ± 6084. From the results, using the Shapiro-Wilk test, $p = 0.715$ ($p > 0.05$), so the data was normally distributed.

The Pearson correlation test of serum level of BDNF and the MoCA-Ina score obtained the result of $p < 0.05$ which showed a correlation between BDNF serum and the MoCA-Ina score. The correlation between MoCA-Ina score and BDNF serum was 0.441 showing a positive, moderate correlation ($r = 0.4 – <0.6$).

4 DISCUSSION

Zhang et al. (2012) state that the neuroprotective effects of BDNF where BDNF plays a key role in modulating synaptic and plasticity transmission and have important factors in long-term induction of potentiation (LTP), continuous synaptic reinforcement associated with learning and memory.

Preclinical studies have shown that LTP is impaired in that the deficient genes BDNF and LTP can be recovered with adenovirus-mediated mutant transfection with the BDNF gene. Simultaneously, these results support a mechanism linking cognitive function and BDNF levels. BDNF may play a role in the pathogenesis of schizophrenia, but it also examines evidence suggesting that it plays a role in the pathophysiology of cognitive deficits.

The results of the study by Zhang et al. in 2012 that examined a group of schizophrenic patients with recurrent episodes found an association between poor BDNF and visuospatial performance variants/construction and attention deficit in schizophrenic patients. They also found that there was a relationship between decreased serum BDNF levels and cognitive impairment in schizophrenic patients depending on BDNF polymorphisms having a significant relationship of $p = 0.023$ i.e. < 0.05.

There was a significant correlation between MoCA-Ina score and serum BDNF level with a correlation value of 0.441, showing a positive, moderate correlation ($r = 0.4 - <0.6$).

REFERENCES

Bath, K.G. & Lee, F.S. (2006). Variant BDNF (Val66Met) impact on brain structure and function. *Cognitive, Affective and Behavioral Neuroscience, 6*(1), 79–85.

Fisekovic, S., Memic, A. & Pasalic, A. (2012). Correlation between MoCA and MMSE for the assessment of cognition in schizophrenia. *Journal of the Society for Medical Informatics of Bosnia and Herzogovina, 20*(3), 186–189.

Niitsu, T., Shirayama, Y., Matsuzawa, D., Hasegawa, T., Kanahara, N., Hashimoto, T., ... Iyo, M. (2011). Associations of serum brain-derived neurotrophic factor with cognitive impairments and negative symptoms in schizophrenia. *Progress in Neuro-psychopharmacology & Biological Psychiatry, 35*(8), 1836–1840.

Rowbotham, I.M., Orsucci, F.F., Mansour, M.F., Chamberlain, S.R. & Raja, H.Y. (2015). Relevance of brain-derived neurotrophic factor levels in schizophrenia: A systematic review and meta-analysis. *AIMS Neuroscience, 2*(4), 280–293.

Zhang, X.Y., Chen, D.C., Tan, Y.L., Luo, X., Zuo, L.J., Lv, M.H., ... Soares, J.C. (2015). Smoking and BDNF Val66Met polymorphism in male schizophrenia: A case-control study. *Journal of Psychiatric Research, 60*, 49–55.

Zhang, X.Y., Chenda, C., Xiu, M.H., Haile, C.N., Luo, X., Xu, K., ... Kosten, T.R. (2012). Cognitive and serum BDNF correlates of BDNF Val66Met gene polymorphism in patients with schizophrenia and normal controls. *Human Genetics, 131*(7), 1187–1195. doi:10.1007/s00439-012-1150-x.

Zhang, X.Y., Xiu, M.H., Chen, D.C., Yang, F.D., Wu, G.Y., Lu, L., ... Kosten, T.R. (2010). Nicotine dependence and serum BDNF levels in male patients with schizophrenia. *Psychopharmacology, 212*(3), 301–307.

Stem Cell Oncology – Adella (Ed.)
© 2018 Taylor & Francis Group, London, ISBN 978-0-8153-9272-9

The effect of hypertonic saline irrigation vs baby shampoo in chronic rhinosinusitis

D. Munir, I.N. Tobing, M. Hasibuan, A. Aboet & P.C. Eyanoer
Department of Otorhinolaryngology Head and Neck Surgery, Faculty of Medicine,
Universitas Sumatera Utara, Medan, North Sumatera, Indonesia

S.V. Hutagalung
Faculty of Tropical Medicine, Mahildo University, Thailand

ABSTRACT: Nasal irrigation is the treatment of choice to relieve symptoms in chronic rhinosinusitis (CRS). Adding a surfactant to the solution may increase its efficacy, but the effects on mucociliary function are unknown. To determine the effect of nasal irrigation with surfactant on the symptoms and Mucociliary Transport Time (MTT) in CRS, 40 patients in the hypertonic saline and the baby shampoo group were evaluated for symptoms and MTT, before and after nasal irrigation, for two weeks. The difference of the average Sino-Nasal Outcome Test 20 (SNOT-20) score in the hypertonic group was statistically significant ($p = 0.01$), but not in the baby shampoo group. The average VAS score in both groups was significantly different ($p = 0.01$ and $p = 0.05$). Neither hypertonic nor baby shampoo solution affects MTT. Nasal irrigation with the baby shampoo solution has not affected the quality of life and MTT in CRS but may affect the severity of the disease.

Keywords: Baby shampoo, Chronic rhinosinusitis, Mucociliary transport time, Nasal irrigation

1 INTRODUCTION

Nasal irrigation using a hypertonic saline solution is the treatment of choice for patients with CRS. Inexpensive and easy to perform, nasal irrigation not only relieves symptoms, but can also decrease the medication required in CRS.

Recent studies reported that saline nasal irrigation given additives such as a surfactant, may increase its efficacy and prevent biofilm formation (Woodworth et al., 2005; Schlosser, 2006; Harvey & Lund, 2007). The surfactant can reduce surface tension on the liquid and increase solubility, mobility, bioavailability and subsequent biodegradation of hydrophobic compounds and insoluble organic compounds (van Hamme et al. 2006).

Baby shampoo may be a useful and well-tolerated surfactant in the treatment of CRS. Chiu et al. (2008) showed that CRS patients experienced improved symptoms based on the SNOT-22 score and the University of Pennsylvania Smell Identification Test (UPSIT). Similarly, Farag et al. (2013) reported improved symptoms based on the Rhinosinusitis Outcome Measure (RSOM-31) and the SNOT-22 questionnaire along with the phenyl ethyl alcohol (PEA) smell threshold test in patients who used baby shampoo solution as nasal irrigation.

Studies of the effects of baby shampoo solution on mucociliary function in CRS have not yet been found. This study aims to compare baby shampoo and hypertonic solutions with symptoms and MTT in CRS patients.

2 METHODS

This study has been approved by the Health Research Ethics Commission at the Faculty of Medicine, Universitas Sumatera Utara. A quasi experimental study was performed from

August 2015 until January 2016 where patients were recruited from the outpatient clinics of a teaching hospital and its satellites in Medan. Inclusion criteria included patients with CRS aged ≥18 years, willing to participate and sign a consent form. The exclusion criteria were pregnant women and patients with hypersensitivity to hypertonic saline or baby shampoo solutions.

Forty patients with CRS were allocated into two groups, a hypertonic saline (H) and a baby shampoo (BS) irrigation group. Before the treatment, patients received an instruction leaflet and an explanation on how to irrigate the nose. Patients were asked to repeat the instructions and perform the nasal irrigation to make sure they understood the task.

Patients conducted nasal irrigation using a prepared irrigation formula. The formula consisted of 1 teaspoon of non-iodised salt and ½ teaspoon of baking soda mixed with 500 cc of previously boiled water. This was given to the H-group while 1 teaspoon of baby shampoo was added to this solution for patients in the BS-group. Patients then irrigated each nostril twice with a 60 cc catheter tip syringe filled with their respective solution, two times a day for two weeks. Patients were also given an oral antibiotic, Ciprofloxacin 2 × 500 mg.

To assess the quality and severity of the nasal symptoms, patients completed SNOT-20 and VAS questionnaires. A saccharin test was also performed.

Patient data was collected before and after the nasal irrigation treatment, but the assessment of the nasal irrigation was carried out every week. If a patient discontinued the use of nasal irrigation, no further data would be collected, and the patient was excluded from the study.

Statistical analysis was conducted to obtain the frequency distribution and mean value of each variable. The dependent t-test was used to compare the proportions. When data was not normally distributed, the Wilcoxon signed-rank test was used for analysis. P values lower than 0.05 were considered significant.

3   RESULTS

The results are presented for 21 patients who used the hypertonic saline solution and 19 patients who used the baby shampoo solution, with a total of 40 patients.

The scores of SNOT-20 are presented in Table 1. The mean SNOT-20 scores in group H before (37.00 ± 20.69) and after (25.71 ± 19.68) treatment are significantly different ($p = 0.01$). As for group BS, the mean SNOT-20 scores decrease from 34.95 ± 25.00 to 28.16 ± 23.23 but it does not differ statistically.

Both groups showed significant difference in mean VAS scores (Table 2). Group BS ($p = 0.05$) showed slight decreases as compared to group H before treatment ($p = 0.01$).

There is a decrease of mean mucociliary transport time in group H and group BS, but it does not differ statistically.

The number of patients who discontinued with the baby shampoo nasal irrigation was higher than those who used the hypertonic saline solution (24% vs 9%). In the baby shampoo group, six patients did not finish the treatment, 5 of whom we could not contact to follow up and one who changed his mind due to nasal burning and headaches. In the hypertonic saline solution group, two patients did not finish the treatment. One felt he had been doing so well that he chose not to continue. The most common side effect complaint by patients in the baby shampoo group were nasal burning and headaches.

Table 1.   Mean and standard deviation of SNOT-20 scores before and after treatment in groups H and BS.

SNOT-20	Pre		Post		
	Mean	SD	Mean	SD	p
Group H	37.00	20.69	25.71	19.68	0.01*
Group BS	34.95	25.00	28.16	23.23	0.07**

*Dependent t-test.

**Wilcoxon signed-rank test.

Table 2. Mean and standard deviation of VAS scores before and after treatment in groups H and BS.

VAS	Pre		Post		
	Mean	SD	Mean	SD	p
Group H	6.24	2.72	4.43	2.71	0.01*
Group BS	6.84	2.85	5.47	3.12	0.05**

*Dependent t-test.
**Wilcoxon signed-rank test.

Table 3. Mean and standard deviation of mucociliary transport time before and after treatment in groups H and BS.

Mucociliary transport time	Pre		Post		
	Mean	SD	Mean	SD	p
Group H	13.92	7.51	12.22	6.29	0.19**
Group BS	15.72	7.47	13.26	5.72	0.09*

*Dependent t-test.
**Wilcoxon signed-rank test.

4 DISCUSSION

There are many studies about hypertonic saline solution being used for nasal irrigation. Many have demonstrated the benefits of surfactant solutions to diseases that fulfil the biofilm bacterial profile (Desrosiers et al., 2007; Chiu, et al., 2008; Farag, et al., 2013). However, there are fewer studies when it comes to adding a surfactant into the nasal irrigation solution. Baby shampoo is a surfactant solution that is believed to decompose the bacterial layer of biofilm in the nasal mucosa of CRS.

Chiu et al. (2008), were the first to describe the use of baby shampoo in nasal irrigation for CRS patients. Farag et al. (2013) did a further research over a longer period. Our study, which was different from these two previous studies, was performed in CRS patients before nasal endoscopic surgery. Administration of nasal irrigation for postoperative patients requires recovery time from postsurgical mucosal changes. Moreover, the goal of nasal irrigation is to clear secretion and relieve symptoms which can be done immediately after a diagnosis of CRS is confirmed.

In their study, Chiu et al. (2008) provided each patient with topical steroids, 10 of whom had an oral antibiotic for two weeks and two who used oral prednisone. For this study, we only gave antibiotics for two weeks as the main treatment.

Farag et al. (2013) studied their patients for four months during which they found decreased SNOT-22 scores both in the hypertonic saline and the baby shampoo groups in the first eight weeks. There was a slight increase of the SNOT-22 scores in the baby shampoo group at the end point, but the score continued to decrease in the hypertonic saline group. At the end of the study, there was an overall improvement over time with both forms of irrigation.

In our study, the average SNOT-20 score in the baby shampoo group began to decrease 6.79 points. Thus, one could infer that the symptoms begin to improve 2 weeks after irrigation. But, given such a short period, this small difference was not statistically significant.

Based on the VAS category, the hypertonic saline group showed better improvement compared to those in the baby shampoo group. This may be due to the side effects that arose after the baby shampoo irrigation. Thus, assessment of the severity of the disease became perplexing. Nevertheless, significant improvement in the VAS scores in the baby shampoo group showed that irrigation with the baby shampoo solution might help to reduce the severity of the disease in CRS patients.

Previous studies have shown variable results about the effects of the hypertonic saline solution on mucociliary transport time. Hauptman & Ryan (2007) and Ural et al. (2009) reported that the hypertonic saline solution improved the mucociliary transport time in CRS. However, Low et al. (2014) found no significant improvement in mucociliary transport time in patients who used either normal saline, Ringer's lactate or hypertonic saline solutions.

Isaacs et al. (2011) provided a surfactant solution to 27 healthy volunteers and evaluated the mucociliary transport time before and after treatment. They found a significant improvement ($p = 0.031$), but this study lacked controls and, thus, cannot specifically address the impact of surfactant on mucociliary transport time.

In our study, both hypertonic saline and baby shampoo solutions have little effect on the mucociliary transport time. Improvement in symptoms can be caused by the nasal irrigation properties which can dissolve the hydrophobic compounds of mucus, thereby reducing its surface tension and viscosity (Rosen et al. 2013). However, it does not seem to be able to fully improve the mucociliary transport time.

The results of this study were not able to prove that baby shampoo solution can be used in the routine management of CRS. However, because of its ability to reduce the severity of the disease, it may considered as an adjunctive treatment when further research is done with more samples over a longer period of time. It is also necessary to modify the surfactant solution in order to reduce the side effects so that it can be widely used as a nasal irrigation.

5 CONCLUSION

Nasal irrigation with a baby shampoo solution does not affect the quality of life and MTT in CRS but it may affect the severity of the disease.

REFERENCES

Chen, M.A. & Davidson, T.M. (2006). Rhinitis in the aging patient. In K.H. Calhoun & D.E. Eibling (Eds.), *Geriatric otolaryngology* (pp. 225–236). Boca Raton: CRC Press.

Chiu, A.G., Palmer, J.N., Woodworth, B.A., Doghramji, L., Cohen, M.B., Prince, A., & Cohen, N.A. (2008). Baby shampoo nasal irrigations for the symptomatic post-functional endoscopic sinus surgery patient. *American Journal of Rhinology, 22*(1), 34–37.

Desrosiers, M., Myntti, M. & James, G. (2007). Methods for removing bacterial biofilms: In vitro study using clinical chronic rhinosinusitis specimens. *American Journal of Rhinology, 21*(5), 527–532.

Farag, A.A., Deal, A.M., McKinney, K.A., Thorp, B.D., Senior, B.A., Ebert, C.S. & Zanation, A.M. (2013). Single-blind randomized controlled trial of surfactant vs hypertonic saline irrigation following endoscopic endonasal surgery. *International Forum of Allergy & Rhinology, 3*(4), 276–280.

Harvey, R.J. & Lund, V.J. (2007). Biofilms and chronic rhinosinusitis: Systematic review of evidence, current concepts and directions for research. *Rhinology, 45*(1), 3–13.

Hauptman, G. & Ryan, M.W. (2007). The effect of saline solutions on nasal patency and mucociliary clearance in rhinosinusitis patients. *Otolaryngology Head and Neck Surgery, 137*(5), 815–821.

Isaacs, S., Fakhri, S., Luong, A., Whited, C. & Citardi, M.J. (2011). The effect of dilute baby shampoo on nasal mucociliary clearance in healthy subjects. *American Journal of Rhinology and Allergy, 25*(1), e27–e29.

Low, T.H., Woods, C.M., Ullah, S. & Carney, A.S. (2014). A double-blind randomized controlled trial of normal saline, lactated Ringer's, and hypertonic saline nasal irrigation solution after endoscopic sinus surgery. *American Journal of Rhinology & Allergy, 28*(3), 225–231.

Rosen, P.L., Palmer, J.N., O'Malley, B.W. & Cohen, N.A. (2013). Surfactants in the management of rhinopathologies. *American Journal of Rhinology & Allergy, 27*(3), 177–180.

Schlosser, R.J. (2006). Surfactant and its role in chronic sinusitis. *Annals of Otology, Rhinology & Laryngology, 196*, 40–44.

Ural, A., Oktemer, T.K., Kizil, Y., Ileri, F. & Uslu, S. (2009). Impact of isotonic and hypertonic saline solutions on mucociliary activity in various nasal pathologies: Clinical study. *The Journal of Laryngology & Otology, 123*(5), 517–521.

van Hamme, J.D., Singh, A. & Ward, O.P. (2006). Physiological aspects. Part 1 in a series of papers devoted to surfactants in microbiology and biotechnology. *Biotechnology Advances, 24*(6), 604–620.

Woodworth, B.A., Smythe, N., Spicer, S.S., Schulte, B.A. & Schlosser, R.J. (2005). Presence of surfactant lamellar bodies in normal and diseased sinus mucosa. *Journal for Oto-rhino-laryngology and its Related Specialities, 67*(4), 199–202.

Stem Cell Oncology – Adella (Ed.)
© 2018 Taylor & Francis Group, London, ISBN 978-0-8153-9272-9

The relationship polymorphism of gene RFC1 A80G and NSCLP in Sumatera Utara, Indonesia

B.Y. Febrianto, U.A. Tarigan, F.B. Buchari & Hidayat
Department of Surgery, Faculty of Medicine, Universitas Sumatera Utara, Medan, North Sumatera, Indonesia

ABSTRACT: The etiology of Non-Syndromic Cleft Lip and Palate (NSCLP) has not yet been defined. Some studies have investigated the involvement of genetic and environmental factors. Some genes involved in the folate metabolism have been recently examined to discover the genetic factors in the cleft lip etiology. This research intends to identify the involvement of polymorphism in the Reduced Folate Carrier 1 (RFC1) A80G with NSCLP in the population of Sumatera Utara. In this case-control study, 62 NSCLP patients and 61 controls underwent DNA isolation and genotyping process using PCR-RFLP. The distribution of genotype and allele variants between the case and control were not significantly different ($p = 0.271$, $p = 0.809$). In the subgroup analysis, the polymorphism of RFC1 A80G showed a significant relationship in the group of CLO + CPO. The data obtained through this research confirms that the RFC1 A80G mutant variant has a relationship with NSCLP.

Keywords: cleft lip, folic acid, NSCLP, polymorphism RFC1

1 INTRODUCTION

The case of cleft lip most frequently found is cleft lip with or without cleft palate, which may be experienced by one in 500 births in the population of Asia and Indian-North American (Wehby & Murray, 2011). The prevalence of cleft lip in the whole of Indonesia according to the data of RISKESDAS 2013 was 0.08%, and in Sumatera Utara, 0.07% (Badan Penelitian Dan Pengembangan Kesehatan Kementerian Kesehatan RI, 2013).

Non-syndromic cleft lip and palate (NSCLP) is a complex result of genetic and environmental factors. Several studies have found that low levels of folic acid are predisposing factors to NSCLP (Langer 2014; Wilcox et al., 2007). This is not only influenced by intake or supplementation of folic acid but also in the process of folic acid metabolism (Cai et al., 2016; De Vos et al., 2008).

Folate undergoes a metabolism consisting of absorption, modification, transport, and interconversion. One of the proteins that plays an important role in the process of folate metabolism is the Reduced Folate Carrier 1 (RFC1) protein that plays a two-way transport of 5-methyltetrahydrololate and thiamine monophosphate into intracellular and red blood cells and maintains folate homeostasis in the event of down-regulation in folate deficiency. The RFC1 protein is coded by the RFC1 gene mapped at the end of the long arm of chromosome 21 (21q22.2-q22.3) (Yee et al., 2010).

Polymorphisms in the RFC1 A80G (rs1051266) are non-synonymous polymorphisms in exon two, which induce histidine substitution into arginine at codon 27 in the protein sequence. In several studies of polymorphism of RFC1 A80G, folic acid levels found in individuals with AA genotype had higher plasma folate levels than individuals variant AG and GG (Wehby et al., 2013), but this relationship was not found in other studies. In another study conducted in India, it was found that children with G alleles were at higher risk of the non-syndromic cleft lip with or without palate compared with the children of A allele ($OR = 1,4$) (Lakkakula et al., 2015). The purpose of this study was to clarify the involvement of polymorphism in the Reduced Folate Carrier 1 A80G with non-syndromic cleft lip and palate (NSCLP) in the population of Sumatera Utara.

2 MATERIAL AND METHOD

2.1 Subjects

This case-control study has earned the approval of the ethics committee. 62 case subjects were NSCLP patients treated for Labiaplasty at the Acuplast Hospital and RSUP Haji Adam Malik Medan from July to September 2017 and 61 control subjects obtained by using a consecutive sampling method who have signed an informed consent for the genotyping examination.

2.2 Genotyping

The DNA of the subject was extracted from a blood sample using the Wizard® Genomic DNA purification kit (Promega Corporation, USA) in accordance with the manufacturer's instructions. Then the DNA was amplified by the PCR method following the procedure used by Lakkakula et al., (2015) with the forward and reverse primer sequences used as follows 5: AGC GGT GA GGT-3 and 5-GGA GGT AGG GGG TGA AG-3. PCR products were cleaved with PCR-RFLP techniques using restriction enzyme HaeII for four hours at 30°C and electrophoresis on agarose gel 3% stained with ethidium bromide.

RFLP products were visualised under UV light to group genotype variants. The fragment 140 bp showed allele A and allele G saw on fragments 76 bp and 64 bp.

2.3 Statistical analysis

Genotype frequencies in the control group and patients were compared using a chi-square test. Analysis of the distribution of genotype and allele varieties in NSCLP subgroups were CLP and CLO + CPO with the control group using chi-square and alternative tests if not qualified.

The risk estimation was calculated by variant AA and allele An as reference category. $P < 0.05$ with two-way hypothesis is considered statistically significant.

3 RESULTS

3.1 Distribution of RFC1 polymorphism

The proportion of RFC1 exon 2 A80G gene polymorphism in case study and control subjects of this study can be seen in Table 1. In genotype distribution group AA 30.6%, AG 51.6%, GG 17.7% compared to control group AA 36.1%, AG 37.7% and GG 26.2%. The genotype distribution between the NSCLP and control cases was not significantly different ($p = 0.271$). The allele G frequency between the control group and the NSCLP cases was also not that different [45.1% (55/67) versus 43.5% (54/70); $p = 0.809$]. However, there were significant differences in genotype distribution between a subgroup of NSCLP and control cases ($p = 0.044$).

To assess the effect of variant genotype RFC1 A80G at risk of NSCLP, an odd ratio (OR) was calculated and 95% confidence interval (Table 2). Genotype AG (OR 0.621; 95% CI: 0.275–1.402) and GG (OR 1.256 95% CI: 0.47–3.357) indicated an increased risk of NSCLP. In AG + GG versus AA model had OR: 1,188; 95% CI: 0,558–2,529 and GG versus AG + AA having OR 1,648; 95% CI 0,693–3,919 indicated that variant A80G did not increase susceptibility of NSCLP because it was statistically insignificant >0.05. Allelic model having OR 1,064; 95% CI: 0.643–1.760 indicated no increased risk of NSCLP in subjects with G allele. In subgroup analysis, variant A80G showed a significant association with CLP group susceptibility in AG + GG versus AA model and allelic model (Table 2).

Table 1. Distribution of genotype and frequency of Allele RFC1 A80G in NSCLP.

	Control %	Overall clefts (%)	CLP (%)	CLO + CPO (%)
Genotype distribution				
AA	22 (36,1)	19 (30,6)	14 (25,5)	5 (71,4)
AG	23 (37,7)	32 (51,6)	30 (54,5)	2 (28,6)
GG	16 (26,2)	11 (17,7)	11 (20,0)	0 (0,0)
P value	0,271*		0,701**	
Alelle frequency				
Aalelle	67 (54,9)	70 (56,5)	58 (52,7)	12 (85,7)
Galelle	55 (45,1)	54 (43,5)	52 (47,3)	2 (14,3)
P value	0,809*		0,044*	

*Tested by chi-square.
**Tested by Mann-Whitney.

Table 2. Results of risk estimating polymorphism RFC1 A80G SNP in cleft lip and palate.

RFC 1 A80G	OR (95% CI)	p-value
Overall cleft		
AA	reference	
AG	0,621 (0,275–1,402)	0,250*
GG	1,256 (0,47–3,357)	0,649*
AG + GG versus AA	1,188 (0,558–2,529)	0,654*
GG versus AG + AA	1,648 (0,693–3,919)	0,256*
A allele	reference	
G allele	1,064 (0,643–1,760)	0,809*
CLP		
AA	reference	
AG	0,786 (0,592–1,043)	0,058**
GG	0,737 (0,563–0,964)	0,082**
AG + GG versus AA	0,773 (0,586–1,019)	0,024**
GG versus AG + AA	0,863 (0,773–0,963)	0,235**
A allele	reference	
G allele	0,860 (0,764–0,969)	0,019*
CLO + CPO		
AA	reference	
AG	4,211 (0,904–19,610)	0,058*
GG	–	
AG + GG versus AA	5,658 (1,203–26,614)	0,024**
GG versus AG + AA	–	–
A allele	reference	
G allele	4,629 (1,081–19,816)	0,019*

*Tested by chi-square.
**Tested by Fisher.

The risk of CLO + CPO increased in subjects AG + GG versus AA (OR: 5.658; 95% CI: 1,203–26,614; P = 0.04) and in subjects with G allele compared to allele A (OR 4.629; 95% CI 1.081–19.816, P = 0.019).

4 DISCUSSION

Nowadays, researchers have investigated the association of Single Nucleotide Polymorphism (SnPs) with the occurrence of a disease or drug side effects due to amino acid substitution caused and affecting the activity of the protein produced (Mostowska et al., 2010; Hasni et al., 2016). This study analyses the relationship of polymorphism of the RFC1 gene on the long arm of chromosome 21 (21q22.2-q22.3) exon 2, which causes the amino acid substitution of histidine to arginine (H27R; rs1051266) due to the substitution of nucleotide 80 adenine to guanine (A80G) (Wang et al., 2009; Yee et al., 2010). These RFC1 proteins play a role in regulating folate transport to red blood cells; in a previous study it was found that subjects with RFC1 alleles G experienced a decrease in plasma folic acid and increased levels of homocysteine due to negative regulation caused by the RFC1 protein in allele G patients (Cai et al., 2016).

Nowadays, researchers have investigated the association of single nucleotide polymorphism (SnPs) with the occurrence of a disease or drug side effects due to amino acid substitution caused and affecting the activity of the protein produced (Mostowska et al., 2010; Hasni et al., 2016). This study analyses the relationship of polymorphism of RFC1 gene on the long arm of chromosome 21 (21q22.2-q22.3) exon two, which causes the amino acid substitution of histidine to arginine (H27R; rs1051266) due to the substitution of nucleotide 80 adenine to guanine (A80G) (Wang et al., 2009; Yee et al., 2010). These RFC1 proteins play a role in regulating folate transport to red blood cells; in a previous study it was found that subjects with RFC1 alleles G experienced a decrease in plasma folic acid and increased levels of homocysteine due to negative regulation caused by the RFC1 protein in allele G patients (Cai et al., 2016).

In this study, we found an association and increased susceptibility of NSCLP in subjects with RFC1 80G alleles. The results of this study support Viera et al.'s research in Brazil that aimed to find the variant association of MTHFR and RFC1 associated with cleft lip incidence, with the results obtained by the variation of RFC-1 over-transmitted to children born with cleft lip. ($p = 0.017$) with the conclusions of Polymorphisms in RFC1 contributed to the incidence of Clef Lip Only (CLO) (Bufalino et al., 2010).

The findings of this study also resemble the results of Lakkakula et al.'s (2015) study in India that examined 142 non-syndromic cleft lip and 141 control subjects, which found a comparison of genotype variant distributions between case and control groups was not statistically different, but there was an increased risk of NSCLP in subjects with G allele (OR: 1.40; 95% CI: 1.00–1.97; $p = 0.005$) (Lakkakula et al., 2015).

The possible role of RFC1 gene polymorphism in NSCLP susceptibility is supported by previous research that the protein encoded by this gene will affect the transport of folic acid to red blood cells and is associated with low levels of folate and elevated levels of homocysteine (Cai et al., 2016; Biselli et al., 2008). In conclusion, in this case-control study, there was a relationship between RFC1 A80G polymorphism with an increased risk of NSCLP in the Population of Sumatra Utara.

REFERENCES

Badan Penelitian Dan Pengembangan Kesehatan Kementrian Kesehatan RI, (2013). *Riset Kesehatan Dasar*, Jakarta.
Biselli, J.M. et al., (2008). A80G Polymorphism of Reduced Folate Carrier 1 (RFC1) and C776G Polymorphism of Transcobalamin 2 (TC2) genes in down's syndrome Etiology. *Sao Paulo Medical Journal*, 126(6), 329–332.
Bufalino, A. et al., (2010). Maternal polymorphisms in folic acid metabolic genes are associated with nonsyndromic cleft lip and palate in the Brazilian population. *Birth Defects Research Part A – Clinical and molecular teratology*, 88(11), 980–986.
Cai, C. et al., (2016). Association of MTHFR, SLC19A1 genetic polymorphism, serum folate, vitamin B12 and HCY status with cognitive functions in Chinese adults. *Nutrients*, 8(10), 1–14.
De Vos, L. et al., (2008). Associations between single nucleotide polymorphisms in folate uptake and metabolizing genes with blood folate, homocysteine, and DNA uracil concentrations. *American Journal of Clinical Nutrition*, 88(4), 1149–1158.
Hasni, D., Siregar, K.B. & Lim, H., (2016). The Influence of Glutathion S-Transferase P-1 Polymorphism A33G Rs1695 on the susceptibility to cyclophosphamide hematologic toxicity in Indonesian patients. *118 Med J Indones @BULLET Med J Indones*, 2525(2), 118–26.

Lakkakula, B., Murthy, J. & Gurramkonda, V.B., (2015). Relationship between reduced folate carrier gene polymorphism and non-syndromic cleft lip and palate in Indian population. *The journal of maternal-fetal & neonatal medicine: the official journal of the European Association of Perinatal Medicine, the Federation of Asia and Oceania Perinatal Societies, the International Society of Perinatal Obstetricians, 28*(3), 329–32.

Langer, (2014). Folic acid deficiency as an etiological factor in cleft lip and palate. *Journal of Cleft Lip Palate and Craniofacial Anomalies, 1*(2), 98.

Mostowska, A. et al., (2010). Associations of folate and choline metabolism gene polymorphisms with orofacial clefts. *Journal of medical genetics, 47*(12), 809–15.

Wang, Y. et al., (2009). Relationship between genetic polymorphisms of RFC1 A80G and nonsymdromic cleft lip with or without palate. *Wei sheng yan jiu = Journal of hygiene research, 38*(3), 276–9.

Wehby, G. & Murray, J.C., (2011). Folic acid and orofacial clefts: A review of the evidence. *Oral Diseases, 16*(1), 11–19.

Wehby, G.L. et al., (2013). High dosage folic acid supplementation, oral cleft recurrence and fetal growth. *International Journal of Environmental Research and Public Health, 10*(2), 590–605.

Wilcox, A.J. et al., (2007). Folic acid supplements and risk of facial clefts: national population based case-control study. *BMJ (Clinical research ed.), 334*(7591), 464.

Yee, S.W. et al., (2010). SLC19A1 Pharmacogenomics summary. *Pharmacogenetics and Genomics, 20*(11), 708–715.

Stem Cell Oncology – Adella (Ed.)
© 2018 Taylor & Francis Group, London, ISBN 978-0-8153-9272-9

Association of Matrix Metalloproteinase 2 (MMP 2) and Tissue Inhibitor Matrix Metalloproteinase 2 (TIMP 2) and bone destruction in atticoantral type of Chronic Suppurative Otitis Media (CSOM)

H.A. Asroel, R.S.P. Wulandari & A. Aboet
Department of Ear, Nose, and Throat, Faculty of Medicine, Universitas Sumatera Utara, Medan, North Sumatera, Indonesia

F. Zaluchu
Epi-Treat, Faculty of North Sumatera, Universitas Sumatera Utara, Medan, North Sumatera, Indonesia

S. Eliandy
Installation of Pathology Anatomy of Haji Adam Malik General Hospital, Medan, North Sumatera, Indonesia

ABSTRACT: To determine an association between Matrix Metalloproteinase 2 (MMP 2) and Tissue Inhibitor Matrix Metalloproteinase 2 (TIMP 2) and bone destruction in atticoantral type Chronic Suppurative Otitis Media (CSOM) in patients at Haji Adam Malik General Hospital. This analytical cross-sectional study included cholesteatoma from atticoantral type CSOM taken and made into paraffin blocks. These tissues were immunohistochemically examined by assessing MMP 2 and TIMP 2 immunoreactivity at the anatomical pathology installation. MMP 2 overexpression (36 sample, 90%), however, samples that overexpressed and did not overexpress TIMP 2 were relatively even, 21 (52.5%) and 19 (47.5%), respectively. MMP 2 expression was not significantly associated with TIMP 2 (p = 0.342). MMP 2 and TIMP 2 expressions were not significantly associated, and TIMP 2 with bone destruction were not significantly associated in atticoantral type CSOM.

Keywords: Chronic Suppurative Otitis Media (CSOM), bone destruction, Matrix Metalloproteinase 2 (MMP 2), Tissue Inhibitor Matrix Metalloproteinase 2 (TIMP 2)

1 INTRODUCTION

CSOM accompanied by cholesteatomas has been known to disturb the balance between bone formation and resorption. This condition is associated with damage to structures of the middle and inner ear, consequently resulting in conductive hearing loss, sensorineural hearing loss, facial nerve palsy, vestibular function disorder, or intracranial complications (Widyatama, 2014). The proteolytic erosion of the temporal bone is the key event in the pathognomonic course of cholesteatoma progression (Schonermark, 1996).

The balance between MMP and TIMP is essential in determining extracellular matrix integrity (Rezende, 2012).

Therefore, this study was conducted to determine the association between MMP 2 and TIMP 2 and bone destruction in atticoantral type CSOM in patients at Haji Adam Malik General Hospital, Medan.

2 MATERIALS AND METHOD

This analytical cross-sectional study included cases of CSOM in which surgery was performed and the cholesteatoma taken and made into paraffin blocks.

Immunohistochemical testing of the paraffin blocks was performed at the anatomical pathology installation of Haji Adam Malik General Hospital, Medan.

2.1 Study sample

Patients diagnosed with the atticoantral type CSOM. The cholesteatomas have been operated upon in these patients and made into paraffin blocks.

2.2 Inclusion criteria

Cholesteatoma samples obtained from a mastoidectomy surgery on patients diagnosed with atticoantral type CSOM.

2.3 Exclusion criteria

Cholesteatoma samples, on which an adequate histopathological or immunohistochemical examination could not be performed due to an unrepresentative or damaged paraffin block based on the assessment of the anatomical, pathological installation, were excluded from this study.

2.4 Operational definition

Cholesteatomas defined as cystic lesions extending to the temporal bone lined by stratified squamous epithelium containing desquamated keratin (Son, 2013).

MMP 2 is a nucleus cell induced protein which is associated with several characteristics such as tumour development consisting of growth, invasion, metastasis and angiogenesis (blood vessel growth), in accordance with Sun & Hemler (2001) who found MMP 2 extracellular interactions. It is described as a proteolytic enzyme with the ability to decrease connective tissue components (Morales, 2007). Furthermore, TIMP 2 was defined as a specific endogenous protein inhibitor that inhibits MMP, especially MMP 2 (Murphy, 2011).

The degree of bone destruction was assessed by observing the damage extent on temporal CT scan, and was classified according to Kuczkowski et al., (2011) with the following degrees; mild degree: scutum and ossicleerotion, moderate degree: tegmen and entire ossicle destruction, severe degree: destruction of the ossicle, labyrinth bone, facial canal, and outer ear (Kuczkowski et al., 2011).

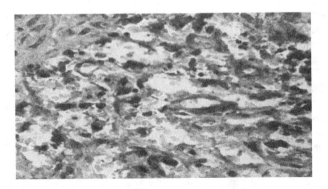

Figure 1.   Overexpression of MMP 2 and TIMP 2.

2.5 Variables

Factors that were presumed to affect bone destruction due to cholesteatoma were set as independent variables. These dependent variables were MMP 2 and TIMP 2. Assessment of MMP 2/TIMP 2 immunoreactivity was also obtained by multiplying the extent score with the intensity score, resulting in the MMP 2/TIMP 2 immunoreactivity score.

2.6 Materials and instruments

Medical records of the patients from which the paraffin blocks were extracted and the immunohistochemistry kit.

2.7 Procedure

Cholesteatoma was taken during a mastoidectomy surgery and then put into formalin 10%. Immunohistochemical images were then assessed using a fluorescence microscope by two anatomical pathology specialists.

2.8 Data management

In this study, the main data comprised secondary data which was paraffin blocks from cholesteatoma tissues. Other secondary data were obtained from patients' medical records.

3 RESULT

A total of 40 paraffin blocks were obtained, retrieved from 27 men and 13 women, during the study period.

The results displayed in Table 1 show that this study was dominated by samples with MMP 2 overexpression (36 sample, 90%). However, samples that overexpressed and did not overexpress TIMP 2 were relatively even, 21 (52.5%) and 19 (47.5%), respectively. Furthermore, based on a degree of bone destruction, 19 samples (47.5%) categorised as moderate bone destruction dominated this study, with only three samples categorised as mild bone destruction (7.5%).

Results from Table 2 showed that MMP 2 expression was not significantly associated with TIMP 2, with p-value = 0.342. Of 36 samples with MMP 2 overexpression, 19 (52.8%) had TIMP 2 overexpression and 17 with no TIMP 2 overexpression.

Table 1. Distribution of atticoantral type CSOM based on the degree of MMP 2, TIMP 2 expression and bone destruction.

Characteristic	(n = 40)	%
Expression MMP2		
Overexpression (Score 4–9)	36	90
No Overexpression (0–3)	4	10
Expression TIMP 2		
Overexpression (Score 4–9)	21	52,5
No Overexpression (0–3)	19	47,5
Bone destruction		
Mild	3	7.5
Moderate	19	47.5
Severe	18	45

Table 2. Association between MMP 2 expression and TIMP 2 in atticoantral type CSOM.

MMP 2	TIMP 2				
	Expression	%	No expression	%	P
Expression	19	52.8	2	50	0,342
No Expression	17	47.2	2	50	
Total	36	100	4	100	

*Fisher Exact Test.

Table 3. Association between MMP 2 expression and bone destruction in atticoantral type CSOM.

TIMP 2	Bone distraction								
	Mild		Moderate		Severe		Total		P
	N	%	N	%	N	%	N	%	
No Expression	2	66.7	11	57.9	8	44.5	21	52.5	0,165
Expression	1	33.3	8	42.1	10	55.5	19	47.5	
Total	3	100	19	100	18	50	40	100	

*Chi-Square.

The proportion of MMP 2 and TIMP 2 expression associated with the degree of bone destruction is displayed in Table 3. Statistical analysis showed that expression of TIMP 2 was not significantly correlated with the degree of bone destruction ($p = 0.165$, $p > 0.05$).

4 DISCUSSION

Inflammations that promote epithelial proliferation is associated with increased expression of lysis enzymes that could further stimulate osteoclast differentiation and maturation or react to bone matrix, therefore exposing the osteoclast.

This could cause bone extracellular matrix degradation resulting in bone erosion and destruction that could further complicate the atticoantral type of CSOM (Frickmann & Zautner, 2012). Matrix metalloproteinases and TIMPs have contradicting functions, therefore a sample that overexpresses MMP should at the same time not overexpress TIMP.

The contradictive results obtained in this study may be because of the different intensity and extent scores that were seen on immunohistochemically examining MMP 2 and TIMP 2, and then maybe we cannot know matrix of cholesteatoma because we used block paraffin of cholesteatoma retrospectively. Also, there are many other cytokines inflammation and inhibitor influence bone destruction in CSOM patients.

REFERENCES

Chole, R.A. & Nason, R. (2009). Chronic otitis media and cholesteatoma. In Snow, J.B. & Ballenger, J.J. (Eds.), *Ballenger's manual of otorhinology head and neck surgery* (pp. 217–27). Connecticut: BC Decker Inc.

Frickmann, H. & Zautner, A.E. (2012). Cholesteatoma—A potential consequence of chronic middle ear inflammation. *Otolaryngology S:5.*

Kuczkowski, J., Sakowicz-Burkiewicz, M., Iżycka-Świeszewska, E., Mikaszewski, B. & Pawełczyk, T. (2011). Expression of tumor necrosis Factor-A, Interleukin-1α, Interleukin-6 and Interleukin-10 in chronic otitis media with bone osteolysis. *Journal for Oto-rhino-laryngology and its Related Specialities, 73*(2), 93–9.

Murphy. (2011). Tissue inhibitors of metalloproteinases. *Genome Biology,* 12, 233.

Orji, F.T. (2013). A survey of the burden of management of chronic suppurative otitis media in a developing country. *Annals of Medical and Health Sciences Research, 3*(4).

Rezende, Souto, Rapoport, Campos, Generato. (2012). Cholesteatoma gene expression of matrix metalloproteinases and their inhibitors by RT-PCR. *Brazilian Journal of Otorhinolaryngology, 78* (3), 116–21.

Schonermark, Mester, Kempf, Blaser, Tschesche, Lenarz. (1996). Expression of matrix-metalloproteinases and their inhibitors in human cholesteatomas. Department of Oto- Rhino-Laryngology, Hannover Medical School, Germany and Department of the Biochemistry University of Bielefeld Germany. *Acta Otolaryngol (Stockh)*, 451–6.

Son, E. (2013). *Cholesteatoma, an overview.* Grand Rounds Presentation Dept. of Otorhinolaryngology Head and Neck Surgery. The University of Texas Medical Branch (UTMB) Health.

Sudiana, I. & Ketut, (2005). *Teknologi ilmu jaringan dan imunohistokimia.* Jakarta: SagungSeto.

Sun, J. & Hemler, M.E. (2001). Regulation of MMP-1 and MMP-2 production through CD147/ extracellular matrix metalloproteinase inducer interactions. *Cancer Research 61*, 2276–2281.

Widyatama, Handoko, Wahyudiono. (2014). Hubungan kadar Interleukin-6 Kolesteatoma dengan derajat kerusakan tulang pendengaran pasien otitis media supuratif kronik. Bagian Ilmu kesehatan Telinga Hidung tenggorok Bedah Kepaladan Leher Fakultas Kedokteran Universitas Brawijaya Malang. ORLI Vol. 44 No. 2 Tahun.

World Health Organization (2004). *Chronic supportive otitis media. The burden of illness and management options.* Geneva, Switzerland: WHO.

Stem Cell Oncology – Adella (Ed.)
© 2018 Taylor & Francis Group, London, ISBN 978-0-8153-9272-9

Anti-EGFR nimotuzumab for DIPG in recurrent or children with high grade glioma: 10 years

U. Bone
Department of Paediatric Hematology/Oncology, University of Bonn Medical School, Bonn, Germany

R. Cabanas
Department of Oncohematology, Juan Manuel Marquez Pediatric Hospital, Havana, Cuba

G. Saurez-Martinez, T. Crombet Ramos & P. Lorenzo-Luaces
Center of Molecular Immunology, Havana, Cuba

M. Massimino
Pediatric Unit, Fondazione IRCCS Istituto Nazionale dei Tumori (INT), Milano, Italy

U. Bartels & E. Bouffet
The Hospital for Sick Children, Toronto, Canada

F. Bach & D. Reuter
Oncoscience GmbH, Hamburg, Germany

R.A. Ilyas, R. Ellerson & N. Iznaga-Escobar
InnoCIMAb Pte Ltd., Singapore

ABSTRACT: Children glioma is a life-threatening condition with a survival rate of less than one year. Nimotuzumab, a unique and affinity differentiated anti-EGFR antibody for the past ten years had been used in combination with radiotherapy or radiochemotherapy. The aim of these studies was to evaluate nimotuzumab in combination with radiotherapy or radiochemotherapy in newly diagnosed children with DIPG. Patients received i.v. infusions of 150 mg/m^2 of nimotuzumab in combination with 54 Gy radiotherapy or radiochemotherapy for DIPG patients or 150 mg/m^2 of nimotuzumab as monotherapy on high-grade glioma, weekly, for 6–8 weeks, and then every 2–3 weeks until disease progression or unacceptable toxicity. A total of 87 newly diagnosed children with DIPG (35 male/52 female), median age 7.6 yr old were recruited. Use of nimotuzumab had been efficacious in newly diagnosis children with DIPG and recurrent or refractory children with high-grade glioma.

Keywords: anti-EGFR, nimotuzumab, DIPG

1 INTRODUCTION

Glioma is a rare but devastating cancer. Although temozolomide is currently the first-line standard of care for the treatment of glioma, temozolomide has shown minimal activity in high-grade glioma of childhood with no convincing evidence of its activity in diffuse intrinsic pontine glioma (DIPG) (Fangusaro, 2012). To date, there is no standard therapy to treat newly diagnosed DIPG or recurrent or relapse high-grade glioma in children and adolescents.

Nimotuzumab, formerly called h-R3, is a genetically engineered humanized mAb that recognizes an epitope located in the extracellular domain of human EGFR. It is an IgG$_1$ isotype that was obtained by transplanting the complementary determining regions (CDR) of the murine anti-EGFR mAb ior egf/r3 (IgG_{2a}) to a human framework assisted by computer modeling (Mateo, 1997).

Nimotuzumab blocks EGF and TGFα binding to the EGFR receptor and inhibits its intrinsic tyrosine kinase activity. In preclinical studies, nimotuzumab showed antiproliferative, proapoptotic, and antiangiogenic effects in tumors that overexpress EGFR, and enhanced radiosensitivity with reduction of tumor blood vessels and proliferation in the human GBM cell line U87MG (Diaz et al., 2009).

The aim of these studies was to evaluate nimotuzumab in combination with radiotherapy or radiochemotherapy in newly diagnosed children with DIPG or as monotherapy in recurrent or refractory children with high-grade glioma, as assessed by overall survival.

2 MATERIAL AND METHODS

2.1 Study objectives

a. **Study OSAG 101-BSC-05:** Multicentre phase III trial to explore the feasibility and efficacy of the h-R3 monoclonal antibody (nimotuzumab) simultaneously to conventionally fractionated local radiotherapy in the treatment of children and adolescents with newly diagnosed DIPG.

b. **Study IIC RD EC-097/EF-090:** To evaluate the efficacy of nimotuzumab in children and adolescents with newly diagnosed brain stem gliomas.

c. **Study BN-001 PED-04:** To evaluate the effectiveness of a humanized EGFR antibody on the treatment of pediatric and adolescents with chemotherapy-resistant high-grade glioma.

d. **Study YMB-1000-013:** to determine the efficacy of the use of the EGF-R antibody nimotuzumab monotherapy in the treatment of recurrent or refractory brain stem glioma.

e. **Expanded Access Program:** to evaluate the effectiveness of the monotherapy treatment of the anti-EGFR monoclonal antibody nimotuzumab in children and adolescents with recurrent or refractory high-grade glioma.

2.2 Inclusion/exclusion criteria

2.2.1 First line treatment on newly diagnosed DIPG patients

Inclusion criteria: pediatric patients with newly diagnosed DIPG which have been documented by conventional imagery methods (MRI, CAT), Age ≥3 years old ≤18 years old, life expectancy ≥12 weeks, laboratory parameters for hematological, liver and renal functions must be within the normal defined limits, and both parents or legal guardian(s) must express in writing the will to allow the patient to participate in the study by signing the informed consent within others.

Exclusion criteria: patients with low grade brain stem glioma (i.e. focal, cerebromedullary, tectal brain stem gliomas), patients previously treated with a monoclonal antibody, patients who previously received some type of cancer treatment including chemotherapy, immunotherapy or radiation therapy, concurrent cancer treatment which is not part of the study protocol, pregnant or nursing patients, patients with a chronic disease (i.e. cardiopathy, diabetes, high blood pressure) at the time of inclusion, patients with hypersensitivity to the drug or to a similar drug, febrile condition, severe septic condition and/or serious or acute allergic condition, patients participating in another clinical study with the intent to treat their tumor at the time of inclusion and presence of a second tumor.

2.2.2 Recurrent or refractory high-grade glioma

Inclusion criteria: histologically verified diagnosis of a high-grade glioma (WHO III and IV) (not applicable or necessary for intrinsic pontine glioma) who were in progression after several lines of treatment, age ≥3 years to ≤20 years, adequate hematological, renal, and hepatic function (CTC grade ≤2), condition is measurable by X-ray in at least one dimension, life expectancy ≥4 weeks and written consent from parents/legal guardian, and, if possible, children, after being informed.

Exclusion criteria: a history of prior use of EGFR-targeting agents (monoclonal antibodies, tyrosine kinase inhibitors), recent introduction of an "alternative" curative treatment method after progressive diagnosis, and during this study, more than one line of treatment (i.e. more than one progression after initial therapy) for the disease, had radiation therapy completed within 12 weeks of enrollment, previous chemotherapy completed ≤2 weeks prior to enrollment, and pregnancy in females of childbearing age.

2.3 Treatment schedule

2.3.1 First line treatment on newly diagnosed DIPG patients

Eligible patients for studies OSAG 101-BSC-05 and IIC RD EC-097/EF-090 were administered i.v. infusion of 150 mg/m^2 of nimotuzumab once a week for 6 weeks and then if patients had stable disease or better response additional 150 mg/m^2 of nimotuzumab every two weeks until disease progression or unacceptable toxicity and radiotherapy 54 Gy based on 1.8 Gy daily for 5 days a week for 6 weeks.

2.3.2 Recurrent or refractory high-grade glioma

Eligible patients from studies BN-001 PED-04, YMB-1000-013, and Expanded Access Program were administered i.v. infusion of 150 mg/m^2 of nimotuzumab once a week for six weeks and them if stable disease or better response additional 150 mg/m^2 every two or three weeks until disease progression or unacceptable toxicity.

2.4 Statistical analysis

Analysis of demography, baseline characteristics, safety, and efficacy were performed on the data set of all treated patients.

Demographics and baseline characteristics: were summarized using descriptive statistics.

Primary efficacy analysis: The primary estimate of median overall survival (OS), progression-free-survival (PFS), overall response rate (ORR) and disease control rate (DCR) was estimated by Intent-To-Treat population.

The primary analysis of survival was conducted using a log-rank test using Kaplan-Meier curves. Median OS, PFS and their 95% confidence interval (CI) were calculated by each tumor localization using a Cox, regression model.

3 RESULT

3.1 Patients demographics

A total of 87 newly diagnosed children with DIPG (35 male/52 female), median age 7.6 yr old were recruited in 2 clinical studies in Brazil, Cuba, Germany, Italy and Russia and 113 recurrent or refractory children with high-grade glioma (60 male/53 female), median age 9.9 yr old were recruited in 2 clinical studies and 2 physician lead studies in Canada, Cuba, Germany and United States (Table 1).

3.2 Clinical response to the treatment

3.2.1 First line treatment on DIPG patients

In the study OSAG 101-BSC-05, there were four patients with partial remissions, 27 stable disease and eight patients progressed. The overall response rate (ORR) in this study was 9.5%, and the disease control rate (DCR) was 73.8%, and in the study IIC RD EC-097/EF-090, there were 20 patients with partial remission, 14 patients with stable disease and 11 patients progressed. The ORR on this study was 44.4%, and the DCR was 75.5% (Table 2).

Table 1. Patient demographic characteristics.

Study number	No. pts	Sex Male	Sex Female	Median age (yr)	Tumor localiz.
OSAG 101-BSC-05	42	16	26	7.6	DIPG
IIC RD EC-097/EF-090	45	19	26	7.9	DIPG
	22	17	5	8.9	DIPG
BN-001 PED-04	13	7	6	12.2	GBM
	12	5	7	10.3	AA
YMB-1000-013	46	21	25	6.0	DIPG
Expanded Access 1	3	0	3	10.8	AA
	9	5	4	10.0	DIPG
Expanded Access 2	5	3	2	10.2	GBM
	3	2	1	8.3	AA

DIPG, diffuse intrinsic pontine glioma, GBM, glioblastoma, AA, anaplastic astrocytoma.

Table 2. Clinical response to the treatment.

Study number	Indication	Treatment	ORR (%)	DCR (%)
OSAG 101-BSC-05	DIPG	RT + nimotuzumab	9.52	73.8
IIC RD EC-097/EF-090	DIPG	RT + nimotuzumab	44.4	75.6
	DIPG	nimotuzumab	4.56	50.0
BN-001 PED-04	GBM	nimotuzumab	0	23.1
	AA	nimotuzumab	8.33	25.0
YMB-1000-013	DIPG	nimotuzumab	4.4	19.6
Expanded Access 1	AA	nimotuzumab	0	0
	DIPG	nimotuzumab	33.3	55.6
Expanded Access 2	GBM	nimotuzumab	0	0
	AA	nimotuzumab	33.3	66.7

RT, radiotherapy, ORR, overall response rate, DCR, disease control rate.

3.2.2 Recurrent or refractory high-grade glioma

In the study BN-001 PED-04 on the DIPG tumors, there was one patient with partial remission, ten stable disease and 11 patients progressed. The ORR was 4.56%, and the DCR was 50.0%. On the GBM tumors, there were three stable diseases, and ten patients progressed. The DCR was 23.1%, and on the AA tumors, there was one patient with partial remission, two stable disease and eight patients progressed. The ORR was 8.33%, and the DCR was 25.0% (Table 2).

On the Expanded Access 1 on the AA tumors, the patient did not receive the response to the treatment.

On the Expanded Access 2 on the DIPG tumors, there were two patients with complete remission, one patients with partial remission, two patients with stable disease and four patients progressed. The ORR was 33.3%, and the DCR was 55.6%.

On the GMB tumors, all five patients did not respond to the treatment, and on the AA tumors, there were one patients with complete remission, one stable disease and one patient who progressed. The ORR was 33.3%, and the DCR was 66.7% (Table 2).

3.3 Progression-Free Survival (PFS) and Overall Survival (OS)

3.3.1 First line treatment on DIPG patients

In the study OSAG 101-BSC-05, DIPG patients following treatment with radiotherapy and nimotuzumab had a median PFS [95% CI] of 5.6 months [5.04, 6.16] and a median OS [95%

254

Table 3. Progression free survival and overall survival.

Parameter	OSAG 101-BSC-05	IIC RD EC-097/EF-090
Treatment	RT + nimotuzumab	RT + nimotuzumab
No of Patients	42	45
PFS (months) [95% CI]	5.60	8.23
	[5.04–6.16]	[6.47–9.99]
one yr PFS rate (%)	5.3	33.3
OS (months) [95% CI]	9.2	9.7
	[7.55–10.85]	[7.99–11.41]
1-yr OS rate (%)	33.3	42.2

CI] of 9.2 months [7.55, 10.85]. The 1-year PFS and OS rate were 5.3% and 33.3% respectively and in the study IIC RD EC-097/EF-090, DIPG patients following treatment with radiotherapy and nimotuzumab had a median PFS [95% CI] of 8.23 months [6.47, 9.99] and a median OS [95% CI] of 9.7 months [7.99, 11.41]. The 1-year PFS and OS rates were 33.3% and 42.2% respectively (Table 3).

3.3.2   Recurrent or refractory high-grade glioma

In the study BN-001 PED-04, the DIPG patients who at the time of the inclusion in the study were in progression and had a life-expectancy of at least 4 weeks following treatment of nimotuzumab monotherapy had a median PFS [95% CI] of 1.53 months [1.04, 2.02] and a median OS [95% CI] of 4.67 months [2.48, 6.85]. The 1-year PFS and OS rates were 4.5% and 9.1% respectively. The GBM patients had a median PFS [95% CI] of 1.67 months [1.61, 1.72] and a median OS [95% CI] of 3.47 months [2.93, 4.00]. The 1-year PFS and OS rate were 0% respectively, and the AA patients had a median PFS [95% CI] of 1.67 months [1.29, 2.04] and a median OS [95% CI] of 6.33 months [1.51, 11.0]. The 0.5-year PFS rate was 16.7%, and the 1-year OS rate was 25.0%. In the study YMB-1000-01, the DIPG patients who at the time of the inclusion in the study were in progression and had a life-expectancy of at least 4 weeks following treatment of nimotuzumab monotherapy had a median PFS [95% CI] of 1.8 months [1.51, 2.10] and a median OS [95% CI] of 3.1 months [1.89, 4.31]. The 0.5-year PFS rate was 4.8%, and the 1-year OS rate was 7.6%, and in the Expanded Access Program 2, patients after receiving nimotuzumab monotherapy had a median OS [95% CI] of 9.17 months [4.28, 14.1] and 1-yr OS rate of 35.3%.

3.4   Safety and tolerability of the treatment

3.4.1   First line treatment on DIPG

In the studies, OSAG 101-BSC-05 and IIC RD-EC-097/EF-090 patients received a median of 20.6 infusions of nimotuzumab (range 1–28). These patients experienced a total of 937 adverse events (AEs) reported in 77 patients (88.5%). Out of 937 AEs, 118 AEs in 35 patients (40.2%) were reported to be possible, probable or definite related to the administration of nimotuzumab and radiotherapy. The most frequently reported related AEs (>5 patients, 5.75%) were vomiting (11 subjects, 12.64%), headache (7 subjects, 8.05%), alopecia (6 subjects, 6.90%), and constipation (5 subjects, 5.75) (Table 4).

3.4.2   Recurrent or refractory high-grade glioma

In the studies, BN-001 PED-04 and YMB-1000-013 these patients experienced a total of 645 adverse events (AEs) reported in 86 patients (94.5%). Out of 645 AEs, 98 AEs in 46 patients (50.5%) were reported to be possible, probable or definite related to the administration of nimotuzumab. The most frequently reported related AEs (>5 patients, 5.49%) were nausea (7 subjects, 7.69%), leukopenia (6 subjects, 6.59%), vomiting (5 subjects, 5.49%), fatigue (5 subjects, 5.49%), and erythema (5 subjects, 5.49%) (Table 5).

Table 4. Percentage of subjects with all grades related AEs occurring in more than 5.0%.

System organ class preferred term	RT (54 Gy) + nimotuzumab (150 mg/m²) (N = 87)
	N[1] (%)
Gastrointestinal disorders	
Constipation	5 (5.75%)
Vomiting	11 (12.64%)
Nervous system disorder	
Headache	7 (8.1%)
Skin and subcutaneous tissue disorders	
Alopecia	6 (6.90%)

[1]Reported number and percentages based on number of patients.

Table 5. Percentage of subjects with all grades related AEs were occurring in more than 5.0%.

System organ class preferred term	Nimotuzumab (150 mg/m²) (N = 91)
	N[1] (%)
Blood and lymphatic system disorders	
Leukopenia	6 (6.59%)
Gastrointestinal disorders	
Nausea	7 (7.69%)
Vomiting	5 (5.49%)
General disorders and administration site conditions	
Fatigue	5 (5.49%)
Skin and subcutaneous tissue disorders	
Erythema	5 (5.49%)

[1]Reported number and percentages based on number of patients.

4 DISCUSSION

Brain tumors are a heterogeneous group of neoplasms, each with its biology, treatment, and prognosis. New therapies are needed, especially for the astrocytic gliomas. In particular brain stem gliomas (BSG) remain the most problematic childhood brain tumor to treat. BSG comprises 10–15% of all pediatric CNS tumors and is uncommon in the adult population. Peak incidence is between 5–9 years of age but may occur anytime in the childhood. These lesions tend to be located in the pons and are termed diffuse intrinsic pontine gliomas (DIPG), which constitute approximately 75–80% of all childhood brain stem gliomas. This DIPG will respond transiently to radiotherapy but have not yet been shown to benefit from the addition of chemotherapy (Paker et al., 1990). After radiotherapy, progressive disease and death will occur in approximately 90% of the patients within 8–10 months of diagnosis.

The treatment of radiotherapy in combination with the anti-EGFR monoclonal antibody nimotuzumab increased the progression-free survival and overall survival of newly diagnosed children and adolescents with DIPG. The addition of nimotuzumab to radiotherapy increased 1-yr OS rate to 38% in newly diagnosed children and adolescents with DIPG.

The use of nimotuzumab monotherapy in recurrent or refractory heavily pretreated children and adolescents with high-grade glioma can achieve an overall response rate (ORR) of 7.1%, and a disease control rate (DCR) of 29.2%.

Nimotuzumab monotherapy in recurrent or refractory heavily pretreated children and adolescents with high-grade glioma increases median PFS to 1.83 months, median OS to 3.90 months, 1-yr PFS rate to 7.1% and 1-yr OS rate to 12.6%.

Use of nimotuzumab had been efficacious in newly diagnosis children with DIPG and in recurrent or refractory children with high grade glioma.

REFERENCES

Diaz-Miqueli A., Rolff J., Lemm M., Fichtner I., Perez R., Montero E. 2009. Radiosensitisation of U87MG brain tumors by anti-epidermal growth factor monoclonal antibodies. British J of Cancer, 100:950–958.

Fangusaro, L. 2012. Pediatric High Grade Glioma: a Review and Update on Tumor Clinical Characteristics and Biology. Front Oncol, 2, 105.

Mateo C., Moreno E., Amour K., Lombardero J., Harris W., Pérez R. 1997. Humanization of a mouse monoclonal antibody that blocks the epidermal growth factor receptor: Recovery of antagonistic activity. Immunotechnology 7;3:71–81.

Packer RJ., Allen JC., Goldwein JL. 1990. Hyperfractionated radiotherapy for children with brain stem gliomas: a pilot study using 7,200 cGy. Ann Neurol; 27:167–173.

Stem Cell Oncology – Adella (Ed.)
© 2018 Taylor & Francis Group, London, ISBN 978-0-8153-9272-9

Diagnostic for TTNA using a thoracic ultrasound guidance for diagnosing lung cancer

N.N. Soeroso, S. Saragih, F.K. Munthe & S.P. Tarigan
Department of Pulmonology and Respiratory Medicine, Faculty of Medicine, Universitas Sumatera Utara, Medan, North Sumatera, Indonesia

F. Zalukhu
The Amsterdam Institute for Social Science Research, University of Amsterdam, Amsterdam, The Netherlands

N. Lubis
Department of Radiology, Faculty of Medicine, Universitas Sumatera Utara, Medan, North Sumatera, Indonesia

ABSTRACT: Transthoracic Needle Aspiration (TTNA) for diagnosing thoracic lesions are usually performed with image guidance, including thoracic computed tomography scan and thoracic ultrasound. The aim of this study is to describe the characteristics of samples, and diagnostic accuracy of TTNA using US guidance compare to CT guidance. Image-guided TTNA were performed in 91 consecutive patients suspected of lung cancer on clinically and radiological work-up. Image guidance was selected randomly. The final diagnosis was based on cytology analysis or clinical follow-up. For thoracic ultrasound guided TTNA, the accuracy, sensitivity, specificity, were 87.8%, 91.6%, and 77.7%, respectively. For thoracic CT-guided TTNA the accuracy, sensitivity, specificity, were 86.84%, 78.3%, and 100%. Thoracic US-guided TTNA had a high sensitivity and specificity in lesions that abut the chest wall.

Keywords: diagnostic accuracy for transthoracic needle aspiration using an Ultrasound thoracic compared thoracic ct scan guided, lung cancer

1 INTRODUCTION

Transthoracic Needle Aspiration (TTNA) was first used for the diagnosis of pulmonary disease in 1883 when Leyden performed the procedure on three patients with pneumonia. In 1886, Menetrier reported the use of TTNA in the diagnosis of lung carcinoma. Since that time, many published series have explained the method of TTNA for the diagnosis of a variety of benign and malignant thoracic lesions (Kern & McLennan, 2008).

The significant indications for TTNA include evaluation of solitary lung nodules and masses, mediastinal and hilar lesions, metastatic disease to the lung from a known extrathoracic malignancy, chest wall invasion by lung carcinoma, and pulmonary consolidation or infiltrates that are likely to be of infectious origin (Kern & McLennan, 2008).

Transthoracic needle aspiration is performed with an image guidance, including Thoracic Computed Tomography (CT) and Thoracic Ultra Sound (US). Several previous published articles for a CT-guided TTNA (Schreiber & McCorry, 2003, ERS/ATS, 2002) and a US-guided TTNA (Saito et al, 1988, Yang et al, 1992, Knudsen et al, 1996, Taviad et al, 2014) have illustrated their role as an active guidance modality for diagnosing intra thoracic lesions. In our facility, a tertiary referral hospital (Adam Malik general hospital, we usually perform TTNA using the CT guidance with good performance, but many other services in our area do not have this equipment, only US. In this paper, our purpose was to describe the characteristics of samples and diagnostic accuracy for transthoracic needle aspiration using the US guidance compared to the CT guidance for diagnosing lung cancer.

2 METHOD

From 1st February 2015 to 29th February 2016, 91 consecutive patients underwent TTNA. All patients were suspected of lung cancer on clinical and radiological work-up. At the time of TTNA, all patients had standard or corrected coagulation parameters (prothrombin time and activated partial thromboplastin time) and platelet count. Written informed consent was obtained in all cases. The image guidance was selected randomly.

The technique for the CT-guided biopsies was as follows: preliminary 5-mm-collimated CT scans were obtained to localize the lesion and select the optimal approach. A CT scan Toshiba asteion slice 4, CXB-400C/1A was used. The skin entry site was marked by using the laser light from the CT gantry and a grid placed on the patient's skin. Additional scans were obtained during a passage of the needle through the chest wall and into the lesion to allow adjustment of the needle direction and to record the position of the needle tip inside the target before sampling.

Our technique for the US-guided TTNA was as follows: preliminary localizing scans were obtained by using 3.5-MHz or 4-MHz multi-frequency sector transducers or a 5-MHz linear transducer (Sonix 01: Ultrasonix Medical Corporation S/N: SX1.1-0809.1841). When necessary, color Doppler was used to detecting potential vessels in the path of the needle. The scans were obtained with the patient in the supine, prone, or decubitus. Frequently, the aspiration was performed by using US transducer with a needle-guide attachment, but in our setting, we used a separate transducer and needle. We marked the location and inserted the needle separately. The transthoracic needle aspiration was performed by using a 25-gauge needle for both images guidance. The aspiration was performed either by one of our pulmonologists with a subspecialty in thoracic oncology or pulmonology residents under the close supervision of the pulmonologist.

The specimens were handled similarly regardless of the guidance modality used: each fine-needle aspirate was immediately smeared onto glass slides, air-dried, fixed by using alcohol 96% and sent to the pathology department for further examination. The diagnostic categories used in cytology of TTNA were inadequate (C1), benign (C2), atypical (C3), suspicious of malignancy (C4), and malignant (C5) according to the National Cancer Institute (NCI) guidelines in 1996 (NCI, 1997).

At the completion of the procedure, all patients were monitored for the signs and symptoms of complication, such as hemoptysis and pneumothorax. The location and size of the lesion, the diagnostic accuracy, and any complications were also recorded.

The success of each procedure was established at a review of the final pathology report and cultures when appropriate. We attempted to obtain a clinical and imaging follow-up in cases where a diagnosis of malignancy was not established.

3 RESULT

During the study period, a total 91 TTNA were done, 46 (50.5%) were performed with the US guidance, and 45 (49.5%) were performed with the CT guidance.

There were no pneumothorax or hemoptysis associated with the US-guided or the CT-guided TTNA.

For the US-guided TTNA, the accuracy, sensitivity, and specificity were 87.87%, 91.6%, and 77.7%, respectively. On the other hand, for the CT-guided TTNA, the accuracy, sensitivity, and specificity were 86.84%, 78.3%, and 100%, respectively.

Table 1. Baseline characteristics of 91 patient underwent TTNA randomised to US guidance or CT guidance.

Characteristics	US-guided TTNA (n = 46)	CT-guided TTNA (n = 45)
Mean (SD) age (years)	54.76 (12.89)	50.46 (16.78)
Age (years)		
18–30	4 (8.7)	9 (20)
31–40	1 (2.2)	1 (2.2)
41–50	10 (21.7)	9 (20)
51–60	15 (32.6)	11 (24.4)
61–70	14 (30.4)	10 (22.2)
71–80	2 (4.3)	5 (11.1)
Male	35 (76.1)	36 (80)
Final diagnosis		
Lung cancer	33 (71.7)	28 (62.2)
Others	13 (28.3)	17 (37.8)
Mediastinal tumor	12 (26.1)	15 (33.3)
Chest wall tumor	1 (2.2)	0 (0)
Aspergilloma	0 (0)	2 (4.4)
Smoking history		
Smoker	37 (80.4)	32 (71.1)
Non-smoker	9 (19.6)	13 (28.9)

Table 2. Comparison of TTNA cytology using different guidance. Values are numbers (percentages).

Smears classification	US-guided TTNA (n = 46)	CT-guided TTNA (n = 45)
C1	7 (15.2)	4 (8.9)
C2	6 (13)	12 (26.67)
C3	1 (2.2)	1 (2.2)
C4	2 (4.3)	0 (0)
C5	30 (65.2)	28 (62.23)

Table 3. Comparison of diameter of lesion, depth of needle insertion, and position of patients in both groups.

	US-guided TTNA (n = 46)	CT-guided TTNA (n = 45)
Diameter of lesion (SD)		
Mean (SD)	9.81 cm (4.1)	6.12 cm (2.76)
Median (min–max)	9.3 cm (3–19)	5.7 cm (3–16)
Depth of needle insertion		
Mean (SD)	3.58 cm (1.11)	5 cm (1.21)
Median (min–max)	4 cm (1.4–6)	5 cm (2–8)
Position of patients (n, %)		
Supine	38 (82.6)	36 (80)
Prone	3 (6.25)	9 (20)
Left Lateral Decubitus (LLD)	2 (4.35)	0 (0)
Right Lateral Decubitus (RLD)	3 (6.25)	0 (0)

4 DISCUSSION

The imaging-guided transthoracic needle aspiration (TTNA) has achieved a great importance in the diagnosis of a variety of thoracic lesions. Due to simplicity, safety, and diagnostic accuracy, this procedure has become a widely used diagnostic technique in the management of lung cancer. This process is performed under the US guidance or the CT guidance (Schreiber & McCorry, 2003, ERS/ATS, 2002).

The National Cancer Institute recommends five categories for a diagnosis of aspiration cytology to bring a degree of uniformity in the diagnostic reports. These types are unsatisfactory (C1), benign lesion (C2), atypical, probably benign (C3), suspicious, probably malignant (C4), and malignant (C5) (NCI, 1997).

Our study found more inadequate smears for the US-guided TTNA compared with the CT-guided TTNA (7/46 [15.2%] versus 4/45 [8.9%]. We used the US with a separate transducer and needle, as we marked the location and inserted the needle separately, we could not evaluate the position of the needle tip directly, inside the tumor or not. Meanwhile, we conducted TTNA under the CT guidance to locate the site of needle insertion and made an additional scan to make sure that the tip of the needle was properly inserted into the lesion.

In terms of position of the patient during the performance of the procedure, we found four different locations in the US-guided TTNA: 38 patients (82.6%) in a supine position, 3 patients (6.25%) in a prone position, 2 patients (4.35%) in a RLD position, and 3 patients (6.25%) in a LLD position. On the other hand, patients under the CT guidance were performed TTNA only in two positions, 36 patients (80%) in a supine position and nine patients (20%) in a prone position. The approach for the needle placement in the CT guidance is usually limited to the axial plane. Angled approaches are more difficult in the CT guidance, and it is an advantage of using the US guidance. The US-guided TTNA allows the use of an oblique, angled approach if necessary (Liao et al., 2013).

In our study, the sensitivity of the US-guided TTNA was higher than the CT-guided (91.6% versus 78.3%). It can be explained by our findings that the average diameter of the lesion in the US group was larger than in the CT group (9.81 cm vs. 6.12 cm). The specificity of the US-guided TTNA was lower than the CT-guided (77.7% vs. 100%). This result can be explained by the fact that we did not use the US with a needle-guide attachment on the transducer to make a real-time visualization during the procedure. Meanwhile, on the CT-guided, the additional scan using the CT was performed to make a documentation of the needle tip's position if it was properly inserted into the mass.

Pneumothorax and minor bleeding are common complications of TTNA. The reported frequency of biopsy associated pneumothorax ranges from 20–35% (Hoffmann, Mauer, and Vokes, 2000). There were no pneumothorax or hemoptysis associated with the US-guided or the CT-guided TTNA in our study. All the lesions in this study were abutted the chest wall.

The limitation of this study was that we assessed complication by signs and symptoms. An immediate posteroanterior chest radiograph was obtained if pneumothorax was suspected clinically.

5 CONCLUSION

The results from our study demonstrated that with proper triaging of patients, the US-guided TTNA might be an attractive and safe alternative compared to the CT-guided TTNA, with a high sensitivity and specificity in lesions that abut the chest wall.

REFERENCES

ERS/ATS. 2002. ERS/ATS statement on interventional pulmonology. Eur Respir J. 19:356–373.
Hoffmann PC, Mauer AM, Vokes EE. 2000. Lung cancer. The Lancet. 355:479–85.

Kern JA, McLennan G. 2008. Genetic and molecular changes of human lung cancer. Dalam: Fishman AP, Elias JA, Fishman JA, editor. Fishman's Pulmonary diseases and disorders. 5th edition. New York: McGraw-Hill Companies. H. 1802–14.

Knudsen DU et al. 1996. Ultrasonographically guided fine-needle aspiration biopsy of intrathoracic tumors. Acta Radiol. 37:327–31.

Liao WC et al. 2013. Ultrasound diagnosis of chest disease. Available from: http://dx.doi.org/10.5772/55419.

NCI. 1997. "The uniform approach to breast fine-needle aspiration biopsy. National Cancer Institute Fine-Needle Aspiration of Breast Workshop Subcommittees" *Diagnostic Cytopathology*. vol. 16, no. 4, pp. 295–311, 1997.

Saito T et al. 1988. Ultrasonically guided needle biopsy in the diagnosis of mediastinal masses. Am Rev Respir Dis. 136:679–84.

Schreiber G, McCorry DC. 2003. Performance characteristics of different modalities for diagnosis of suspected lung cancer: Summary of Published Evidence. Chest. 123:115S-128S.

Taviad DS et al. 2014. Diagnostic value of ultrasound-guided transthoracic fine needle aspiration cytology in bronchogenic carcinoma. Int J Med Sci Public Health. 3:1007–10.

Yang PC et al. 1992. Ultrasonographically guided biopsy of thoracic tumors. A comparison of large-bore cutting biopsy with fine-needle aspiration. Cancer. 69(10):2553–60.

Stem Cell Oncology – Adella (Ed.)
© 2018 Taylor & Francis Group, London, ISBN 978-0-8153-9272-9

The CYP2A13 Arg257Cys polymorphism and its relationship to lung cancer

N.N. Soeroso & B.Y.M. Sinaga
Department Pulmonology and Respiratory Medicine, Faculty of Medicine, Universitas Sumatera Utara, Medan, North Sumatera, Indonesia

R. Zain-Hamid
Department of Pharmacology, Faculty of Medicine, Universitas Sumatera Utara, Medan, North Sumatera, Indonesia

A.H. Sadewa
Department of Biochemistry, Faculty of Medicine, Universitas Gadjah Mada, Yogyakarta, Indonesia

E. Syahruddin
Department Pulmonology and Respiratory Medicine, Faculty of Medicine, Universitas Indonesia, Medan, North Sumatera, Indonesia

ABSTRACT: A common polymorphism, Arg257Cys of CYP2A13 gene, is associated with lung cancer in several populations. The aim of this study was to analyse the relationship between this polymorphism and lung cancer in several ethnics of the Indonesia population. Consecutive sampling and case-control study were applied. The PCR-RFLP assay was employed to genotype. The chi-square test with $p < 0.05$ considered as significant. Of all 50 subjects, 26 (13%) individuals were heterozygotes, and 37 (74%) were homozygote for the 257Cys allele. The frequency distributions among ethnics were Acehnese two (5.4%) homozygote, Malay two (5.4%) homozygote, Chinese one (7.7%) heterozygote, 20 (54%) homozygote and six (46.1%) heterozygotes in Batak, 13 (35.1%) homozygote and six (46.1%) heterozygotes in Javanese. The CYP2A13 Arg257Cys variant represents a common polymorphism in Batak and Javanese ethnics. There is no association between Arg257Cys polymorphism of CYP2A13 and lung cancer.

Keywords: CYP2A13 gene, PCR-RFLP, lung cancer, Indonesia population

1 INTRODUCTION

Lung cancer is the most common cancer in the world, representing approximately 1.2 million lung cancer patient annually, which is leading cause of cancer death (Parkin et al., 2001). Lung cancer deaths contribute to more than 1 million deaths with the prediction of approximately 1.4 million people (Globocan, 2012). Since 1950, tobacco smoke has been recognised as the main cause of lung cancer and smoking has also become a life style. Lung cancer will be the health problem in the future (Medical Research Council, 1957). In Indonesia, tobacco smoke and smokeless tobacco is used by approximately 67.4% of the male and 4.5% of the female population. It means Indonesia has the most common tobacco use, approximately 61.4 million people (31.1% of the population), (Global Adult Tobacco Survey, 2011).

Cytochrome P450 2 A13 (CYP2A13) is expressed in the highest level in the human respiratory tract, in the nasal mucosa, lung, and trachea (Su et al., 2000). Several genetic polymorphisms of CYP2A13 Single Nucleotide Polymorphism (SNP) C3375T were identified. Polymorphism C3375T in exon 5 of CYP2A13 and changes in Arg257Cys are functionally important. The Arg-257Cys polymorphism provides some protection against xenobiotic toxicity to individuals who are homozygous for the Cys257 allele because the Cys257 variant had a > 2-fold less catalytic efficiency for Nicotine-derived Nitrosamine Ketone (NNK). However, this relationship is still controversial, and further study is needed in several ethnics (Cheng et al., 2004).

So far, there is still limited data regarding the Arg257Cys polymorphism of CYP2A13 in the Indonesia population. Therefore, the aim of this study is to identify this polymorphism and its relationship to lung cancer in the Indonesia population.

2 METHOD

2.1 Subjects

50 male subjects with a history of cigarette smoking were recruited in the study, 25 subjects with lung cancer compared with 25 healthy subjects. All subjects were patients in Adam Malik General Hospital. This study was approved by the Ethical Committee of Faculty of Medicine, Universitas Sumatera Utara, and obtained informed consent from each participant.

2.2 Blood acquisition and DNA isolation

3 ml of venous blood was collected from the mediana cubiti vein in a sterile tube containing EDTA and stored at 4°C in the refrigerator (Sambrook et al., 1989).

2.3 PCR-RFLP assay for genotyping

Exon 5 of the CYP2A13 gene was amplified using a forward primer 5'- CCTGGACAGAT-GCCTTTAACTCCG-3' paired with a reverse primer 5'- TGGCTTTGCACCTGCCT-GCACT-3'. PCR amplification was performed in a Bio-Rad DNA Model T-100 thermal cycler in a total volume of 25 μl containing approximately 200 ng of genomic DNA, 2.5 μl × PCR buffer 2 mmol/l MgCl2, 0.2 mmol/l of each dNTP, 0.28 μmol/l of each primer, and 2 U of Taq DNA polymerase. The PCR conditions involved an initial denaturation at 95°C for three minutes, followed by 35 cycles of denaturation at 95°C for 30 seconds, annealing at 63°C for 45 seconds, and extension at 72°C for 30 seconds, with a final extension at 72°C for five minutes. After amplification, the PCR products (332 bp) were digested with *HhaI* restriction. Endonuclease at 37°C for at least four hours. Digested products were analysed by electrophoresis on a 2% agarose gel in the presence of ethidium bromide (Zhang et al., 2003).

2.4 Statistical analysis

The chi-square test was used to compare genotypic frequencies between the case and control. The OR and 95% CI were calculated to determine the association between variables and the risk of lung cancer regarding the Arg257Cys polymorphism in both cases and controls. Statistical analyses were conducted using statistical software SPSS 17.0 for PC A p-value of < 0.05 was required for statistical significance.

3 RESULT

The characteristic of subject is shown in Table 1. Of all 50 participants, the overall frequency of genotype CC, CT and TT was 72%, 26%, and 2% respectively. The frequency of allele homozygote was 74%, while the heterozygote was 26%. Genotype distribution based on six groups of ethnicity revealed that Javanese and Batak had the highest frequency of CT genotype, 31.5%, and 23% respectively of Chinese participated in this study. The TT genotype was detected in one sample only (Table 2). The genotype distribution was in Hardy-Weinberg equilibrium.

This research failed to confirm the association between genetic polymorphism of CYP2A13 Arg257Cys and lung cancer susceptibility. Of all 25 cases and 25 controls, the combined genotype frequency of CT and TT was found to be 32% and 24% respectively (Table 2). Chi-square analysis revealed that there was no significant association between genetic polymorphism CYP2A13 Arg257Cys and lung cancer susceptibility (OR 0.67; 95% CI 0.19–2.32; $p = 0.52$). Figure 1 shows that the Arg257Cys mutation eliminates an *HhaI* cleavage site (Cheng et al., 2004).

Table 1. The characteristics of the subjects.

Subjects		Case n	Case %	Control n	Control %
Age	25–34 years old	–	–	19	76
	35–44 years old	1	4	5	20
	45–54 years old	3	12	1	4
	55–64 years old	15	60	–	–
	> 65 years old	6	24	–	–
Type of cigarette	Kretek	14	56	1	4
	Mild	8	32	22	88
	Kretek Mild	3	12	2	8
Brinkman Index	Mild	1	4	15	60
	Moderate	–	–	9	36
	Severe	24	96	1	4
Lung cancer	Adenocarcinoma	19	76	–	–
	Squamous cell ca	5	20	–	–
	Large cell ca	1	4	–	–
Ethnicity	Batak	16	64	10	40
	Javanese	4	16	15	60
	Acehnese	2	8	–	–
	Malay	2	8	–	–
	China	1	4	–	–
	Total	25	100	25	10

Table 2. CYP2A13 polymorphism and lung cancer.

	Case n	Case %	Control n	Control %	*p-value*	OR	95% CI
CC	17	34.0	19	38.0	0.529	0.671	0.193–2.329
CT&TT	8	16.0	6	12.0			
Total	25	100	25	100			

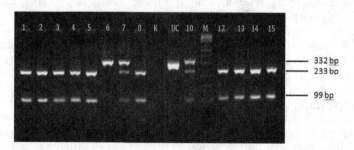

Figure 1. PCR-RFLP analysis of the *CYP2A13* Arg257Cys polymorphism with *Hha I*. M: DNA Marker, lane 6 was genotype with Cys/Cys at 257; lanes 7 and 10 were genotype with Arg/Cys at 257; lanes 1–5, 8, 12–15 were genotype with Arg/Arg at 257.

267

Table 3. CYP2A13 polymorphism and histologic type of lung cancer.

	Adenocarcinoma		Squamous cell carcinoma		Large cell carcinoma		
	n	%	n	%	n	%	p-value
CC	14	70	3	75	0	0	
CT	5	25	1	25	1	100	0.471
TT	1	5	0	0	0	0	
Total	20	100	4	100	1	100	

Furthermore, we evaluated the association of genetic polymorphism CYP2A13 Arg-257Cys and histologic type of lung cancer. Of the 25 lung cancer patients, the highest rate of type was adenocarcinoma, in which the frequency of CC, CT, and TT was 70%, 25% and 5% respectively (Table 3). There was no relationship between genetic polymorphism of CYP2A13 Arg257Cys and histologic type of lung cancer ($p = 0.42$).

4 DISCUSSION

We found that the most predominant ethnicity in this study was Batak (52%) compared with four other ethnics in Indonesia. There is a tradition in Batak culture to serve cigarettes in several traditional ceremonies, and smoking habits are very common among the Batak population. Furthermore, Batak ethnics are well known to have a pure genetic heritance due to its culture in marriage and thus will provide a better model for genetic polymorphism to identify its effect on Tobacco-Specific Nitrosamine (TSNA) contained in cigarettes.

Each cigarette contains a mixture of carcinogen, including a small dose of Polycyclic Aromatic Hydrocarbons (PAH) and 4-(methylnitrosamino)-1-(3-pyridyl)-1 butanone (NNK/Nicotine-derived Nitrosamine Ketone) among other lung carcinogens, tumour promoters and co-carcinogens. The metabolism of TSNA needs a CYP2A13 in phase 1 metabolism (Su et al., 2000, Wang et al., 2003).

Arg257Cys CYP2A13 variant has been detected at frequencies of 1.9%, 14.4% and 7.7% in the white, black and Asian population respectively. Functional analysis has shown that the Cys257 variant is some 37–56% less active than the wildtype Arg257 form of the CYP2A13 protein in all subtracts tested. Heterozygosity and homozygosity for the Cys257 variant have been found to be associated with the Chinese population with the significantly reduced risk of lung adenocarcinoma (OR 0.41, 95% CI 0.23–0.71). On this basis, it might seem reasonable to surmise that individuals possessing a significantly reduced level of CYP2A13 may manifest sensitivity reduction to xenobiotic toxicity resulting from the CYP2A13 mediated metabolic activation of procarcinogens in the respiratory tract (Zhang et al., 2003).

CYP2A13-catalysed metabolic activation *in situ* may play a critical role in human lung carcinogenesis related to cigarette smoking. It is reasonable to further speculate that functional genetic polymorphisms of CYP2A13 may have a significant impact on human susceptibility to lung cancers related to NNK. Single nucleotide polymorphism CYP2A13 in 5 exons with the variant of C/T had been identified with Arg257Cys amino acid alteration in this study. This study found wild-type Arg257 allele could be cut to yield two fragments of 99 and 233bp in length, whereas the variant Cys257 allele gave only a 332bp band, C/C about 36 persons (72%), C/T about 13 persons (26%) and T/T about one person (2%). Genetic polymorphism analysis of CYP2A13 in lung cancer patients revealed C/T in about seven persons (58.8%), C/C in about 17 persons (47.2%) and T/T in about one person (1%). In contrast to Zhang et al., (2003), statistical analysis of this study showed that there was no significant relationship between CYP2A13 gene with lung cancer, OR = 0.67 (95% CI = 0,193–2,329).

5 CONCLUSION

The CYP2A13 Arg257Cys variant represents a common polymorphism in the Indonesia population, particularly in Batak and Javanese ethnics. There is no association between Arg-257Cys polymorphisms of CYP2A13 and lung cancer.

REFERENCES

Cheng, X.Y., Chen, G.L., Zhang, W.X, Zhou, G., Wang, D. & Zhou, H.H. (2004). Arg257Cys Polymorphism of CYP2 A13 in a Chinese population. *Clinica chimica acta; International Journal of Clinical Chemistry, 343*, 213–216.

Global Adult Tobacco Survey. Indonesia Report, (2011). *World National Institute of Health Research and Development Ministry of Health.*

Globocan. (2012). Estimated cancer incidence. Mortality and prevalence worldwide in 2012.

Medical Research Council. (1957). Tobacco smoking and cancer of the lung. *British Medical Journal, 1* (5034), 1523–1524.

Nakajima, M., Yamamoto, T., Nunoya, K., Yokoi, T, & Nagashima, K. (1996). Role of human cytochrome P4502 A6 in C-oxidation of nicotine. *Drug metabolism and disposition: The Biological Fate of Chemicals, 24*, 1212–1217.

Parkin, D.M., Bray, F.I. & Devesa, S.S. (2001). Cancer burden in the year 2000. The global picture. *European Journal of Cancer, 37*(8), 54–66.

Sambrook, J., Fritsch, E.F. & Maniatis, T. (1989). *Molecular cloning: A laboratory manual* (2nd ed). Cold Spring Harbor, NY: Cold Spring Harbor Laboratory, pp. 16–19.

Su, T., Bao, Z., Zhang, Q.T., Smith, T.J/, Hong. J/Y. & Ding, X. (2000). Human cytochrome p450 CYP2 A13: predominant expression in the respiratory tracts and its high-efficiency metabolic activation of a tobacco-specific carcinogen, 4-(Methylnitrosamino)-1-(3-Pyridyl)-1-butanone. *Cancer Research, 60*(18), 5074–5079.

Wang, H., Tan, W.M., Hao, B., Miao, X., Zhou, G. & He, F. (2003). Substantial reduction in risk of lung adenocarcinoma associated with genetic polymorphism in CYP2A13, the most active cytochrome p450 for the metabolic activation of tobacco-specific carcinogen NNK (Nicotine- derived Nitrosamine Ketone), *Cancer Research, 63*(22), 8057–8061.

Zhang, X., Chen, Y., Liu, Y., Ren, X., Zhang, Q.Y., Caggana, M., et al. Single nucleotide polymorphism of the human CYP2A13 gene: Evidence for a null allele. *Drug Metab Dispos., 31*, 1081–1085.

Stem Cell Oncology – Adella (Ed.)
© *2018 Taylor & Francis Group, London, ISBN 978-0-8153-9272-9*

L858R EGFR mutant expressions in triple negative, luminal and HER2 breast cancer

D. Budhiarko, T.P. Putra, A.T. Harsono, N. Masykura, G. Widjajahakim &
A.R.H. Utomo
Kalbe Genomics Laboratory, Stem-cell and Cancer Institute, Jakarta, Indonesia

D. Tjindarbumi
Dharmanugraha Hospital, Rawamangun, Jakarta, Indonesia

ABSTRACT: The presence of EGFR mutation L858R conferring sensitivity to Tyrosine Kinase Inhibitor (TKI) in primary breast cancer has been unclear. An anti L858R EGFR mutant protein specific antibody was used to screen EGFR mutations in 174 Formalin Fixed Paraffin Embedded (FFPE) specimens. Immunohistochemistry revealed strong reactions to the L858R antibody in 16 out of 174 specimens. The proportion of positive staining was highest in HER2 (11 of 16), followed by the triple negative (2 of 55) and luminal (3 of 103) subtypes. However, upon DNA isolation and analyses, there were six L858R mutations, four L861Q mutations, and the remaining six had no mutations. HER2 had the highest proportion of confirmed EGFR L858R and L861Q mutations (31%; n = 16), followed by the triple negative (3.6%; n = 55), and Luminal (1.9%; n = 103) cancer subtypes. While EGFR mutation was rare, HER2 subtype had the highest frequency of TKI sensitising EGFR mutations.

Keywords: EGFR, HER2 breast cancers, L858R

1 INTRODUCTION

Breast cancer has been categorised into three major types, namely Luminal or hormone receptor positive (expressing estrogen and/or progesterone receptors, and HER2 negative), HER2 (hormone receptors negative and HER2 positive), and Triple Negative Breast Cancer (TNBC, expressing neither hormone receptors nor HER2) subtypes (Allison, 2012). TNBC constitutes approximately 10–20% of all breast cancer and demonstrates the high histological grade of invasive carcinoma with poor prognosis (Dent et al., 2007). Notably, TNBC patients are responsive to chemotherapy but succumb to rapid relapse as shown by having visceral metastases. Therefore, TNBC patients have poor overall survival and high mortality rates (Kumar & Aggarwal, 2016).

Lung adenocarcinoma patients bearing mutations in L858R in exon 21 of Epidermal Growth Factor Receptor (EGFR) gene have shown good responses to TKIs, such as gefitinib, erlotinib and afatinib treatments, and have reduced the hazard risk of Progression-Free Survival (PFS) (Petrelli et al, 2012; Morgenztern et al, 2015). Recently, some publications have described genetic alterations of the EGFR gene in breast cancer including TNBC. 30–50% of TNBC patients have overexpressed EGFR proteins (Masuda et al., 2012), which has been associated with gene copy numbers caused by gene amplification (Shao et al., 2011). Also, there are contrasting reports describing either presence (Teng et al., 2011; Ly et al., 2011) or absence of EGFR mutations in Asian (Cao et al., 2015) and Caucasian (Secq et al., 2014) TNBC.

In this study, we wish to report the presence of TKI sensitive L858R EGFR mutant proteins in different subtypes of breast cancer, namely Luminal, HER2 and TNBC subtypes. We used the antibody against L858R EGFR mutant protein followed by direct DNA sequencing and Restriction Fragment Length Polymorphism (RFLP) to confirm the presence of bona fide mutations.

2 MATERIALS AND METHOD

2.1 *Patients samples*

174 FFPE breast cancer samples from Dharmanugraha Hospital were sent to Kalgen Laboratory between 2011 and 2015. Using a protocol approved by the Research Ethics Board at Stem Cell and Cancer Institute, we anonymised patient identity and categorised samples into three breast cancer subtypes, namely Luminal (Estrogen receptor (ER) and/or Progesterone Receptor (PR) positive), HER2 (positive for HER2 and negative for both ER and PR expression), and TNBC (ER/PR/HER2 negative). HER2 was positive when tumour cells scored 2+ and 3+ for the degree of membrane staining. Hormone ER and PR positive were defined as positive when at least 1% of tumour cells had expressed hormone (estrogen or progesterone) receptors.

2.2 *Immunohistochemistry*

Immunohistochemical staining was performed on 4 μm thick sections cut from FFPE blocks. Antigen epitopes were retrieved using heat method by boiling the tissues for 10 minutes in 0.01 M Tris-EDTA pH9 using the microwave. Tissues were then incubated for 1.5h with EGFR mutation-specific antibody L858R (43B2, Cell Signaling Technology, Inc.) that were diluted at 1:100 at room temperate. The antibody was detected using Envision Detection Systems Peroxidase/DAB (Dako). Immunohistochemical staining results were scored as described previously (Fan et al., 2012). We did not pursue screening of exon 19 deletion mutation of EGFR because we could not get consistent immunopositive staining in FFPE samples that had known status of exon 19 deletion mutation.

2.3 *DNA extraction*

Tumour areas were identified and marked by the pathologist. Tissues were then scraped, and DNA was extracted using High Pure PCR Template Preparation Kit (Roche) or QIAamp DNA Micro Kit (Qiagen) according to the manufacturer's protocol. DNA yield and purity were quantified using Nanodrop (Thermo Fisher Scientific).

2.4 *DNA sequencing*

PCR was performed in 25 μl PCR reaction volume containing 1 × PCR buffer, 0.2 mM dNTP, 400 nM forward and reverse primers, and 1.25U Taq DNA polymerase. The PCR protocol was set as follows: one cycle of denaturation at 95°C for 15 minutes, then 40 cycles of 95°C for 40 seconds, 58°C for 40 seconds, and 72°C for 40 seconds (Y. Nagai et al., 2005). PCR products were purified using High Pure PCR Product Purification Kit (Roche) and cycle sequencing reaction performed using BigDye Terminator v.3.1 (Applied Biosystems). The cycle sequencing reactions were then purified with ethanol precipitation methods and then sequenced using ABI 3500 Genetic Analyzer (Applied Biosystems).

2.5 *Restriction Fragment Length Polymorphism (RFLP)*

We had used this method as routine lung cancer genotyping and had passed routine proficiency examination of EGFR mutation testing organised by the European Molecular Genetic Quality Network (EMQN). Briefly, restriction enzymes MscI and PvuII were used to differentiate between L858R and L861Q point mutation in exon 21 of EGFR gene as described. MscI enzyme digested TGGCCA sequence within wild-type allele of PCR amplicons. The mutant allele (L858R) was not digested due to the base substitution of T to G at the first base of TGGCCA. On the other hand, *PvuII* enzyme digested mutant allele in the CAGCTG sequence. We then ran the RFLP method on 4 μl of PCR products and analysed on 2.5% agarose gel (Kawada et al., 2008).

3 RESULT

174 breast cancer samples categorised as Luminal A (n = 103), HER2 (n = 16), and triple negative (n = 55) breast cancer subtypes were screened for EGFR mutant proteins using the L858R mutant specific antibody as shown in the following diagnostic algorithm (Figure 1). Samples that showed positive results were then followed up by sequencing and RFLP method to confirm DNA mutations.

Expressions of L858R EGFR mutant proteins were found in 11 of 16 HER2 (68.8%), 3 of 103 Luminal A (2.9%), and 2 of 55 triple negatives (3.6%) breast cancer subtypes. Representative results of immunohistochemistry staining with anti L858R EGFR mutant antibody were shown in Figure 2.

Samples showing L858R positive staining results were then submitted for independent DNA mutation analyses using direct DNA sequencing (examples are shown in Figure 3) and RFLP (data not shown). In HER2 breast cancer subtypes, DNA mutations were found in 5 out of 11 L858R immunohistochemistry positive samples. Three samples had consistent L858R mutations, while one sample had L861Q and one sample had the complex mutation (L858R and L861Q). In Luminal subtype, L858R DNA mutation was not found in spite of positive L858R immunohistochemistry in two samples. Instead of L858R, we detected L861Q mutations in those two samples.

Lastly, within TNBC subtype, two samples that were L858R immunohistochemistry positive was associated with one sample showing DNA mutation of L858R, and the other sample showed L861Q mutation. The false positive rate was also not seen in TNBC, while both luminal and HER2 demonstrated a high false positive rate. Therefore, using stepwise screening of L858R mutation with immunohistochemistry followed by a sequencing method, we observed L858R EGFR mutation frequency is 25%, 1.8% and 0% in HER2, triple negative and luminal breast cancer subtypes, respectively.

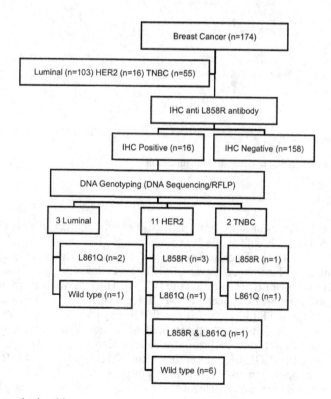

Figure 1.   Diagnostic algorithm.

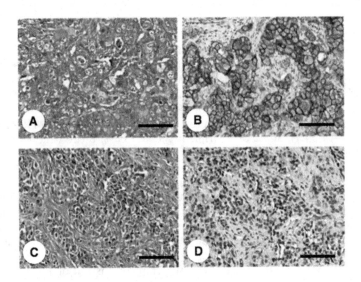

Figure 2. A representative of positive (B) and negative (D) expressions of EGFR L858R proteins. A&C were corresponding tissues stained with Hematoxylin/Eosin.

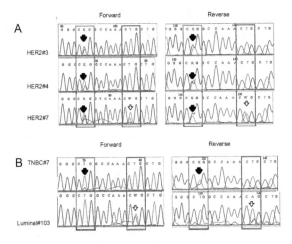

Figure 3. Sanger sequencing to detect EGFR mutations.

4 DISCUSSION

EGFR mutation L858R is an important predictive genetic marker of sensitivity to TKIs, such as gefitinib, erlotinib, and afatinib in lung cancer. The prevalence of TKI sensitive EGFR mutation tends to be higher in Asian (30–55%) than Caucasian lung cancer patients (5–15%). In contrast to lung cancer, several EGFR TKI clinical trials in breast cancer have shown minimal efficacy or disappointing result [15–17]. The relatively rare frequency of TKI sensitising mutations in breast cancer (Y.H.-F. Teng et al., 2011; N. Ly et al., 2011) may explain poor response to TKI in trials that enrolled largely Caucasian and unselected breast cancer. Interestingly, few Caucasian patients had been shown to harbour T790M EGFR mutation that is known to confer TKI resistance (Bemanian et al., 2015).

Our study showed that EGFR mutation, specifically TKI sensitising L858R in exon 21 of EGFR gene was found in certain breast cancer subtypes such as HER2 (25%) and TNBC (1.8%) using combined immunohistochemistry and direct DNA sequencing. However, there are two caveats when using immunohistochemistry to genotype EGFR mutations in breast cancer. The first caveat was the issue of cross-reactivity. While anti-mutant EGFR antibodies have shown excellent sensitivity in lung cancer specimens, there are studies including ours in which these antibodies have shown high cross-reactivity in HER2 overexpressing breast cancer samples (Verdu et al., 2015). It is thought that amplification of HER2 genes causes cross-reactivity between HER2-epitope and EGFR L858R mutant-specific antibody. The mutation site of EGFR exon 21 was located near the C-terminus as well as the position of HER2-epitope, making the high chance of cross-reactivity between them (Verdu et al., 2015). A previous study using highly sensitive ARMS PCR was not able to demonstrate L858R mutations in HER2 breast cancer showing strong immunostaining to anti L858R (Verdu et al., 2015). Although the cause of discrepancy was not clear, we speculate that differences may be due to different ethnic and geographical location as shown in lung cancer.

The second caveat was the issue of non-specific binding to EGFR mutations other than L858R. We showed that anti L858R antibodies apparently showed non-specific binding to antigens that were coded by L861Q mutation instead of L858R of EGFR gene especially in the luminal subtype of breast cancer. In lung cancer, L861Q mutations are rare, yet several groups have shown some sensitivity of L861Q patients to TKI (Peng et al., 2014). In spite of these two caveats, we had confirmed EGFR mutations in HER2 and TNBC when both immunohistochemistry and DNA sequencing were used in stepwise manners. Consistent mutations of L858R that were in agreement with positive immunohistochemistry results were 25% in HER2 (N = 16) and 1.8% in TNBC samples (N = 55).

Teng et al. (2011) reported that the frequency of EGFR mutation was 11.4% upon screening four exons of EGFR gene (18, 19, 20 and 21) in TNBC population in Singapore using sequencing method (Teng et al., 2011). Mutation prevalence of L858R was 1.5% in TNBC (n = 70) population in Singapore (Teng et al., 2011), which is similar to our cohort (1.8%, N = 55).

Contrary to our study, Chao et al. (2015) reported that there was no mutation found in EGFR gene in 50 frozen specimens of TNBC patients in China. They screened for 25 EGFR-activating mutations (G719S, G719A, G719C, S768I, L858R and L861Q and 19 mutations of exon 19-Del) using Amplification Refractory Mutation Systems (ARMS) and sequencing assay. The study of EGFR in TNBC was also carried out on Japanese patients. There was no mutation found in 108 of primary breast cancer patients that were analysed with mutant-allele specific amplification assay (Uramoto et al., 2010). Jacot et al. (2011) also reported there was no mutation in 229 frozen tumours of European TNBC patients that were analysed with High-Resolution Melting (HRM) and sequencing method.

Variations in the frequency of EGFR mutations in breast cancer, particularly in TNBC, potentially were caused by geographic and ethnic variations. Specific environmental carcinogenic factors were seen to play a role in NSCLC and TNBC in East Asian patients (Broet et al., 2011). It is necessary to do the specificity and sensitivity analysis in breast cancer patients according to IHC methods as detection assay of EGFR mutation and also to have genomic profiles related to ascertaining the geographic and ethnic variations, as was done in lung adenocarcinoma and NSCLC cases (Brevet et al., 2010).

To summarise, the anti-EGFR L858R mutation antibody may be prone to false positive in HER2 breast cancer and requires the additional genotyping method to confirm. However, the rate of false positive was low in TNBC and luminal subtypes making immunohistochemistry a cost-effective method to screen low prevalence rates of EGFR mutation in breast cancer patients. A future clinical trial involving EGFR TKI is warranted to assess the impact of EGFR L858R mutations in breast cancer. Moreover, immunohistochemistry may be useful to select Asian breast cancer patients for future clinical trials to test the efficacy of EGFR TKI.

ACKNOWLEDGEMENT

Dini Budhiarko wrote manuscript, generated and analysed key data of immunohistochemistry and direct DNA sequencing
Teguh Pribadi Putra generated and validated immunohistochemical data
Audi Tri Harsono generated key data for PCR based method

Najmiatul Masykura validated EGFR genotyping method
Grace Widjajahakim performed pathology review
Didid Tjindarbumi reviewed manuscript
Ahmad Rusdan Handoyo Utomo designed the project, analysed data and wrote the manuscript.

REFERENCES

Allison, (2012). Molecular pathology of breast cancer: what a pathologist needs to know. *American Journal of Clinical Pathology, 138*, 770–780. doi:10.1309/AJCPIV9IQ1MRQMOO.

Baselga, J., Albanell, A., Ruiz, A., Lluch, P., Gascón, V., Guillém, et al., (2005). Phase II and tumor pharmacodynamic study of gefitinib in patients with advanced breast cancer. *Journal of Clinical Oncology, 23*, 5323–5333. doi:10.1200/JCO.2005.08.326.

Bemanian, T., Sauer, J., Touma, B.A., Lindstedt, Y., Chen, H.P., Ødegård, et al., (2015). The Epidermal Growth Factor Receptor (EGFR/HER-1) gatekeeper mutation T790M is present in European patients with early breast cancer. *PLoS ONE, 10 e0134398-11*. doi:10.1371/journal.pone.0134398.

Brevet, M., Arcila, M., Ladanyi, (2010). Assessment of EGFR mutation status in lung adenocarcinoma by immunohistochemistry using antibodies specific to the two major forms of mutant EGFR. *Journal of Molecular Diagnosis, 12*, 169–176. doi:10.2353/jmoldx.2010.090140.

Broët, C., Dalmasso, E.H., Tan, M., Alifano, S., Zhang, J., Wu, et al., (2011). Genomic profiles specific to patient ethnicity in lung. *Adenocarcinoma, Clinical Cancer Research, 17*, 3542–3550. doi:10.1158/1078-0432.CCR-10-2185.

Cao, Y. & Gao, X.-J. Wang, (2015). Lack of Epidermal Growth Factor Receptor (EGFR)-Activating Mutations in Triple-negative Breast Cancer in China, *Breast Cancer Research, 17*, 115. doi:10.1186/s13058-015-0628-6.

Dent, M., Trudeau, K.I., Pritchard, W.M., Hanna, H.K., Kahn, C.A., Sawka, et al., (2007). Triple-negative breast cancer: Clinical features and patterns of recurrence. *Clinical Cancer Research. 13*, 4429–4434. doi:10.1158/1078-0432.CCR-06-3045.

Dickler, M.A., Cobleigh, K.D., Miller, P.M., Klein, E.P. & Winer, (2009). Efficacy and safety of erlotinib in patients with locally advanced or metastatic breast cancer. *Breast Cancer Research and Treatment, 115*, 115–121. doi:10.1007/s10549-008-0055-9 1096-1103 doi:10.1097/JTO.0b013e318186fadd.

Fan, B., Liu, H., Xu, B., Yu, S., Shi, J., Zhang, et al., (2013). Immunostaining with EGFR mutation-specific antibodies: A reliable screening method for lung adenocarcinomas harboring EGFR mutation in biopsy and resection samples. *Human Pathology, 44*, 1499–1507. doi:10.1016/j.humpath.2012.12.002.

Harbeck, C.-S., Huang, S., Hurvitz, D.-C., Yeh, Z., Shao, S.-A., Im, et al., (2016). Afatinib plus vinorelbine versus trastuzumab plus vinorelbine in patients with HER2-overexpressing metastatic breast cancer who had progressed on one previous trastuzumab treatment (LUX-Breast 1): An open-label, randomised, phase 3 trial. *The Lancet Oncology, 17*, 357–366. doi:10.1016/S1470-2045(15)00540-9.

Jacot, E., Lopez-Crapez, S., Thezenas, R., Senal, F., Fina, F., Bibeau, et al., (2011). Lack of EGFR-activating mutations in european patients with triple-negative breast cancer could emphasize geographic and ethnic variations in breast cancer mutation profiles. *Breast Cancer Research, 13*, R133. doi:10.1186/bcr3079.

Kawada, K., Soejima, H., Watanabe, I., Nakachi, H., Yasuda, K., Naoki, et al., (2008). An alternative method for screening EGFR mutation using RFLP in non-small cell lung cancer patients. *Journal of Thoracic Oncology, 3*.

Kumar, R. Aggarwal, (2016). An overview of triple-negative breast cancer. *Archives of Gynecology and Obstetric, 293*, 247–269. doi:10.1007/s00404-015-3859-y.

Lv, X., Xie, Q., Ge, S., Lin, X., Wang, Y., Kong, et al., (2011). Epidermal growth factor receptor in breast carcinoma: Association between gene copy number and mutations. *Diagnostic Pathology, 6*(18). doi:10.1186/1746-1596-6-118.

Masuda, D., Zhang, C., Bartholomeusz, H., Doihara, G.N., Hortobagyi, N.T., Ueno, (2016). Role of epidermal growth factor receptor in breast cancer. *Breast Cancer Research and Treatment, 136*, 331–345. doi:10.1007/s10549-012-2289-9.

Morgensztern, K. & Politi, R.S. Herbst, (2015). EGFR mutations in non-small-cell lung cancer: find, divide, and conquer. *JAMA Oncology 1*, 146–148. doi:10.1001/jamaoncol.2014.278.

Nagai, H., Miyazawa, Huqun, T., Tanaka, K., Udagawa, M., Kato, et al., (2005). Genetic heterogeneity of the epidermal growth factor receptor in non-small cell lung cancer cell lines revealed by a rapid and sensitive detection system, the peptide nucleic acid-locked nucleic acid PCR clamp. *Cancer Research, 65*, 7276–7282. doi:10.1158/0008-5472.CAN-05-0331.

Peng, Z.-G., Song, S.-C., Jiao, (2014). Efficacy analysis of tyrosine kinase inhibitors in rare non-small cell lung cancer patients harboring complex EGFR mutations. *Science Reports, 4*, 6104. doi:10.1038/srep06104.

Petrelli, K., Borgonovo, M. Cabiddu. S. & Barni, (2012). Efficacy of EGFR tyrosine kinase inhibitors in patients with EGFR-mutated non–small-cell lung cancer: A meta-analysis of 13 randomized trials. *Clinical Lung Cancer, 13*, 107–114. doi:10.1016/j.cllc.2011.08.005.

Secq, J., Villeret, F., Fina, M., Carmassi, X., Carcopino, S., Garcia, et al., (2014). Triple negative breast carcinoma egfr amplification is not associated with EGFR, Kras or ALK mutations. *British Journal of Cancer, 110*, 1045–1052. doi:10.1038/bjc.2013.794.

Shao, F., Zhang, G., Meng, X.-X., Wang, H., Xu, X.-W., Yu, et al., (2011). Epidermal growth factor receptor gene amplification and protein overexpression in basal-like carcinoma of the breast. *Histopathology, 59*, 264–273. doi:10.1111/j.1365-2559.2011.03921.x.

Teng, W.-J., Tan, A.-A., Thike, P.-Y., Cheok, G.M.-K., Tse, N.-S., Wong, et al., (2011). Mutations in the epidermal growth factor receptor (egfr) gene in triple negative breast bancer: possible implications for targeted therapy. *Breast Cancer Research, 13*(R35). doi:10.1186/bcr2857.

Uramto, H., Shimokawa, Y., Nagata, K., Ono, T., Hanagiri, (2010). EGFR-activating mutations are not present in breast tumors of Japanese patients. *Anticancer Research, 30*, 4219–4222.

Verdu, I., Trias, R., Roman, N., Rodon, C., Pubill, N., Arraiza, et al., (2015). Cross-reactivity of EGFR mutation-specific immunohistochemistry assay in HER2-positive tumors. *Applied Immunohistochemistry & Molecular Morphology, 23*, 565–570. doi:10.1097/PAI.0000000000000129.

Wen, E., Brogi, A., Hasanovic, M., Ladanyi, R.A., Soslow, D., Chitale, et al., (2013). Immunohistochemical staining with egfr mutation-specific antibodies: High specificity as a diagnostic marker for lung adenocarcinoma. *Modern Pathology, 26*, 1197–1203. doi:10.1038/modpathol.2013.53.

Stem Cell Oncology – Adella (Ed.)
© *2018 Taylor & Francis Group, London, ISBN 978-0-8153-9272-9*

Expression of p53 as a potential marker of muscle invasiveness in bladder cancer

S.M. Warli

Department of Urology, Faculty of Medicine, Universitas Sumatera Utara, Medan, North Sumatera, Indonesia

L.I. Laksmi

Department of Pathology, Faculty of Medicine, Universitas Sumatera Utara, Medan, North Sumatera, Indonesia

F. Safriadi

Department of Urology, Faculty of Medicine, Padjajaran University, Bandung, Indonesia

R. Umbas

Department of Urology, Faculty of Medicine, University of Indonesia, Jakarta, Indonesia

ABSTRACT: To analyse the association of p53 and muscle invasiveness in bladder cancer. The samples of this study are patients with bladder cancer. The samples were then classified into Non-Muscle Invasive Bladder Cancer (NMIBC) and Muscle Invasive Bladder Cancer (MIBC). All samples then underwent immunohistochemistry assay for p53, and then group analysed. p53 was expressed in 29 (96.7%) patients with MIBC and 23 (76.7%) patients with NMIBC. There was a significant difference in the expression of p53 between both groups (OR 8.8; 95% CI: 1.012- 76.96). The expression of p53 was significantly associated with muscle invasiveness of bladder cancer. Prospective study is needed to determine its potential in predicting muscle invasiveness of bladder cancer.

Keywords: Bladder cancer, predictive factors, p53

1   INTRODUCTION

Bladder cancer is the ninth most common malignancy in the world, with more than 380,000 cases and 150,000 deaths annually (Witjes et al., 2014). More than 90% of bladder cancers are Urothelial Cell Carcinoma (UCC). Most of all new cases (75–80%) from UCC are classified as non-muscle-invasive or superficial. This tumour has a recurrence rate of 50–70% and 10–15% progress to muscle invasion over a five year period (Shariat et al., 2008).

The high incidence causes special attention became necessary after the initial management. Progression and metastasis are the main problems after initial therapy (Cheng et al., 2009). Staging, grading, size, and multifocality, which are conventional prognostic factors, could not predict clinical outcome in the majority of patients with bladder cancer. Marking could predict recurrence, progression, therapeutic response, and survival (Malats et al., 2005; Schrier et al., 2004).

UCC has various biological and functional characteristics. Recurrence, progression into a higher grade and stage tumours and metastasis are the most common risks in patients with clinically diagnosed UCC. Bladder cancer prognostic could not be predicted by current available prognostic markers that to newly discovered molecular markers. Molecular changes caused phenotype alterations, thus immunohistochemistry could be used as an early detection tool for bladder cancer.

2 METHODS

The expression of p53, which indicates the muscle invasion in bladder cancer, were analysed in this case-control study, which included patients with muscle-invasive bladder cancer while patients with non-muscle invasive bladder cancer were used as controls. The study was conducted in Haji Adam Malik Hospital – Faculty of Medicine, Sumatera Utara University in conjunction with the Pathology Department, Haji Adam Malik Hospital in Medan, Indonesia from January 2012 to December 2015. Histopathologically diagnosed bladder cancer and good condition of paraffin block. Meanwhile, the exclusion criteria patients with bladder cancer who chemotherapy or radiotherapy and other malignancy.

Changes in brownish colour in epithelial cell cytoplasm or stroma for p53, which is seen the light microscope and will be assessed as intensity positivity and classified into four levels: Negative = 0; Weak = +1, Moderate = +2, Strong = +3. The positive value of p53 immunohistochemistry is defined as a quantitative value in the brown intensity distribution percentage per one field of view of the light microscope with a magnitude of 400 times. Positivity of value is classified into three levels: Negative (0): IHC negative; Focal (1): coloured cells < 50%; Diffuse (2): coloured cells > 50%. These two positivity value combined nH-score value. H-score value is determined based on McCarty criteria, which are: intensity positivity value with the addition of 1 multiplied with the quantity positivity value; [HS = (i+1) x k] (McCarty, 1986) thus the cut-off point is determined at 3. Therefore, the samples were divided into two groups, with H-score 3 or greater, and below 3.

The negative value is acquired by determining the cut-off point involving cases with colour intensity and negative control, cases with weak, moderate, and strong positive colour, with focal quantity positivity. Further analyses were done using SPSS version 20.0. Any statistical test which has p-value < 0.05 is considered statistically significant.

3 RESULT

A total of 60 subjects were involved. This study consisted of 30 cases and 30 controls. Characteristics of the subjects are presented in Table 1.

The mean age in the cases and controls group were 57.07 years and 55.9 years respectively theten. ladder cancer occur in men. Both age and gender were not significantly correlated with muscle invasiveness of bladder cancer (p > 0.05). The example result of IHC of p53 is shown in Figure 1.

p53 was significantly correlated with muscle invasiveness of bladder cancer. The probability of positive expression of p53 was 8.8 times higher in MIBC (p = 0.026; OR 8.8; 95% CI: 1.012–76.96).

Table 1. Frequency of age and sex results based on p53 expression.

Variable	Group Cases n = 30	Controls n = 30	p-value
Age			
Mean	5.9 ± 10.37	55.9 ± 11.91	0.687
Gender			
Male	26 (86.7%)	26 (86.7%)	0.647
Female	4 (13.3%)	4 (13.3%)	

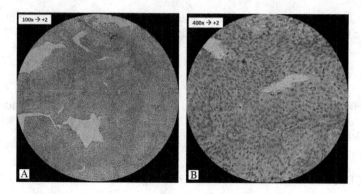

Figure 1. A) Moderate intensity positivity; B) Diffuse quantity positivity > 50% coloured cells.

Table 2. Correlation of p53 expression with MIBC and NMIBC.

Variable p53	Group		p-Value	OR	95%CI
	MIBC n = 30	NMIBC N = 30			
Positive	29 (96.7%)	23 (76.7%)	p = 0.026	8.8	1.012–76.96
Negative	1 (3.33%)	7 (23.3%)			

4 DISCUSSION

A total of 96.7% of MIBC patients in this study showed a positive p53 expression. To find the relationship between the expression of IHC p53 with the occurrence of muscle invasion in bladder cancer, we performed bivariate analysis using a chi-square test. The chance of IHC p53 positive appearing in MIBC is 8.8 times higher than the negative p53 IHC. This indicates that p53 contributes to muscle invasion in bladder cancer.

The result in this study is in accordance with some previous studies (Schrier et al., 2004; Esrig et al., 1994; Serdar et al., 2005), which also concluded that overexpression of p53 was higher in group invasive tumours. This study also discovered that overexpression of p53 with tumour progression does not depend on the grading, the presence or absence of vascular invasion, or the presence of carcinoma *in situ* (Sarkis et al., 1993).

Grosmann Barton et al. (1998) recommend allocating bladder cancer patients stratification of pT1 based on the status of p53 and RB.10 as results suggest that patients whose normal expression of these two genes can be managed conservatively. However, if there is a change in any of the two genes, aggressive management to prevent disease progression into invasive is recommended (Grossman et al., 1998; Van Rhijn et al., 2001).

A meta-analysis that was performed by Malats et al. (2005) in 117 studies had shown different results. Four showed that changes in p53 are a weak predictor factor of recurrence, progression, and mortality in bladder cancer. This result might be caused by the long period of patient recruitment, thus causing a heterogeneity, variability of immunohistochemistry, either in the antibody or the scoring system used, or the absence of a uniform definition to determine the limits of positive staining so that it can give different results due to differences in the cut-off (Malats et al., 2005). p53 has an important role for cell response to various stress and to maintain the stability of the gene. Because of its critical role in tissue homeostasis, p53 is the most commonly mutated gene in malignancy. p53 mutation causes the accumulation of p53 in the cell nucleus. Generally, overexpression in cell nuclei associates with p53 inactivation. In addition, overexpression can also be caused by the physiological response to DNA damage. The instability of these genes can also be caused by their bond with other molecules, such as MDM2 oncogenes, and viral genes, or even mutations that cause damage to the protein due to the insertion of a stop codon prematurely.

5 CONCLUSION

Expression of p53 was significantly associated with muscle invasiveness of bladder cancer. Prospective study is needed to investigate further its potential in predicting muscle invasiveness of bladder cancer.

REFERENCES

Cheng, L., Zhang, S., Davidson, D.D., MacLennan, G.T., Koch, M.O., Montironi, R., et al. (2009). Molecular determinants of tumor recurrence in the urinary bladder. *Future Oncology (London, England), 5*(6), 843–57.

Esrig, D., Elmajian, D., Groshen, S., Freeman, J.A., Stein, J.P., Chen, S.C., et al. (1994). Accumulation of nuclear p53 and tumor progressioniin bladder cancer. *The New England Journal of Medecine, 331*(19), 259–64.

Grossman, H.B., Liebert, M., Antelo, M., Dinney, C.P., Hu, S.X., Palmer, J.L., et al. (1998). p53 and RB expression predict progression in T1 bladder cancer. *Clinical Cancer Research: An Official Journal of the American Association for Cancer Research, 4*(4), 829–34.

Malats, N., Bustos, A., Nascimento,. C.M., Fernandez, F., Rivas, M., Puente, D., et al. (2005). p53 as a prognostic marker for bladder cancer: A meta-analysis and review. *The Lancet. Oncoogy, 6*(9), 678–86.

McCarty, K.S. Jr., Szabo, E., Flowers, J.L., Cox, E.B., Leight, G.S., Miller, L., et al. (1986). Use of a monoclonal anti-estrogen receptor antibody in the immunohistochemical evaluation of human tumors. *Cancer Research, 46*(8), 4244s–8s.

Sarkis, A.S., Dalbagni, G., Cordon-Cardo, C., Zhang, Z.F., Sheinfeld, J., Fair, W.R., et al. (1993). Nuclear overexpression of p53 protein in transitional cell bladder carcinoma: A marker for disease progression. *Journal of National Cancer Institute, 85*(1), 53–9.

Schrier, B.P., Hollander, M.P., van Rhijn, B.W., Kiemeney, L.A., Witjes, J.A. (2004). Prognosis of muscle-invasive bladder cancer: difference between primary and Progressive tumours and implications for therapy. *European Urology, 45*(3), 292–6.

Serdar, A., Turhan, C., Soner, G., Cem, S.N., Bayram, K., Damla, B.E., et al. (2005). The prognostic importance of e-cadherin and p53 gene expression in transitional bladder carcinoma patients. *International Urology and Nephrology, 37*(3), 485–92.

Shariat, S.F., Margulis, V., Lotan, Y., Montorsi, F., Karakiewicz, P.I. (2008). Nomograms for bladder cancer. *European Urology, 54*(1), 41–53.

Van Rhijn, B.W., Lurkin, I., Radvanyi, F., Kirkels, W.J., van der Kwast, T.H., Zwarthoff, E.C. (2001). The fibroblast growth factor receptor 3 (FGFR3) mutation is a strong indicator of superficial bladder cancer with low recurrence rate. *Cancer Research, 61*(4), 1265–8.

Witjes, J.A., Comperat, E., Cowan, N.C., De Santis, M., Gakis, G., Lebret, T., et al. (2014). EAU guidelines on muscle-invasive and metastatic bladder cancer: Summary of the 2013 guidelines. *European Urology, 65*(4), 778–92.

Stem Cell Oncology – Adella (Ed.)
© 2018 Taylor & Francis Group, London, ISBN 978-0-8153-9272-9

Human Epididymis Protein 4 immunohistochemistry expression in benign ovarian cysts

M. Rusda, D. Lutan, A. Gafur, M.F. Sahil, T.M. Ichsan & H.L. Haryono
Department of Obstetrics and Gynecology, Faculty of Medicine, Universitas Sumatera Utara, Medan, North Sumatera, Indonesia

Z.Z. Tala
Department of Nutrition, Faculty of Medicine, Universitas Sumatera Utara, Medan, North Sumatera, Indonesia

M.I. Sari
Department of Biochemistry, Faculty of Medicine, Universitas Sumatera Utara, Medan, North Sumatera, Indonesia

ABSTRACT: This study seeks to determine the characteristics of the patient with benign ovarian cysts, the histopathologic distribution of benign ovarian cysts, Human Epididymis Protein 4 (HE4) expression in various benign ovarian cyst tissues and normal ovaries, and to determine an HE4 expression base from histopathologic type. This analytic observational study was performed with a case-controlled design. In this study, HE4 immunohistochemistry staining was performed for various benign ovarian cysts (n = 20), and normal ovaries (n = 20) and interpretation was performed by a pathologist using Allred scoring. There is a statistically significant relationship between benign ovarian cysts and HE4 expression. However, there is no significant difference between histopathologic subtype of the benign ovarian cyst and HE4 expression.

Keywords: benign ovarian cyst, normal ovaries, Human Epididymis Protein 4 (HE4)

1 INTRODUCTION

Ovarian cysts are sacs filled with fluid or semi-liquid material derived from ovarian tissue. Ovarian cysts often appear at reproductive age and are benign. Ovarian cysts may vary in size, and in most cases are harmless; there are even types of cysts that can disappear by themselves. Nevertheless, ovarian cyst findings can cause anxiety among women with potential malignancies (American College of Obstetricians and Gynecologists, 2015; Grabosch & Karjane, 2017).

The overall incidence of symptomatic ovarian cysts in premenopausal women which are malignant is 1:1000 and increases to 3:1000 at 50 years of age. About 7% of women worldwide develop ovarian cysts during their lifetimes. A screening test carried out in Europe showed an incidence of 21.2% of ovarian cysts among healthy postmenopausal women. Data from the National Cancer Institute's Surveillance, Epidemiology, and End Results Program (SEER) (2003) indicated that the lifetime risk for the development of ovarian cancer was 1 in 70. An estimated 22,430 new ovarian cancer cases occurred in the US that year. The SEER data also showed an increased incidence of ovarian cancer annually among women aged 65 and under (Kaloo et al., 2011).

Increased expression of HE4 tissue occurs in some malignant tumours, especially those from gynaecological or respiratory tracts. A large study has reported serum HE4 as a putative tumour marker which can be used to distinguish between benign gynaecologic tumours and ovarian cancer, suggesting that HE4 is as good as CA-125 as a tumour marker. So far there has been no comprehensive review of HE4-expressing tissues and conditions associated with elevated serum HE4 (Karlsen et al. 2014).

In addition to the mitogen-activated protein kinase (MAPK) pathway, the extracellular matrix (ECM) receptor interaction pathway is also involved in the regulation of the HE4 protein (Zhu et al. 2015; Jinping, 2013). Expression of HE4 protein, as in other ovarian markers, can be identified by gene expression analysis and related processes found in cortical inclusion cyst formation and Mullerian metaplasia. So far, the study of HE4 is still relatively limited, and the authors are therefore interested in research to increase the understanding of benign ovarian tumours by means of immunohistochemistry (IHC).

2 METHOD

This research is an observational analytic study with a case-controlled design. The IHC expression of HE4 in paraffin blocks of benign ovarian cysts is compared with normal ovaries. The study was conducted at the Department of Obstetrics and Gynecology, Faculty of Medicine Universitas of Sumatera Utara, and immunohistochemical examination was performed at the Laboratory of Anatomy Pathology Department of the Universitas Sumatera Utara Medical School Medan during May and June 2017.

The case group comprises paraffin blocks of benign ovarian cyst tissue obtained from gynaecological surgery of benign ovarian cysts. The control group is composed of normal ovarian tissue paraffin blocks obtained from non-ovarian cyst gynaecological surgery.

The sample size of the groups is n1 = n2 = 18.63 rounded to 19 samples (the number of samples of each case and control), so the total sample size in this study is 38. However, in this study, HE4 IHC examination was carried out for 20 paraffin blocks each of benign ovarian cysts and normal ovarian tissue, giving a total sample size of 40.

Data analysis and statistical tests were computerised, and the results are presented in frequency distribution tables. The relationship between variables was analysed by chi-square testing with 95% confidence interval and $p < 0.05$ was considered significant. This research has received approval from the Ethics Committee of the Faculty of Medicine, Universitas Sumatera Utara.

3 RESULTS

Table 1 shows that in the benign ovarian cysts group the majority are in the age range 20–50 years (14 people, 70%).

Table 2 shows the histopathologic distribution of benign ovarian cysts. The most common types are epithelial (85%), subtype cystadenoma mucinosum (40%).

Table 3 shows that the benign cyst ovarian group has predominantly positive HE4 expression (12 people, 60%) with a negative result for eight people (40%). Statistically, there was a significant correlation between the group of study subjects with HE4 expression with $p < 0.05$, with an odds ratio for the possibility of negative HE4 expression of 0.4 (CI 95% 0.23–0.68) which means the probability of negative HE4 expression is approximately 0.4.

Table 4 shows that the highest positive HE4 expression was found in the cystadenoma mucinosum group (two samples, 66.7%) while negative HE4 expression was found most frequently in the cystadenoma serosum and endometriotic cyst subtypes. Statistically, it was concluded that there was no correlation between the subtype of benign ovarian cyst in HE4 immunohistochemical expression ($p > 0.05$).

Table 1. Characteristics of research subjects by age, age of menarche, parity and body mass index.

Characteristics	Benign ovarian cyst n (%)	Normal ovarium n (%)
Age (years)		
<20	3 (15)	0 (0)
20–50	14 (70)	8 (40)
>50	3 (15)	12 (60)
Age of menarche (years)		
≤12	17 (85)	15 (75)
>12	3 (15)	5 (25)
Parity		
Virgo	4 (20)	0 (0)
Nullipara	2 (10)	0 (0)
1	14 (70)	20 (100)
Body Mass Index (BMI)		
Normoweight	14 (70)	15 (75)
Overweight	4 (20)	5 (25)
Obese	2 (10)	0 (0)

Table 2. Distribution of benign ovarian cyst histopathology.

Histopathology of benign ovarian cyst	Total n	(%)
Epithelial		
Cystadenoma mucinosum	8	40
Cystadenoma serosum	7	35
Endometriotic cyst	2	10
Non-epithelial		
Dermoid cyst	3	15

Table 3. Expression of immunohistochemistry HE4 in benign ovarian cysts and normal ovaries.

Research subject	HE4 expression (Allred score) Positive n (%)	Negative n (%)	Total n (%)	p^*	OR	CI 95%
Benign ovarian cyst	12 (60)	8 (40)	20 (100)	*0,001*	*0,4*	*0,23–0,68*
Normal ovarium	0 (0)	20 (100)	20 (100)			

Chi-square test.

Table 4. HE4 immunohistochemical expression in benign ovarian cyst tissue based on histopathologic subtypes.

	HE4 expression Positive n	%	Negative n	%	p-value*
Cystadenoma mucinosum	2	66.7	1	33.3	0.98
Cystadenoma serosum	5	62.5	3	37.5	0.77
Endometriotic cyst	4	57.1	3	42.9	0.89
Dermoid cyst	1	50.0	1	50.0	0.71

*Logistic regression test.

4 DISCUSSION

The results show that the benign ovarian cyst group are mostly in the age range of 20 to 50 years (14 people, 70%), with the remaining samples split equally between the 20 and under and the 50 and over age groups (3 people (15%) in each group). In the normal ovary group, 12 people (60%) are over 50 and eight people (40%) are aged from 20 to 50 years.

The risk factors associated with ovarian cysts are increasing age, premature menarche and late menopause. The ageing process will allow an extended time to cause random genetic changes in the ovarian surface epithelium. Repeated stimulation of the ovarian surface epithelium will cause changes. The pathogenesis theory of ovarian cysts is known as the 'incessant ovulation' hypothesis. The process of repairing the epithelial tissue of the ovaries during repeated and cyclic periods of ovulation causes frequent cellular proliferation. This will lead to the mutation of the p53 gene in the DNA phase, and this occurrence is considered to contribute to the process of ovarian cyst tumourigenesis (Kumar, 2010).

The majority of the benign ovarian cyst group presented with positive HE4 expression, (12 people, 60%) with only eight people (40%) having negative HE4 expression. Meanwhile, the normal ovarian group all had negative HE4 expression (100%). Statistically, there was a significant correlation between the group of study subjects with HE4 expression with $p < 0.05$. Expression of HE4 in cortical inclusion cysts with epithelial Mullerian and ovarian carcinomas showed that expression of HE4 could be raised in early-stage ovarian carcinomas. Immunofluorescence studies show that HE4 is distributed in the region of the cytoplasm with a perinuclear pattern of endoplasmic reticulum and Golgi apparatus. HE4 existence with positive findings in benign ovarian cysts is not in line with several previous research studies, such as that of Escudero et al. (2011), which show that HE4 is less affected by gender or menopausal status than CA-125. HE4 levels did not increase in benign conditions when compared with CA-125, including in benign gynaecological conditions.

From the results shown in Table 4 it was concluded that there was no correlation between subtypes of benign ovarian cysts with HE4 immunohistochemical expression ($p > 0.05$). However, since HE4 expression increases in the benign ovarian cyst, this might show that HE4 plays a role in the process of benign ovarian cyst formation. The expression of HE4 in the progression of benign neoplasms is not fully understood. Findings at histopathological examination levels show that HE4 is not only expressed in malignant ovarian tumours, but also in various benign ovarian lesions. Previous findings have shown that HE4 shows strong expression in serous carcinomas and endometrioid tumours. Georgakopoulos et al. (2012) found strong HE4 expression in clear-cell carcinomas, borderline serous tumours, endometriosis and ovarian mucinous cystadenomas. In fallopian tubes, carcinomas showed elevated HE4 expression levels. HE4 was strongly expressed in primary carcinomas of the fallopian tubes, cortical inclusion cysts and in mesothelial cells.

5 CONCLUSION

There is a significant association between benign ovarian cysts and HE4 expression. But there is no significant association between histopathologic subtypes of benign ovarian cysts and HE4 expression. More studies are needed to determine the role of HE4 in the pathogenesis of benign ovarian cysts.

REFERENCES

American College of Obstetricians and Gynecologists. (July 2015). Frequently Asked Question FAQ075: Gynecologic problem. Retrieved from https://www.acog.org/patients/FAQs/Ovarian-Cysts.

Escudero, J.M. (2011). Comparison of serum human epididymis protein 4 with cancer antigen 125 as a tumor marker in patients with malignant and nonmalignant diseases. *Clinical Chemistry, 57*(11), 1534–1544.

Georgakopoulos, P., Mehmood, S., Akalin, A. & Shroyer, K.R. (2012). Immunohistochemical localization of HE4 in benign, borderline, and malignant lesions of the ovary. *International Journal of Gynecological Pathology, 31*(6), 517–523.

Grabosch, S.M. & Karjane, N.W. (January 2017) Ovarian cysts. Retrieved from http://emedicine.medscape.com/article/255865-overview.

Jinping, L. (2013). HE4 (WFDC2) promotes tumor growth in endometrial cancer cell lines. *International Journal of Molecular Sciences, 14*, 6026–6043. doi:10.3390/ijms14036026.

Kaloo, P.D. Louden, K.A., Khazali, S., Hoy, D. and Sadoon, S. (2011). Management of suspected ovarian masses in premenopausal women. *Royal College of Obstetricians and Gynaecologists Green-top Guideline No. 62.* November 2011. Retrieved from https://www.rcog.org.uk/globalassets/documents/guidelines/gtg_62.pdf.

Karlsen, N.S., Karlsen, M.A., Høgdall, C.K. & Høgdall E.V.S. (2014). HE4 tissue expression and serum he4 levels in healthy individuals and patients with benign or malignant tumors: A systematic review. *Cancer Epidemiology, Biomarkers & Prevention, 23*(11), 2285–2295.

Kumar, V., Abbas, A.K., Fausto, N., and Aster, J.C. (2010) Ovarian cysts, *Robbins & Cotran Pathologic Basis of Diseases.*

National Cancer Institute. (Please insert publication date here). *SEER cancer statistics review* (1975–2003). Retrieved from http://seer.cancer.gov.

Zhu, L., Zhuang, H. Wang, H., Tan, M., Schwab, C.L., Deng, L. ... Lin, B. (2015). Overexpression of HE4 (human epididymis protein 4) enhances proliferation, invasion and metastasis of ovarian cancer. *Oncotarget, 7*(1), 729–744. doi: 10.18632/oncotarget.6327.

Stem Cell Oncology – Adella (Ed.)
© 2018 Taylor & Francis Group, London, ISBN 978-0-8153-9272-9

The accuracy of the Paediatric Appendicitis Score (PAS) based on age group in cases of acute appendicitis

D. Paramitha, E. Fikri & I. Nasution
Surgical Department, Faculty of Medicine, Universitas Sumatera Utara, Medan, North Sumatera, Indonesia

ABSTRACT Acute appendicitis in children is one of the leading causes of abdominal emergencies that require immediate surgery. The authors conducted research to determine the accuracy of the Paediatric Appendicitis Score (PAS) based on age group in acute appendicitis patients. Data were analysed by bivariate analysis with appropriate hypothesis testing. The results were then reanalysed by dividing the PAS value according to age group, and the sensitivity of the PAS to the histopathological outcomes found in the appendix tissue was then calculated to assess the accuracy of the PAS in each age group. There was no statistically significant relationship between PAS and outcomes in the <5 years age group. Overall, PAS accuracy was higher, at 77.6%, in the 13–18 age group. There is no statistically significant relationship between PAS value and appendicitis diagnosis in the under 5 age group.

Keywords: Appendicitis, child, Paediatric Appendicitis Score (PAS)

1 INTRODUCTION

Acute appendicitis in children is one of the causes of abdominal emergencies requiring immediate surgical action (Kong et al., 2012; Ballester et al., 2009; Huckins et al., 2013). The world incidence of acute appendicitis in children ranges from 1% to 8% of all paediatric patients attending emergency departments with acute abdominal pain (Jangra et al., 2013). In 2006, acute appendicitis was ranked as the fourth most common reason (28,949 cases) for hospitalisation in Indonesia, after dyspepsia, duodenitis and other gastrointestinal diseases (Eylin, 2009). In the city of Medan, there is no data on the incidence of acute appendicitis in children. However, in 2009 there were 60 cases of acute appendicitis at Rumah Sakit Umum Pusat (RSUP) Haji Adam Malik Medan (Ivan, 2013).

Acute appendicitis is common in young adults: 40% of patients with acute appendicitis are between the ages of 10 and 30, while the condition is very rare in infants. Ratios of males to females are 3:2 in adolescence, becoming 1:1 after the age of 25 years. The incidence of appendicitis in children and young people of one to two cases per 10,000 children aged one day to four years increases to 25 cases for every 10,000 children aged 10–17 years (Schwartz, 2009).

2 RESEARCH METHODS

This study comprises a diagnostic test with a cross-sectional design. The research was conducted at RSUP Haji Adam Malik Medan (RSUP HAM) from April to November 2016. The population of this study was composed of paediatric patients who attended RSUP HAM with complaints of abdominal pain and who were diagnosed with appendicitis, thus fulfilling the inclusion criteria. Sampling was consecutive. The collected data was presented descriptively in a frequency distribution table. Data for PAS components and histopathologic results were then analysed by bivariate analysis with appropriate hypothesis testing. The results were then reanalysed by dividing the PAS value according to age group and then calculating the sensitivity of the PAS in relation to the histopathological outcomes of the appendix tissue, to assess the accuracy of the PAS in each age group. The hypothesis testing performed on PAS (ordinal), and the histopathological result (ordinal) was carried out using the Mann-Whitney test. The study included toddlers, children and adolescent patients as reference points for PAS groupings, which were then used to assess PAS accuracy in predicting the histopathological results of postoperative appendix tissue.

3 RESULTS

A total of 135 patients, including 70 males (51.9%), were included in the study after patients with a PAS that could not be assessed were excluded from the study. All patients had appendectomies, with pathology results showing that 86 (63.7%) of them had complicated appendicitis. The mean ± SD age of the patients was 15.4 ± 1.73 years, with the most populated group being for children aged 6–12 years, numbering 62 patients (45.9%). Detailed data for patient characteristics are presented in Table 1.

Complete components of PAS are then presented by age group in Table 2. Most history-taking components (pain during coughing, nausea/vomiting, lower right abdominal pain and pain migration) were difficult to assess in the <6 years age group, thus giving small numbers for these components. Lower right abdominal pain was the most common component in all age groups.

The researchers then performed an analysis of PAS and its relationship to the diagnosis of appendicitis. The PAS was grouped into three ranges of values: ≤ 5, 6–8, and ≥ 9. The PAS did not have a statistically significant relationship in the < 5 years age group (Table 3).

Table 1. Subject characteristics.

Characteristic		n	%
Sex	Male	70	51.9
	Female	65	48.1
Appendicitis diagnosis	Simple	49	36.3
	Complicated	86	63.7
Age	Mean ± SD (y/o)*	15.4 ± 1.73	
	Infant and toddler (<5 y/o)	15	11.1
	Child (6–12 y/o)	62	45.9
	Adolescent (13–18 y/o)	58	43.0
PAS	≤ 5	18	13.3
	6–8	81	60
	≥ 9	36	26.7

*years old.

Table 2. PAS by age group.

| Diagnostic indicator | Age group (y/o) | | |
	< 5	6–12	> 12
Pain during coughing/percussion/jumping	4 (26.7%)	44 (71%)	44 (75.9%)
Decreased appetite	9 (60%)	34 (54.8%)	22 (37.9%)
Increased body temperature	15 (100%)	46 (74.2%)	33 (56.9%)
Nausea/vomiting	11 (73.3%)	49 (79%)	38 (65.5%)
Lower right quadrant abdominal pain	5 (33.3%)	60 (96.8%)	57 (98.3%)
Leukocytosis (≥ 10,000/mm³)	13 (86.7%)	54 (87.1%)	39 (67.2%)
Neutrophilia (≥ 70/mm³)	12 (80%)	55 (88.7%)	39 (67.2%)
Migration of pain	1 (6.7%)	39 (62.9%)	40 (69%)
Total	15 (100%)	62 (100%)	58 (100%)

Table 3. PAS and appendicitis diagnosis.

Age Group (y/o)	PAS	Simple	Complicated	p*
< 5	≤ 5	2 (18.2%)	9 (81.8%)	0.382
	6–8	0	2 (100%)	
	≥ 9	0	2 (100%)	
6–12	≤ 5	2 (100%)	0 (0)	<0.0001
	6–8	10 (27.8%)	26 (72.2%)	
	≥ 9	0 (0)	24 (100%)	
13–18	≤ 5	4 (80%)	1 (20%)	<0.0001
	6–8	31 (72.1%)	12 (27.9%)	
	≥ 9	0 (0)	10 (100%)	

*Mann-Whitney Test.

Table 4. PAS sensitivity.

	Child (6–12)	Adolescent (13–18)
Sensitivity	52%	45.8%
Specificity	91.7%	100%
Accuracy	59.7%	77.6%

The <5 age group was then excluded from the assessment as a diagnostic tool. The value of PAS and its relationship with the complications of appendicitis diagnosis was then assessed for sensitivity and specificity based on the value of PAS in the ≥ 9 range for complicated appendicitis. The diagnostic test values of PAS in both age groups are presented in Table 4.

4 DISCUSSION

Of all PAS components, the most frequently occurring was found to be the fever component which was present in all the children in the <5 years of age (n = 15; 100%). This was followed by leukocytosis (≥ 10,000/mm^3) as the second most common finding (n = 13; 86.7%). In the age groups 6–12 years and >12 years, the lower right quadrant abdominal pain component was the most frequent finding, at 96.8% and 98.3% respectively. The second and third most common components in this group were leukocytosis (87.1%) and neutrophilia (88.7%). In the >12 group, pain migration and nausea/vomiting were jointly the second and third most frequent complaints (69% and 65.5%). Researchers suspect that this is a result of the improved communication skills of older children. Almost all children <6 years have PAS components that can hardly be assessed in terms of history-taking. In the 6–12 year group children begin to describe their perception of and the location of pain more accurately.

In previous studies, the authors found that the PAS in the <5 years age group always has a value of below 5. PAS values begin to vary in children aged 6 years and over. This results from older children indicating more severe appendicitis levels. PAS has a lower sensitivity in the younger age group (Rao & Galani, 2015).

The PAS value of 5 has a higher sensitivity value in detecting appendicitis in children younger than four years when compared with the use of 6 as the cut-off point in PAS as a diagnosis of appendicitis. In the 2008study by Goldman et al. it is suggested that PAS scores of <2 had high validity in excluding appendicitis diagnosis, whereas a value of >7 was effectively predictive in the diagnosis of appendicitis. Children with a PAS score of 3 to 6 should undergo further assessment, in the form of observation, ultrasonography or CT scanning, before a diagnosis of appendicitis can be established. In this study, all children were diagnosed with appendicitis by a 'gold standard' postoperative histopathologic examination.

In this study, the researchers used PAS 6 as the cut-off point to establish the diagnosis of appendicitis and found a low sensitivity value, but a high specificity value. This means that the PAS value > 6 may include a child with complicated appendicitis, but values of <6 are not sufficient to exclude complicated appendicitis.

5 CONCLUSION

The study found that PAS sensitivity was higher in patients aged 6–12 years than in the 12–18 age group (52% vs 45.8%), but the specificity of PAS was higher in the 12–18 age group (91.7% vs 100%). Overall, PAS accuracy was higher in the age 13–18 group, at 77.6%, compared with 59.7% at age ≤ 12 years. This study also analysed PAS and appendicitis diagnosis in the <5 years age group and found no statistically significant relationship between PAS value and appendicitis diagnosis at that age. Thus, PAS should not be used at ages of ≤ five years.

REFERENCES

Adibe, O.O, et al. (2011). Severity of appendicitis correlates with the pediatric appendicitis score. *Pediatric Surgery International*, 27, 655–658. doi 10.1007/s00383-010-2744-9.

Alder, A.C. & Minkes, R.K. (2017). Pediatric appendicitis. Retrieved from http://emedicine.medscape.com/article/926795.

Appendicitis. (2013). In DynaMed [database online]. EBSCO Information Services. Retrieved from http://search.ebscohost.com/login.aspx?direct=true&site=DynaMed&id=115548.

Aschraff, K.W. (2000). *Pediatric Surgery* (3rd ed.). Philadelpia: WB Saunders Company.

Ballester, J.C.A., Sanchez, A.G. & Ballester, F. (2009). Epidemiology of appendectomy and appendicitis in the Valencian community (Spain) 1998–2007. *Digestive Surgery*, 26, 406–412. doi 10.1159/000235956.

Bhatt, M. (2008). Prospective validation of the pediatric appendicitis score in a Canadian pediatric emergency department (Thesis). McGill University, Montreal.

Eylin. (2009). Karakteristik pasien dan diagnosis histologi pada kasus apendisitis berdasarkan data registrasi depatremen patologi anatomi FKUI RSUPN Cipto Mangunkusumo pada tahun 2003–2007. Jakarta. Skripsi, FK Universitas Indonesia.

Goldman, R.D., Carter, S., & Stephens, D., et al. (2008). Prospective validation of pediatric appendicitis score. *Journal of Pediatrics*. 153, 278–282. doi 10.1016/j.jpeds.2008.01.033.

Goulder, F. & Simpson, T. (2008). Pediatric appendicitis score: a retrospective analysis. *Journal of Indian Association of Pediatric Surgeons*, 13(4), 125–127. doi 10.4103/0971-9261.44761.

Hermanto. (2011). Apendisitis pada Anak, emergency department diagnosis & management. Artikel Kesehatan.

Huckins, D.S., et al. (2013). A novel biomarker panel to rule out acute appendicitis in pediatric patients with abdominal pain. *American Journal of Emergency Medicine*, 31(9), 1368–1375. Retrieved from http://search.proquest.com/docview/1430634945?accountid=50257.

Ivan, C.P. (2009). Karakteristik penderita apendisitis di RSUP Haji Adam Malik Medan pada tahun. Retrieved from http://repository.usu.ac.id/handle/123456789/21908.

Jangra, Babita, Jangra, et al. (2013). Seasonal and day of week variations in acute appendicitis in north Indian children. *Journal of Indian Association of Pediatric Surgeons*, 18(1), 42–43. Retrieved from http://search.proquest.com/docview/1317919106?accountid=50257.

Kong, V.Y., Bulajic, B., Allorto, N.L., Handley, J. & Clarke, D.L. (2012). *World Journal of Surgery*, 36, 2068–2071. doi 10.1007/s00268-012-1629-9.

Lee, S.L. (2013). Inflammation of vermiform appendix. Retrieved from http://emedicine.medscape.com/article/195652-overview.

Robbins and Cotran: Pathologic Basic of Disease, 8th ed Philadelpia: by Saunders, an imprint of Elsevier Inc, 2004.

Santacrose, R., & Craig, S. (2006). Appendicitis. Retrieved from http://www.emedicine.com/topic41.

Saucier, A. Huang, E.Y. et al. (2013). Prospective evaluation of a clinical pathway for suspected appendicitis. *Pediatrics*, e88-e95. doi 10.1542/peds.2013-2208.

Schwartz, S.I. (2009) Appendix. In *Principles of Surgery* (8th ed. pp. 1307–1330). New York: Mc Graw Hill Inc.

Wesson, D.E. (2014). Acute appendicitis in children. Retrieved from https://www.uptodate.com/contents/acute-appendicitis-in-children-clinical-manifestations-and-diagnosis.

Stem Cell Oncology – Adella (Ed.)
© 2018 Taylor & Francis Group, London, ISBN 978-0-8153-9272-9

Proportion of ameloblastoma subtypes based on location, size and radiological imaging appearance

M.M. Christin, T.I. Alferally & Betty

Department of Anatomical Pathology, Faculty of Medicine, Universitas Sumatera Utara, Medan, North Sumatera, Indonesia

ABSTRACT: Ameloblastoma is the most common odontogenic tumour of odontogenic epithelial origin. The objective of this study is to investigate if there is any dominant subtype at a specific location, size or radiological imaging appearance. This is a descriptive study with a cross-sectional approach. The samples for this study were determined by histopathological subtype and then correlated with location, size and radiological appearance from medical records. Based on data from 25 samples, this study showed that in the mandible the most frequent subtype has the follicular pattern. In terms of tumour size, the smallest group (<5 cm) was dominated by the plexiform pattern while the largest size (>5 cm) was dominated by the follicular pattern. Tumours with multilocular appearance were dominated by the follicular pattern while those with unilocular appearance contained follicular and plexiform patterns in equal proportions. The follicular pattern was the most frequently found in the mandible, in large size tumours and in multilocular radiological appearance.

Keywords: ameloblastoma, histopathological subtype, location, tumour size, radiological imaging appearance

1 INTRODUCTION

Ameloblastomas are the most common odontogenic tumours of odontogenic epithelial origin. They are slow-growing but locally invasive (Neville et al., 2002; Soames & Southam, 2005; Slootweg, 2007; Sapp et al., 2004; Burciaga et al., 2015; Setiady, 2013; Singh, 2010; Gardner, 2005). Global incidence is about 0.5/1,000,000 of the population per year, with occurrence in Indonesia of approximately 115 cases per year (Setiady, 2013; Rudiana et al., 2011). The treatment of ameloblastomas consists of enucleation, curettage and resection (Dandrigal et al., 2011; Filizzola, 2014). Inadequate treatment results in high rates of recurrence, and some studies suggest that this could be a factor in the malignant transformation of ameloblastomas (Slootweg, 2007; Soames & Southam, 2005; McClary et al., 2005). The mapping of a proportion of the histological subtypes of ameloblastomas based on their location, size and radiological appearance can assist pathologists and clinicians in diagnosis and in deciding on the optimal treatment for patients. Up to now, there has been no study of the proportion of histopathological subtypes of ameloblastomas in terms of their specific locations, tumour sizes and radiological appearance.

2 MATERIALS AND METHODS

2.1 Location

This study was carried out at Haji Adam Malik General Hospital in Medan, Indonesia.

2.2 Method

This study was a retrospective descriptive study with a cross-sectional approach. It was carried out over ten months, from December 2016 to September 2017, with consecutive sampling.

The medical records of ameloblastoma patients were selected using inclusion and exclusion criteria, and slides and paraffin blocks for the chosen cases were collected for review. Broken and inadequate slides from the paraffin blocks were reprocessed. These samples were then reviewed by the researchers and two pathologists without the identity of the patients being known. The sample slides were stained by haematoxylin-eosin, categorised according to histological subtypes and then correlated to medical record data of location, size and radiological imaging appearance. This study was approved by the Ethical Committee of the Medical Faculty of University of Sumatera Utara Medan.

3 RESULTS

In this study, 40 cases of ameloblastomas from Haji Adam Malik General Hospital from between 2012–2016 were identified, but only 25 of them met the inclusion criteria (i.e. had location, tumour size and radiological imaging records). The results of this study are presented in the following tables.

Of the samples, 12 (48%) were from female patients and 13 (52%) from males (Table 1).

It was found that ameloblastomas most frequently occurred in the 28–37 age range (eight cases; 32%), with fewer found in the 48–57 range (1 case; 4%). The mean age was 34.04 years with standard deviation of 13.23 years (Table 2).

Most of the ameloblastomas in this study were found in the mandible (18 cases; 72%) compared to the maxilla (six cases; 28%). In the mandible, the most frequent histopathological subtype was follicular (66.67%) followed by plexiform (27.77%) and extraosseous (5.56%), while in the maxilla the most frequent histopathological subtype was plexiform (57.14%), followed by follicular (38.57%) and unicystic (14.29%) (Table 3).

Table 1. Distribution by sex of ameloblastoma cases.

Sex	Sum (n)	Percentage (%)
Male	13	52
Female	12	48
Total	25	100

Table 2. Distribution of ameloblastomas based on patient's age.

Patient age (years)	Sum (n)	Percentage (%)
10–18	3	12
19–27	5	20
28–37	8	32
38–47	6	24
48–57	1	4
58–67	2	8
Total	25	100

Table 3. Proportion of histopathological subtypes of ameloblastomas based on tumour location.

Ameloblastoma subtype	Location			
	Maxilla	Percentage (%)	Mandible	Percentage (%)
Follicular	2	28.57	12	66.67
Plexiform	4	57.14	5	27.77
Extraosseous	0	0	1	5.56
Plexiform	1	0	0	0
Unicystic	7	14.29	18	0
Total		100		100

Table 4. Proportion of histopathological subtypes of ameloblastomas based on their radiological appearance.

Ameloblastoma subtype	Radiological appearance			
	Uni-locular	Percentage (%)	Multi-locular	Percentage (%)
Follicular	3	42.86	11	61.11
Plexiform	3	42.86	6	33.33
Extraosseous	0	0	1	5.56
Desmoplastic	0	0	0	0
Unicystic	1	14.28	0	0
Total	7	100	18	100

Table 5. Proportion of histopathological subtype of ameloblastoma based on tumour size.

Amelo-blastoma subtype	Tumour size					
	5 cm	Percentage (%)	5–10 cm	Percentage (%)	>10 cm	Percentage (%)
Follicular	2	8	9	36	3	12
Plexiform	4	16	4	16	1	4
Extraosseous	1	4	0	0	0	0
Desmoplastic	0	0	0	0	0	0
Unicystic	1	4	0	0	0	0
Total	8	32	13	52	4	16

Multilocular lesions were more frequent than unilocular ones (multilocular: 18 cases; unilocular: 7 cases). The most frequently found subtype in multilocular lesions was follicular, followed by plexiform and extraosseous subtypes. In unilocular lesions it was found that follicular and plexiform subtypes were the most frequent, followed by the unicystic subtype (Table 4).

Ameloblastomas with follicular subtype was the most numerous tumour type in this study, with three cases measuring >10 cm and nine cases measuring 5–10 cm. Tumours of <5 cm in size were dominated by the plexiform subtype followed by the follicular, extraosseous and unicystic subtypes (Table 5).

4 DISCUSSION

In this study, 40 cases of ameloblastoma were found at Haji Adam Malik General Hospital between 2012 and 2016, of which 25 met the inclusion and exclusion criteria. Of these samples, males were slightly more frequent than females. This result is similar to studies by Singh et al. (2010), Setiady (2013) and Gardner et al. (2005). This can be correlated to information from the literature review identifying that ameloblastoma is closely related to tooth development, which is not differentiated by sex (Neville et al., 2002). In this study, peak incidence occurred in the 28–37 age group. This reflects the results of studies by Setiady (2013) and Singh et al. (2010), although in the latter study the incidence began in a younger age group (the second decade). This can be correlated to the eruption of the third molars in the second to third decades of life that is often correlated to the formation of ameloblastomas (Gardner et al., 2005; Neville et al., 2002). Histologically, ameloblastomas present with four subtypes: solid (follicular and plexiform), unicystic, desmoplastic and extraosseous. The unicystic type has the cystic structure of the ameloblastomatous epithelium; the extraosseous type could present with follicular or plexiform patterns, while the follicular pattern shows islands of palisading columnar cells with displaced nuclei away from the basal membrane, and with reticulum stellate-like cells in the centre of the island. The plexiform pattern shows basal cells arranged in anastomosing strands. The desmoplastic type appears as islands that are pinched by the dominant fibrous stroma (Gardner et al., 2005; Neville et al., 2002; Cui et al., 2011).

As is known, ameloblastoma can occur in the maxilla or mandible, but when found on other sites such tumours would be classified as adamantinomas. Ameloblastomas are mainly found in the mandible rather than the maxilla (Gardner et al., 2005; Slootweg, 2007; Neville et al., 2005). The radiographic appearance of ameloblastomas can be unilocular or multilocular, and the multilocular appearance can be further subdivided into honeycomb and soap-bubble patterns (Gumgum & Hosgoren, 2005; Figueiredo et al., 2014; Li et al., 2012; Neville et al., 2002). In this study, the ameloblastomas which were most commonly found in the mandible had the follicular pattern, and this pattern was also mostly found in larger tumours and in those with multilocular appearance. These results were similar to studies carried out be Singh et al. (2010) and Neville et al. (2002). This characteristic of this pattern would need further research if it had a higher proliferation index. The result would be very useful for clinicians in deciding to resection this type of tumour. It is expected that adequate treatment of this tumour would reduce its recurrence.

5 CONCLUSION

Based on location, the most frequent histological subtype of ameloblastomas was follicular for those located in the mandible and plexiform for the maxilla. The follicular subtype dominated the larger size tumours, while smaller tumours were dominated by the plexiform subtype. The type most frequently found in those with multilocular appearance was the follicular subtype, while in those with unilocular appearance both follicular and plexiform subtypes were found in the same proportion.

REFERENCES

Burciaga, R.G.C., Gonzalea, R.G., Frechero, N.M. & Molina, R.B. (2015). Immunoexpression of Ki-67, MCM2, and MCM3 in ameloblastoma and ameloblastic carcinoma and their correlations with clinical and histopathological patterns. *Disease Markers*, 2015, Article ID 683087.
Cui, D., Naftal, J.P., Daley, W.P., Lynch, J.C., Haines, D.E. & Yang, G. (2010). *Atlas of histology with functional & critical correlations*. Philadelphia: Lippincott, Williams and Wilkins.
Dandrigal, R., Gupta, A. & Baweja, H.H. (2011). Surgical management of ameloblastoma: Conservative or radical approach. *National Journal of Maxillofacial Surgery*, 2(1), 22–27.
Figueiredo, N.R., Dinkar, A.D., Meena, M., Satoskar, S. & Khorate, M. (2014). Ameloblastoma: A clinicoradiographic and histopathologic correlation of 11 cases seen in Goa during 2008–2012. *Contemporary Clinical Dentistry, 5*(2), 160–165.
Gardner, D.G., Heikinheimo, K., Shear, M., Philipsen, H.P. & Colewan, H. (2005). Ameloblastoma. In Barnes L, Eveson JW, Reichart P, Sidransky D, (Eds.) *World Health Organization classification of tumours pathology and genetics head and neck tumours* (pp. 297–301). France: IARC Press.
Gumgum, S. & Hosgoren, B. (2005). Clinical and radiologic behaviour of ameloblastoma in 4 cases. *Journal of the Canadian Dental Association, 71*(7), 481–484.
Li, Y., Han, B. and Jiang-Li L. (2012). Prognostic and proliferative evaluation of ameloblastoma based on the radiographic boundary. *International Journal of Oral Science, 4*, 30–33.
McClary, A.C., West, R.B., Pollack, J.R., Fischbein, N.J., Holsinger, C.F., Sunwoo, J., ... Sirjani, D. (2005). Ameloblastoma: a clinical review and trends in management. *European Archives of Oto-Rhino-Laryngology, 273*(7), 1649–61. doi 10.1007/s00405-015-3631-8.
Neville, B.W., Damm, D.D., Allen, C.M. & Bouquot, J.E. (2002). *Oral & maxillofacial pathology* (2nd ed., pp. 611–620). Philadelphia: WB Saunders Company.
Rudiana, Sandini, S.U., Vitria, E.E. & Santosa, T.I. (2011). Profile of ameloblastoma from a retrospective study in Jakarta, Indonesia. *Journal of Dentistry Indonesia, 18*(2), 27–32.
Sapp, J.P., Eversole, L.R., & Wysocki, G.P. (2004). *Contemporary oral and maxillofacial pathology* (2nd ed., pp. 134–143). Missouri: Mosby.
Setiady, D.R. (2013). Kajianprevalensiameloblastomaberdasarkanusia, regio, Jenis kelamin, type histopathology anatomic dan penatalaksanaannya di RSD DR. Soebandijembertahun 2008–2012.
Singh, V., Dhasmana, S., Mohammad, S. & Dwivedi, C. (2010). Clinicopathological study and treatment outcome of 40 cases of ameloblastoma—A seven-year retrospective report. *World Articles in Ear, Nose and Throat, 3*(2).
Slootweg, P.J. (2007). *Dental pathology. A practical introduction* (pp. 59–61). Berlin: Springer.
Soames, J.V. and Southam, J.C. (2005). *Oral pathology* (4th ed). Oxford: Oxford University Press.

Stem Cell Oncology – Adella (Ed.)

Correlation of subjective global assessment with resting metabolic rate and fat free mass as measured by bioelectrical impedance analysis in non-Hodgkin lymphoma

D. Gatot, A.I. Maria & Safrian
Department of Internal Medicine, Faculty of Medicine, Universitas Sumatera Utara, Medan, North Sumatera, Indonesia

ABSTRACT: Subjective global assessment is used as a simple way to assess malnutrition without the use of complete body composition analysis. Increased metabolism, characterised by increased resting metabolic rate, is often found in patients with cancer. The aim of this research is to identify the correlation between subjective global assessment, resting metabolic rate and fat free mass in patients with Non-Hodgkin lymphoma. Correlation between resting metabolic rate and fat free mass are measured by bioelectrical impedance analysis and subjective global assessment and then assessed and analysed. A sample of 27 non-Hodgkin lymphoma patients was used, consisting of approximately 60% men and 40% women. Of the subjects, 7.4% were found to be well nourished, 63% were malnourished and 29.6% were severely malnourished. The mean resting metabolic rate and fat free mass were 1346.3 ± 145.7 kcal and 44.5 ± 6.8 kg respectively. Only 3% of the patients were found to have above-normal resting metabolic rates. No correlation was found between subjective global assessment and resting metabolic rate (p = 0.275) or fat free mass (p = 0.850). There was no correlation between subjective global assessment and resting metabolic rate or fat free mass as measured by bioelectrical impedance analysis in non-Hodgkin lymphoma patients.

Keywords: BIA, free fat mass, resting metabolic rate, SGA

1 INTRODUCTION

Non-Hodgkin Lymphoma (NHL) is the most commonly found haematopoietic neoplasm, ranking as the seventh most frequent of all cancers. NHL is found five times more frequently than Hodgkin lymphoma. The number of patients with NHL is increasing, and this may be related to early detection or to increased HIV infection (Sanjay, 2015; Lin & Guan, 2008).

Patients with haematologic malignancies and breast cancer rarely experience significant weight loss, unlike most patients with solid tumours, who frequently suffer from weight loss. It is estimated that the incidence of malnutrition in cancer patients ranges from 40–80% (Filipovic et al., 2010). When diagnosed, 80% of patients with upper gastrointestinal cancer and 60% of lung cancer patients have experienced obvious weight loss (Akio, 2002). In cancer patients, weight loss can be caused by increasing energy expenditure and reduced food intake. Some studies have shown an increase in energy expenditure at rest in patients with malignancies (Fredrix et al., 1991). Many methods have been developed to assess nutritional status to identify malnourished patients or patients who are at risk of malnutrition, including the Subjective Global Assessment (SGA). SGA was first introduced by Baker et al. in 1982, and is used to assess malnutrition in patients without the need for comprehensive analysis of body composition (Detsky et al., 1987).

Malnutrition can be detected earlier from the evidence provided by the changes in cell membranes and fluid imbalances that precede changes in anthropometric measurements and biochemical markers, and which can be analysed by Bioelectrical Impedance Analysis (BIA). BIA analyses the composition of body fluid indirectly by noting the change in impedance of electrical current in parts of the body. BIA examination is quick, non-invasive and does not require active participation by patients (Fredrix et al., 1990).

BIA reflects the volume of body fluids, such as total body water, extracellular water and intracellular water, as well as total body potassium and the nutritional status of the body. These measurements are provided as Body Cell Mass (BCM), Fat Free Mass (FFM), Fat Mass (FM), Resting Metabolic Rate (RMR), total protein, mineral and glycogen and phase angle (Gudivaka et al., 1999). FFM is a combination of BCM and extracellular mass or body mass minus FM. RMR is used to determine how quickly calories are burned in the body. Burning more calories than consumed will lead to weight loss, and hypermetabolism is common in cancer patients, who present with increased of metabolism of up to 50% higher than patients without cancer (Liedtke, n.d.).

Therefore, this study aims to determine whether there is any correlation between nutritional status, as measured by SGA, and RMR and FFM, as measured by BIA, in NHL patients who have not received chemotherapy.

2 METHOD

This study was conducted using a cross sectional approach at RSUP Adam Malik Hospital, Medan. The study population consisted of 27 patients with NHL in whom evidence for correlation between SGA and RMR and/or FFM was assessed and analysed. RMR and FFM were measured by BIA. Patients had to meet inclusion and exclusion criteria. The inclusion criteria for this study were NHL patients who were newly diagnosed and had not received chemotherapy. The exclusion criterion was those unwilling to participate in the study.

All NHL diagnoses were confirmed by histopathology examination, and nutritional status was investigated using SGA. BIA equipment (Maltron Bio Scan 916) made by Maltron International Ltd, Essex, UK, was used at room temperature, with a frequency of 50 kHz and an amplitude of 800 μA. Electrodes were placed on each patient's feet and hands. BIA examination was conducted by the researchers themselves.

3 RESULTS

This study involved a total of 27 NHL patients who were newly diagnosed and had not received chemotherapy. The patients consisted of 16 (59.3%) men and 11 (40.7%) women with a mean age of 44.7 ± 12.5 years, with the youngest being 22 years and the oldest 75 years. Of the subjects, 7.4% were found to be well nourished, 63% were malnourished and 29.6% were severely malnourished. The mean RMR and FFM were 1346.3 ± 145.7 kcal and 44.5 ± 6.8 kg respectively (Table 1).

Table 1. Characteristics of the study population.

Characteristic	Patients (n: 27)
Age (in years)	44.7 ± 12.5
Gender	
Male	16 (59.3%)
Female	11 (40.7%)
SGA	
Well nourished	2 (7.4%)
Malnourished	17 (63%)
Severely malnourished	8 (29.6%)
BIA nutrition status parameter	
FFM (kg)	44.5 ± 6.8
RMR (kcal)	1346.3 ± 145.7

Table 2. Correlation between SGA and RMR as well as FFM on BIA nutrition parameter.

Parameter	p
RMR	0.275
FFM	0.850

Only 1 (3%) patient with NHL was found to have RMR above normal. No correlation was found between SGA and RMR (p = 0.275) or FFM (p = 0.850) (Table 2).

4 DISCUSSION

BIA is the analysis of electrical resistance and reactance in the human body (Paeratahuls et al., 1999). There are several factors that can affect BIA measurements, including sex, age and ethnicity/race. In the study by Bailey et al. (2004) it is stated that there is a difference in total body mass between men and women, with men having a total body mass 8% higher than women. Liebelt et al. (1999) present that there are different patterns of fat distribution between men and women: the pattern of fat distribution in men tends to be in the area of the upper body and abdominal areas (upper body–abdominal pattern), whereas in women the pattern of fat distribution tends to be in the gluteal and femoral regions (gluteal–femoral pattern). RMR is lower in women than in men. In men, RMR is found to be 194 kcal/day compared to 125 kcal/day in women. RMR in women is lower than in men of the same age due to premenopausal and postmenopausal processes (Dehghan & Merchant, 2008).

A decrease in FFM has a correlation with RMR in elderly subjects. Reductions in organ/tissue mass due to ageing and organ metabolic rates contribute to a decrease in RMR, an increase in FM and a decrease in FFM (Aapro et al., 2014).

SGA is a subjective, simple, inexpensive and effective method for assessing the nutritional status of cancer patients. SGA is also a tool that can assess the functional capacity or energy level of patients. Following anamnesis and physical examination patients are classified as follows: well nourished (SGA A), moderately malnourished or suspected malnourished (SGA B), or severely malnourished (SGA C). SGA has generally been used to assess malnutrition because it is simple, does not require any medical instruments and can be the first assessment tool for assessing functional capacity. Well nourished patients (SGA A) were found in 7.4% of the subjects in this study; 63% were moderately malnourished (SGA B) and 29.6% were severely malnourished (SGA C) (Table 1). Dewys et al. (1980) found a frequency of weight loss of about 31% in patients with high-risk NHL (Aapro et al, 2014).

Research in Australia by Bauer et al. (2002) using SGA scores showed that 42 out of 71 cancer patients under treatment (59%) suffered from moderate malnutrition, and 12 patients (17%) suffered from severe malnutrition. Weight loss and decreased appetite are problems that occur in cancer patients. In research by Hopkinson et al. (2006), the prevalence of weight loss as a symptom ranged from 39% to 82%, while a decrease in appetite ranged from 30% to 80%. These conditions can be related to the absence of feedback regulation caused by products of the tumour that affect the activity of enzymes. Most cancer patients are not able to meet their calorie needs, possibly as a secondary factor related to metabolic changes, fatigue or decreased appetite as a result of treatment for cancer (Susetyowati et al., 2010).

In this study, the mean RMR was 1346.3 ± 145.7 kcal and only 1 patient (3%) with NHL was found to have a RMR above normal. It may be that this may reflect ethnic RMR differences, as normal RMR in Indonesian people has not been studied. The lack of correlation between SGA and RMR (p = 0.275) and FFM (p = 0.094) (Table 2) is likely to be due to the absence of information on normal values of RMR and FM in Indonesia.

The first weakness of this study is that it does not differentiate the stages of NHL, a factor which allegedly affects nutritional status parameters. The second weakness is that the normal

FFM and RMR values used refer to the normal value of the general population worldwide, not to the normal values for the Indonesian population specifically.

5 CONCLUSION

There was no correlation between SGA and RMR or FFM as measured by BIA in NHL patients who were newly diagnosed and had not received chemotherapy.

REFERENCES

Aapro, M., Arends, J., Bozzetti, F., Fearon, K., Grunberg, S.M. Herrstedt, J., ... Strasser, F. (2014). Early recognition of malnutrition and cachexia in the cancer patient: A position paper of a European School of Oncology Task Force. *Annals of Oncology*, 25(8), 1492–1499.

Akio, I. (2002). Cancer anorexia-cachexia syndrome: Current issues in research and management. *CA: A Cancer Journal for Clinicians*, 52, 72–91.

Dehghan, M. & Merchant, A. (2008). Is bioelectrical impedance accurate for use in large epidemiological studies? *Nutrition Journal*, 7(1), 26.

Detsky, A.S., McLaughlin, J.R., Baker, J.P., Johnston, N., Whittaker, S., Mendelson, R.A. & Jeejeebhov, K.N. (1987). What is subjective global assessment of nutritional status? *Journal of Parenteral and Enteral Nutrition*, 11(1), 8–13.

Filipovic, B., Gajic, M. (2010). Comparison of two nutritional assessment methodes in gastroenterology patients. *World Journal of Gastroenterology*, 16(16), 1999–2004.

Fredrix, E., Soeters, P., (1990). Estimation of body composition by bioelectrical impedance analysis in cancer patients. *European Journal of Clinical Nutrition*, 44, 749–752.

Fredrix, E., Soeters, P., (1991) Effect of different tumor types on resting energy expenditure. *Cancer Research*, 51, 6138–6141.

Gudivaka, D., Schoeller, A., (1999). Single and multifrequency model for bioelectrical impedance analysis of body water compartments. *Journal of Applied Physiology*, 87, 1087–1096.

Liedtke R. (n.d.) Bioimpedance analysis. Retrieved from http://rjlsystems.com.

Lin, T. & Guan, Z. (2008). Limfoma malignum. Buku Ajar Onkologi Klinis. Edisi 2 (pp. 547–563). Jakarta: Balai Penerbit FK UI, hlm.

Paeratahuls, S., Adair. L.S., Zhai, F., Ge, K. and Popkin, B.M. (1999). Sex difference in measures of body fatness and the possible difference in the effect of dietary on body fatness in men and women. *European Journal of Clinical Nutrition*, 53, 865–871.

Sanjay V. (2017). Non-Hodgkin Lymphoma. Retrieved from http://emedicine.medscape.com/article/203399-overview.

Susetyowati, S. Yenita, Y. & Kurnianda, J. (2010). Status Gizi Awal Berdasarkan Patient Generated Subjective Global Assessment Berhubungan Dengan Asupan Zat Gizi dan Perubahan Berat Badan Pada Penderita Kanker Rawat Inap di RSUP. DR. Mohammad Hosein Palembang. *Jurnal Gizi Klinik Indonesia*, 7(2), 80–4.

Stem Cell Oncology – Adella (Ed.)
© *2018 Taylor & Francis Group, London, ISBN 978-0-8153-9272-9*

Apoptotic effect of gentamicin in cochlea ototoxic rat model (preliminary study)

T.S.H. Haryuna & A.H.W. Purba
Department of Otorhinolaryngology Head and Neck Surgery, Faculty of Medicine, Universitas Sumatera Utara, Medan, North Sumatera, Indonesia

ABSTRACT: This study aimed to show the potency of gentamicin in increasing the apoptotic index in the cochlea lateral wall of ototoxic rat models. Eight *Rattus norvegicus* were divided into two groups: 1) control and 2) gentamicin administered. The rats were terminated to measure the apoptotic index using TUNEL assay of the fibroblasts of the cochlea lateral walls. Data were analysed by using ANOVA, with p <0.05 used as the cut-off for statistical significance. Administration of gentamicin showed increased apoptotic index which was statistically significant ($p < 0.05$). This study demonstrates that gentamicin is a pro-apoptotic and demonstrates its potency.

Keywords: apoptotic, cochlea, gentamicin, ototoxic

1   INTRODUCTION

Gentamicin is one of the aminoglycoside antibiotics which is important in challenging Gram-negative bacteria (Mouedden et al., 2000), however, it is often criticised because of its nephrotoxicity and ototoxicity (Sardana et al., 2015; Huth et al., 2011; Petersen & Rogers, 2015).

Aminoglycoside usage induces reactive oxygen species (ROS) and caspase formation, and can lead to apoptosis (Glutz et al., 2015).

The patterns and mechanisms of hearing loss which are caused by aminoglycosides are not fully understood (Selimoglu, 2007). The aim of this research was to assess gentamicin as a pro-apoptotic in the cochlea lateral wall in ototoxic rat models.

2   MATERIALS AND METHODS

Eight male *Rattus norvegicus* of 150–250 grams in weight were used. They were separated into two equal-sized groups. The rats were anesthetised using 10 mg/kg of xylazine and 90 mg/kg of ketamine intraperitoneally (Toydemir et al., 2015). Injections of gentamicin (40 mg/ml) 0.03–0.05 cc (Sagit et al., 2013), guided using a microscope, were placed anterosuperior to the tympanic membrane. Group 1 was the control group which was not treated, while group 2 was injected with gentamicin. Ad libitum food, and comfortable lightning, humidity and room temperatures of between 20°C to 26°C were provided. The rats were terminated 18 hours after being injected (Suzuki et al., 2008).

Temporal bone tissues were fixated with 10% formalin buffer solution and EDTA for four weeks and it was then possible to evaluate the apoptotic index of fibroblasts on the cochlea lateral wall.

The following procedural steps were carried out: the apoptotic index was evaluated using an Olympus XC 10 microscope with 40x magnification. Brown-stained TUNEL-positive markers were seen in the nuclei of cells, and counted in a masked manner. The researchers evaluated two fields which were randomly selected (Zhang et al., 2013).

The data were analysed using one-way ANOVA by using IBM SPSS statistical software with a significance level of 0.05.

3 RESULTS

Figure 1 shows the lateral wall of the cochlea and Figure 2 shows the role of gentamicin in the lateral wall of the cochlea of *Rattus norvegicus*, observed by using the TUNEL assay method. Using this method the researchers assessed the fragmentation of DNA in the cell nucleus as indicated by brown colouration. In group 2, in which the rats were given gentamicin, the cell nuclei are mostly brown, compared to group 1 where far fewer are seen.

Table 1 shows significant differences ($p < 0.05$) between the control group and group 2. Gentamicin administration increased the apoptotic index in group 2.

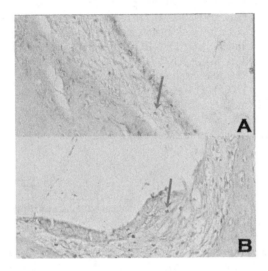

Figure 1.   Apoptosis index in each group (40x magnification). The arrows indicate TUNEL (+) cells. A: Group 1; B: Group 2.

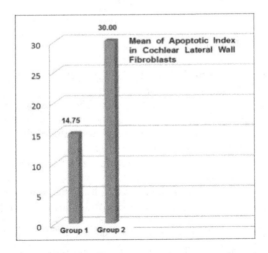

Figure 2.   Average number of cells undergoing apoptosis in cochlea lateral wall fibroblasts for each treatment group.

Table 1. ANOVA test results for apoptotic index.

Group		Mean difference ± standard deviation	p-value
1	2	−15.250 ± 3.433	0.000*

*Denotes statistically significant.

4 DISCUSSION

The lateral wall of the cochlea is the first the part of the cochlea in which histological change occurs (Fujioka et al., 2014), and this led the researchers to investigate this site for this research.

In this study, the pro-apoptotic role of gentamicin as shown in the apoptotic index of the fibroblasts of ototoxic rat models was evaluated. Gentamicin at a dosage of 40 mg/ml was enough to increase the apoptotic index in lateral cochlear wall fibroblasts. Gentamicin toxicity enhances stress markers (caspase 12), pro-apoptotic BAX, released caspase 3 and blocked anti-apoptotic Bcl-2 (Jaikumkao et al., 2016). In chinchillas exposed to gentamicin it was found that cochlea cell death markers increased (Ding et al., 2010). In this present study the method of intratympanic gentamicin injection dose to a Wistar rat used in other research (Sagit et al., 2013) was followed. The chosen termination time of 18 hours after exposure was based on the results of a study of the round window membrane in guinea pigs, which gave the best TUNEL results (Suzuki et al., 2008).

After exposure, aminoglycoside binds to ferric iron (Fe^{III}) (Fetoni et al., 2012; Kurasawa and Steyger, 2011) leading to Fe^{II}-aminoglycoside complexes and forming ROS. ROS activate BAX which in turn triggers apoptosis (Kurasawa and Steyger, 2011).

5 CONCLUSION

This study showed that gentamicin is able to increase the index of apoptosis in rat models.

REFERENCES

Fetoni, A.R., Eramo, S.L.M., Rolesi, R., Troiani, D. & Paludetti G. (2012). Antioxidant treatment with coenzyme Q-ter in prevention of gentamycin ototoxicity in an animal model. *Acta Otorhinolaryngologica Italica*, *32*(2), 103–110.

Fujioka, M., Okamoto, Y., Shinden, S., Okano, H.J., Okano, H., Ogawa K. & Matsunaga T. (2014). Pharmacological inhibition of cochlear mitochondrial respiratory chain induces secondary inflammation in the lateral wall: A potential therapeutic target for sensorineural hearing loss. *PLOS ONE*, *9*(3).

Glutz, A., Leitmeyer, K., Setz, C., Brand, Y. & Bodmer, D. (2015). Metformin protects auditory hair cells from gentamicin-induced toxicity in vitro. *Audiology and Neurotology*, *20*(6), 360–369.

Huth, M.E., Ricci, A.J. & Cheng A.G. 2011. Mechanism of aminoglycoside ototoxicity and targets of hair cell protection. *International Journal of Otolaryngology*, 937861. doi: 10.1155/2011/937861.

Jaikumkao, K., (2016). Amelioration of renal inflammation, endoplasmic reticulum stress and apoptosis underlies the protective effect of low dosage of atorvastatin in gentamicin-induced nephrotoxicity. *PLOS ONE*. doi.org/10.1371/journal.pone.0164528.

Kurasawa, T. & Steyger, P.S. (2011). Intracellular mechanism of aminoglycoside-induced cytotoxicity. *Integrative Biology*, *3*, 879–886.

Mouedden, M.E., Laurent, G., Mingeot-Leclerq, M.P. & Tulkens, P.M. (2000). Gentamicin-induced apoptosis in renal cell lines and embryonic rat fibroblasts. *Toxicological Sciences*, *56*(1), 229–239.

Petersen L. & Rogers C. 2015. Aminoglycoside-induced hearing deficits—a review of cochlea ototoxicity. *South African Family Practice*, *57*(2), 77–82.

Sagit, M., Somdas, M.A., Korkmaz, F. & Akcadag, A. (2013). The ototoxic effect of intratympanic terbinafine applied in the middle ear of rats. *Journal of Otolaryngology—Head and Neck Surgery*, *42*(1), 13.

Sardana, A., Kalra, S., Khanna, D. & Balakumar, P. (2015). Nephroprotective effect of catechin on gentamicin-induced experimental nephrotoxicity. *Clinical and Experimental Nephrology*, *19*(2), 178–184.

Selimoglu, E. (2007). Aminoglycoside-induced ototoxicity. *Current Pharmaceutical Design*, *13*(1) 119–126.

Suzuki, M., Ushio, M. & Yamasoba, T. (2008). Time course of apoptotic cell death in guinea pig cochlea following intratympanic gentamicin application. *Acta Otolaryngologica*. *128*(7), 724–731.

Toydemir, T., Kanter, M., Erboga, M., Oguz, S. & Erenoglu, C. (2015). Antioxidative, antiapoptotic and proliferative effect of curcumin on liver regeneration after partial hepatectomy in rats. *Toxicology and Industrial Health,* 31(2), 162–172.

Zhang, W., Feng, H., Gao Y., Sun L., Wang, J., Li, Y., ... Sun, D. (2013). Role of pigment epithelium-derived factor (PEDF) in arsenic-induced cell apoptosis of liver and brain in a rat model. *Biological Trace Element Research*, 151(2), 269–276.

Stem Cell Oncology – Adella (Ed.)
© 2018 Taylor & Francis Group, London, ISBN 978-0-8153-9272-9

Increased expression of TGF-β in the cochlear fibroblast of diabetic model rats

T.S.H. Haryuna & T. Melinda
Department of Otorhinolaryngology, Faculty of Medicine, Universitas Sumatera Utara, Medan, Indonesia

ABSTRACT: The cochlea, as a microvascular organ, is very susceptible to conditions that result in a disruption of vascularisation. Transforming Growth Factor-β (TGF-β) plays a role in diabetic complication process, especially in microangiopathy, due to its role in thickening the basal membrane of the vessel. This study aims to see the TGF-β expression in cochlear fibroblasts diabetic model rats. Eight male *Rattus norvegicus* were divided into two groups> Group 1: control, rats were injected only with a single dose of sodium citrate intraperitoneally and then terminated on day 5. Group 2: rats were injected with intraperitoneal single-dose Streptozotocin (STZ) and terminated on day 5. Samples were terminated and necropsied for the removal of their cochlear tissue and their TGF-β expression determined by immunohistochemical examination. There was a significant difference ($p < 0.05$) in TGF-β expression in group 1 compared to group 2.

Keywords: Cochlea, Diabetes, Transforming Growth Factor-β

1   INTRODUCTION

The hyperglycaemia that happens in this disease can induce the occurrence of inflammation in the cells of the body (Romero, Sadidi & Feldman, 2008). This plays a role in the emergence of diabetic microvascular complications (Navarro and Mora, 2004), wherein inflammation that occurs can be through the Protein Kinase C (PKC) pathway along with Transforming Growth Factor-β (TGF-β) (Romero et al., 2008).

2   METHODS

Male *Rattus norvegicus* Wistar strain (150–250g), treated at controlled temperature ($25 \pm 2°C$) with a 12-hour light/12-hour dark cycle with free access to water and food and handled following the standard guide for the care and use of laboratory animals.

Streptozotocin (STZ) at 60 mg/kg BW dissolved in sodium citrate (22.5 mg STZ/ml) was injected in a single dose intraperitoneally. Blood sugar levels were examined in peripheral blood taken from the rats' tails daily using a glucometer. Forty-eight hours after the STZ injection, hyperglycaemia was positive if rats had blood sugar levels greater than 200 mg/dl (Patterson et al., 2015).

In this study, there were two groups with each consisting of four rats. Group 1 was the control group where they were injected only with a single dose of sodium citrate intraperitoneally and then terminated on day 5. In group 2, the rats were injected with an intraperitoneal single dose of STZ and terminated on day 5. Tissue samples were taken and fixed with a 10% formalin buffer solution and decalcified with EDTA for four weeks and continued by cutting the tissue until it became a slide preparation.

Immunohistochemistry (IHC) staining used Polyclonal Anti-TGF-β1. Examined using a light microscope with 100x magnification, the TGF-β expression was identified by IHC

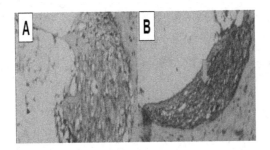

Figure 1.

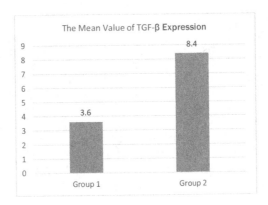

Figure 2.   The mean value of TGF-β expression in each group.

Table 1.   The test results for TGF-β expression values.

Group	Group	Mean difference ± standard error	P value
Group 1	Group 2	−4.800 ± 1.099	0.004*

(*: p<0,05).

imaging showing cytoplasmic colour changes to brown. The TGF-β expression ratings were assessed by multiplication of intensity with extend of staining score (Tan and Putti, 2004), and the data collected was analysed with SPSS 21 (SPSS Inc., NY, USA).

3 RESULT

TGF-β expression, characterised by a brown colour on the cytoplasm, was higher in the diabetic group (Figure 1B) compared to the control group (Figure 1A).

The following graph shows the average TGF-β expression in each group. TGF-β is higher in group 2 (8.4).

The table above shows a significant result of TGF-β expression (p < 0,05) when comparing the control group (group 1) with the diabetic model group (group 2).

4 DISCUSSION

Hyperglycaemia is a characterised condition in diabetes as a group of chronic disease that can cause macrovascular (coronary artery disease, peripheral arterial disease, and stroke) and microvascular complications (diabetic nephropathy, neuropathy, and retinopathy) where aldose reductase pathway and oxidative stress, and TGF-β may play an important role in the cellular injury that is caused by hyperglycaemia (Fowler, 2008).

As a multi-functional cytokine, TGF-β was also increased the synthesis of extracellular matrix, and the increase in TGF-β expression is also known to be in line with the severity of glomerulosclerosis in diabetics (Chang et al., 2016). In 2013, a study showed that TGF-β serum level in patients suffering from diabetes with diabetic retinopathy was significantly higher compared to diabetic patients without diabetic retinopathy (Zorena et al., 2013).

Haemodynamic changes and microcirculation disorders that are often found in diabetic conditions also happened in the cochlea. The studies showed that, especially in *stria vascularis*, vascular changes in the cochlea including thickening of the capillary walls (Xipeng et al., 2013). The increase in extracellular matrix accumulation through the stimulation of type IV collagen and the production of fibronectin (Russo et al., 2007), and the increase in Connective Tissue Growth Factor (CTGF), as well as Vascular Endothelial Growth Factor (VEGF) (Lee, 2013), all known to be induced by TGF-β. In 2013, a study showed that the TGF-β serum level in patients suffering from diabetes with diabetic retinopathy was significantly higher compared to diabetic patients without diabetic retinopathy (Zorena et al., 2013).

In this preliminary study, we wanted to compare the expression of TGF-β in the cochlear fibroblast in diabetic model rats to the non-diabetic control group and found that the TGF-β expression was significantly higher in the cochlear of the diabetic group (p <0,05). This result is similar to the study which stated that TGF-β renal expression is increased after induction of STZ diabetes in rats (Hill et al., 2000).

ACKNOWLEDGEMENT

This research received funding from the Directorate of Research Service to the Community, Universitas Sumatera Utara.

REFERENCES

Chang, A.S., Hathaway, C.K., Smithies, O. & Kakoki, M. (2016). Transforming growth factor-β1 and diabetic neuropathy. *American Journal of Physiology-Renal Physiology, 310*, F689–F696.

Fowler, M.J. (2008). Microvascular and macrovascular complications of diabetes. *Clinical Diabetes, 26*(2), 77–82.

Hill, C., Flyvbjerg, A., Gronbaek, H., Petrik, J., Hill, D.J., Thomas, R., Sheppard, M.C. & Logan, A. (2000). The renal expression of transforming growth factor-b isoforms and their receptors in acute and chronic experimental diabetes in rats. *Endocrinology, 141*(3), 1196–1208.

Lee, H.S. (2013). Pathogenic role of TGF-β in diabetic nephropathy. *Journal of Diabetes and Metabolism,* doi.org/10.4172/2155-6156.S9-008.

Navarro, J.F. & Mora, C. (2005). Role of inflammation in diabetic complications. *Nephrology, Dialysis, Transplantation, 20*, 2601–2604.

Patterson, E., Marques, T.M, O'Sullivan, O., Fitzgerald, P., Fitzgerald, G.F., Cotter, P.D., Dinan, T.G., Cryan, J.F., Stanton, C. & Ross, R.P. (2015). Streptozotocin-induced type-1-diabetes disease onset in Sprague–Dawley rats is associated with an altered intestinal microbiota composition and decreased diversity. *Microbiology, 161*, 182–193.

Romero, C.F., Sadidi, M. & Feldman, E.L. (2008). Mechanism of disease: The oxidative stress theory of diabetic neuropathy. *Reviews in Endocrine & Metabolic Disorders, 9*, 301–304.

Russo, L.M., Re, E.D., Brown, D. & Lin, H.Y. (2007). Evidence for a role of transforming growth factor (TGF)-β1 in the induction of postglomerular albuminuria in diabetic nephropathy amelioration by soluble TGF-β type II receptor. *Diabetes, 56*, 380–388.

Tan, K.B. & Putti, T.C. (2004). Cyclooxygenase 2 expression in nasopharyngeal carcinoma: immunohistochemical findings and potential implications. *Journal of Clinical Pathology, 58*, 535–538.

Xipeng, L., Ruiyu, L., Yanzuo, Z., Kaosan, G. & Liping, W. (2013). Effects of diabetes on hearing and cochlear structures. *Journal of Otology, 8*(2), 82–87.

Zorena, K., Malinowska, E., Raczynska, D. & Mysliwiec, M., Raczynska, K. (2013). Serum concentrations of transforming growth factor-beta 1 in predicting the occurrence of diabetic retinopathy in juvenile patients with type 1 diabetes mellitus. *Journal of Diabetes Research.* doi.org/10.1155/2013/614908.

Stem Cell Oncology – Adella (Ed.)
© 2018 Taylor & Francis Group, London, ISBN 978-0-8153-9272-9

Effect of fluticasone furoate on metalloproteinase matrix expression-9 in nasal polyps

S.V. Hutagalung
Department of Parasitology, Mahidol University, Thailand

F. Sofyan, Suriyanti & D. Munir
Department of Otorhinolaryngology Head and Neck Surgery, Faculty of Medicine, Universitas Sumatera Utara, Medan, North Sumatera, Indonesia

ABSTRACT: MMP-9 enhances vascular permeability resulting in oedema and the displacement of inflammatory cells. Fluticasone furoate has a receptor affinity for glucocorticoid receptors. The objective is to find out the effect of fluticasone furoate on the expression of MMP-9 in nasal polyps. The research was with an experimental quasi-design of 16 nasal polyps. Examination of MMP-9 expression in nasal polyps was performed with immunohistochemistry. MMP-9 expression before fluticasone furoate showed an overexpression of 75%, but after therapy it was 37.5%. There was a significant decrease in MMP-9 expression after fluticasone furoate therapy.

Keywords: fluticasone furoate, metalloproteinase-9 matrix, nasal polyp

1 INTRODUCTION

Nasal polyps are a chronic inflammatory disease of the nasal mucosa and paranasal sinuses, with a distinctive feature of oedematous mass, having 'bodies' and 'stalks' with slippery surfaces and a more yellow colour than the mucous membranes in the rice cavity and paranasal sinuses. The disease is known to have a high recurrence rate despite progress in its management (Chi & Annete, 2005; Mygind & Lund, 2009).

The formation of nasal polyps is assumed to be closely related to infiltration of inflammatory cells, loose connective tissue, reduced collagen, and pseudocyst formation with albumin and oedema accumulation. Excessive production and accumulation of extracellular matrix has been reported to contribute to the formation of nasal polyps (Bachert, 2005; Cincik et al., 2013; Callejas et al., 2015).

Corticosteroids can inhibit interstitial collagen synthesis such as blocking the production of degranulation of the proteinase matrix in some parts of the body (Bachert, 2005; Cincik et al., 2013; Callejas et al., 2015).

2 METHOD

This research is analytic with the quasi experimental design. This study will examine the expression of MMP-9 in nasal polyps before and after using a nasal spray of fluticasone furoate.

The research was conducted in the Department of THT-KL RSUP H. Adam Malik Medan. The immunohistochemical examination was conducted in the Department of Anatomical Pathology, Faculty of Medicine, Universitas Sumatera Utara.

Table 1. The differences in MMP-9 expression in nasal polyps before and after treatment with fluticasone furoate.

Expression of MMP-9	Before		After		P
	N	%	n	%	
Negative	4	25	10	625	0.027
Positive	12	75	6	37.5	
Total	16	100	16	100	

Table 2. The differences in MMP-9 expression before and after treatment with fluticasone furoate, based on stage of nasal polyp.

Nasal polyp stage	Before				After				P
	Negative		Positive		Negative		Positive		
	n	%	n	%	n	%	n	%	
I	0	0	1	100	3	75	1	25	0.511
II	3	50	3	50	7	58	5	42	
III	1	11	8	89	0	0	0	0	

3 RESULT

The research data is from all cases of nasal polyps performed biopsy and treatment at RSUP H. Adam Malik Medan from July 2013 to January 2015 that is as many as 16 subjects.

There was a significant difference between MMP-9 expression in nasal polyps before and after treatment with fluticasone furoate, $p = 0.027$.

There was no significant difference in MMP-9 expression in nasal polyps before or after therapy with fluticasone furoate, based on polyp stage, $p = 0.511$.

4 DISCUSSION

Immunoreactive MMP-9 scores were obtained in patients with nasal polyps before fluticasone furoate therapy was the group of overexpression (positive expression) with the total number of 12 people (75%) and negative expression group with the amount of 4 (25%). Lechapt-Zalcman et al. (2001) reported an increase in the expression of MMP-9 in glandular and blood vessel nasal polyps. Kahveci et al. (2008) and Guerra et al. (2012) obtained high MMP-9 expression and low TIMP-1 expression in nasal polyps. Pawankar et al. (2004) found high MMP-9 in nasal polyp tissue, and Lee et al. (2003) states that the ratio imbalance of MMP-9 and TIMP-1 contributes to the inflammatory process of nasal polyps. After getting over expression therapy group (positive expression) was as many as 6 people (37.5%) meanwhile the negative expression group was 10 people (62, 5%). There was a significant correlation ($p = 0.027$) in MMP-9 expression before and after fluticasone furoate therapy decreased. The results of this research comply with Callejas et al. (2014) who examined the effect of corticosteroids on mucosal remodelling on chronic rhinosinusitis with nasal polyps and found that MMP-9 expression significantly decreased ($p<0.01$) at week 2 and week 12 compared with those not obtaining intranasal budesonide therapy.

Hoshino et al. (1999) reported that corticosteroid therapy would lead to a decrease of subepithelial collagen accumulation in asthma patients by decreasing MMP-9 and increasing TIMP-1 expression.

In this research, the clinical stages of the nasal polyps were obtained before fluticasone furoate therapy was performed based on overexpression view of the highest MMP-9 group stage 1 is 100%, after obtaining fluticasone furoate therapy of negative expression of MMP-9 in the highest stage 1 group of 75%. Polyps stage 1 and two have decreased stages after therapy. There was no significant difference ($p = 0.51$) in changes in MMP-9 expression in nasal polyps before and after treatment of fluticasone furoate based on the polyp stage. There are other factors that have an important role in the formation of nasal polyps, such as changes in epithelial structure, angiogenesis, and extracellular matrix degradation caused by low levels of TGF-β. Some inflammatory mediators and differentiation factors are also growth factors of nasal polyps (Cohen et al., 2011).

Naclerio and Mackay (2001) reported that using nasal spray corticosteroids for 4-6 weeks effectively reduces the size of nasal polyps. In this research, researchers used fluticasone furoate 110 μg once daily given in two sprays (27.5 μg/spray) for each nasal polyp.

5 CONCLUSION

In this research, there is MMP-9 overexpression in nasal polyps before fluticasone furoate therapy and a significant decrease in MMP-9 expression in nasal polyps after therapy. There was no significant difference in MMP-9 expression in nasal polyps before and after treatment with fluticasone furoate based on polyp stage.

REFERENCES

Assanasen, P. & Naclerio, R.M. (2001). Medical and nasal surgical management of nasal polyps in current opinion in otolaryngology and head and neck surgery. Lippincott Williams and Wilkins Inc, 27–36.

Bachert, C. (2011). Evidence-based management of nasal polyposis by intranasal corticosteroid: from the cause to the clinic. *International Archives of Allergy and Immunology, 155*, 309–321.

Callejas, F,B. et al. (2014). Corticosteroid treatment regulates mucosal remodelling in chronic rhinosinusitis with nasal polyps. *The Laryngoscope*, 25147.

Chi, A.H. & Annette. (2005). Nasal polyposis: an immunohistochemical study of cell cycle regulator proteins in epithelial proliferation. A thesis submitted for the degree of master of science.

Cincik, H. et al. (2013). Evaluation of MMP-9 and TIMP-1 levels of the patients with nasal polyposis after corticosteroid therapies. *Indian Journal of Otolaryngology and Head & Neck Surgery, 65*, s445–s449.

Cohen, S., Ben Efraim, A.N., Levi-Schaffer, F. & Eliashar, R. (2011). The effect of hypoxia and cyclooxygenase inhibitors on nasal polyp-derived fibroblasts. *American Journal of Otolaryngology—Head and Neck Medicine and Surgery, 32*, 564–573.

Guerra, G., Testa, D., Marcuccio, G., D'Errico, Cianchetta, M.R., Cinelli, M., Russo, A. & Montagnani, S. (2012). TIMPs and MMPs expression in nasal polyps. *Italian Journal of Anatomy and Embryology, 117*(2), 87.

Hoshino, M., Takahashi, M., Takai, Y., Sim, J. & Aoike, N. (1999). Inhaled corticosteroids decrease subepithelial collagen deposition by modulation of the balance between matrix metalloproteinase-9 and tissue inhibitor of metalloproteinase-1 expression in asthma. *Journal of Allergy and Clinical Immunology, 104*, 356–363. doi: 10.1016/S0091-6749(99)70379-9.

Kahveci, O.K., Derekoy, F.S., Yilmaz, M.D., Serteser, M. & Altuntas, A. (2008). The role of MMP-9 and TIMP-1 in nasal polyp formation. *Swiss Medical Weekly, 138*(45-46), 684–688.

Lee, Y.M., Kim, S.S., Kim, H.A., Suh, Y.J., Lee, S.K., Nahm, D.H. & Park, H.S. (2003). Eosinophil inflammation of nasal polyp tissue: Relationships with matrix metalloproteinases, tissue inhibitor of metalloproteinase-1, and transforming growth factor-β1. *Journal of Korean Medical Science, 18*, 97–102.

Lechapt-Zalcman, E., Coste, A., d'Ortho, M.P., et al. (2001). Increased expression of matrix metalloproteinase-9 in nasal polyps. *Journal of Pathology, 193*, 233–241.

Mygind, N. & Lund, V.J. (2008). Nasal polyposis. In Scott-Brown, *Otorhinolaryngology, Head and Neck Surgery* (pp 1549–1557) (7th Ed, vol 2). London, England: Hodder Arnold.

Pawankar, R., Watanabe, S., Nonaka, M., Ozu, C., Aida, M. & Yagi, T. (2004). Differential expression of matrix metalloproteinase 2 and 9 in the allergic nasal mucosa and nasal polyps. *Journal of Allergy and Clinical Immunology, 113*, 1229. doi: 10.1016/j.jaci.2004.01.701.

Pearlman, A.N., Chandra, R.K., Conley, D.B. Kern, R.C. (2010). *Epidemiology of nasal polyps in nasal polyposis*. Berlin, Germany: Springer-Verlag.

Stem Cell Oncology – Adella (Ed.)
© 2018 Taylor & Francis Group, London, ISBN 978-0-8153-9272-9

Multiplex testing of *BCR-ABL1* and *JAK2* V617F in suspected MPN using RT-PCR RDB method

N. Masykura, F. Albertha & A.R.H. Utomo
Kalbe Genomics Laboratory, Stem Cell and Cancer Institute, Jakarta, Indonesia

U. Habibah, M. Yunus & Suharsono
Department of Biotechnology, Institut Pertanian Bogor, Bogor, West Java, Indonesia

F. Selasih & A. Bowolaksono
Universitas Indonesia, Depok, West Java, Indonesia

ABSTRACT: The presence of the *BCR-ABL1* transcript is essential in establishing a diagnosis of Chronic Myeloid Leukaemia (CML). In the absence of *BCR-ABL1*, *JAK2* V617F mutation testing is performed to support the diagnosis of *Polycythemia Vera* (PV), Essential Thrombocythemia (ET), and primary myelofibrosis (MF). We wanted to test the feasibility of multiplex detection of *BCR-ABL1* transcript variants and *JAK2* V617F mutation simultaneously using the Reverse Dot-Blot Hybridisation (RDB) method. The Limit of Detection (LOD) or analytical sensitivity of the RDB method using cDNA specimens was 0.5% and 6.25% in detecting *BCR-ABL1* and *JAK2* mutant transcripts, respectively. Diagnostic specificity and sensitivity to detect BCR ABL1 and JAK2 were 100% and 85.7%; 92% and 100%, respectively. RDB also detected *BCR-ABL1* transcripts in 22% of *JAK2* V617F mutation positive samples (N = 36). RT-PCR RDB is a promising qualitative multiplexing method to detect simultaneous *BCR-ABL1* and *JAK2* mutant transcripts.

Keywords: *BCR-ABL1*, *JAK2* V617F, RT-PCR RDB

1 INTRODUCTION

Myeloproliferative Neoplasms (MPN) is a group of blood disorders consisting of Chronic Myeloid Leukaemia (CML), *Polycythemia Vera* (PV), essential thrombocythemia (ET), primary myelofibrosis (PMF), chronic neutrophilic leukaemia, chronic eosinophilic leukaemia, hypereosinophilic syndrome, mast cell disease, and another unclassifiable disease (Tefferi & Vardiman, 2008). CML is caused Philadelphia Chromosome (Ph), a reciprocal translocation of *BCR* and *ABL1* genes that increases tyrosine kinase activation (Järås et al., 2010). *BCR-ABL1* translocation is comprised of four groups based at the translocation breakpoint; major, minor, micro and nano (Burmeister & Reinhardt, 2008). Reverse Transcript RT-PCR is a common method to detect the presence of *BCR-ABL1*(Gutiérrez et al., 2010) in samples obtained from either peripheral blood or bone marrow of suspected MPN patients (Burmeister et al., 2010).

Mutation of *JAK2* V617F has been found in and may contribute to etiology of 95%, 50%, and 40% of PV, ET, and MF, respectively (Vannuchi et al., 2010). Substitution of phenylalanine for valine at codon 617 of *JAK2* gene causes loss of autoinhibitory control leading to constitutive activation of *JAK2* tyrosine kinase. In 2008, WHO incorporated molecular genetic testing of *JAK2* V617F mutation into MPN diagnostic algorithm (Tefferi et al., 2009). To follow up *BCR-ABL1* negative MPN, many laboratories use different PCR methods of *JAK2* mutation testing such as direct DNA sequencing, ARMS, RFLP, pyrosequencing, real-time and melting curve analyses (Didone et al., 2016; Cankovic et al., 2009).

A recent survey suggests upfront determination of *BCR-ABL1* and *JAK2* would be desirable (Gong et al., 2013). However, performing *en masse* screening of both *BCR-ABL1* and *JAK2* using existing methods is not encouraged for the following reasons. First, the chance to find concomitant mutation is extremely rare (McCarron et al., 2012). Second, most existing methods do not allow simultaneous testing, especially when *BCR-ABL1* testing cDNA conversion from mRNA *JAK2* tests requires genomic DNA. Here we describe a simple multiplex method to test both *BCR-ABL1* and *JAK2* cDNAs using Reverse Transcription PCR (RT-PCR) followed by Reversed Dot Blot hybridisation (RDB).

To develop a feasible RT-PCR RDB test, we aimed to meet two criteria. First, the test should use cDNA isolated from peripheral blood. Second, the test should recognise at least four variants of *BCR-ABL1* (M-Bcre13a2 (b2a2), M-Bcre14a2 (b3a2), m-Bcr e1a2 and μ-Bcr c3a2 (e19a2)) and *JAK2* V617F with high specificity.

2 MATERIALS AND METHOD

2.1 *Materials and patient samples*

Oligonucleotides were synthesised by IDT, and the negatively charged membrane was purchased from Biodyne (Pall Corporation).

RNA of K562 (*BCR-ABL1* positive e14a2/b3a2 variant) and HL60 (*BCR-ABL1* negative) cell lines were used as control materials. Random archived RNA was obtained from 155 suspected MPN patients who had been referred to Kalbe Genomics Laboratory between 2014 and 2015 for routine clinical testing of qualitative *BCR-ABL1* (41 patients), quantitative *BCR-ABL1* (49 patients), *JAK2* V617F genotyping (29 patients), combined *BCR-ABL1* and *JAK2* V617F (36 patients). Archived human clinical specimens were anonymised and studied within the ethical policies of the Stem-Cell and Cancer Institute (SCI) IRB and by the Declaration of Helsinki.

Qualitative *BCR-ABL1* was performed according to RT-PCR gel electrophoresis protocol (Burmeister & Reinhardt, 2008) and had been validated by successful participation in Leukocyte Immunophenotyping proficiency testing programme organised by UKNEQAS (United Kingdom National External Quality Assessment Scheme). The quantitative test protocol was conducted using the commercial kit (Molecular MD, Portland) expressing results of major *BCR-ABL1* transcript levels on international scales (IS). *JAK2* V617F genotyping was done using direct DNA sequencing as described (Gonzales et al., 2014).

RT reverse transcriptase cDNA conversion. Isolated RNAs were converted into cDNA with reverse transcriptase enzyme and random hexamer primers using Transcriptor First Strand cDNA Synthesis (Roche).

PCR. BCR-ABL1 amplification used a multiplex PCR method with six primers in one reaction mix based on Zhang et al. (1991). *JAK2* V617F PCR amplification followed the method described previously (Gonzales et al., 2014). All PCR primers were biotinylated.

Gel electrophoresis. Five μL of PCR amplification products were mixed with one μL loading dye loaded into 2.5% agarose gel for 60 minutes at 95 volts.

Probe Immobilisation. Membranes were washed with HCl 0.1 N, then incubated with 10% EDC for 15 minutes while shaken at 60 rpm. Membranes were washed with ddH$_2$O, dried at room temperature, spotted with 2 μM of each probe (diluted with NaHCO$_3$ at 0.5 M), and incubated for 15 minutes. Membranes were then washed with TBS 0.1% Tween for 2 minutes and shaken at 60 rpm, then incubated with 0.1 N NaOH to quench the reaction. Lastly, membranes were rinsed with H$_2$O twice. Each spot on membranes had different probe concentrations, i.e., two μM for *JAK2* WT, ten μM for *JAK2* V617F probe and two μM for biotin probe, and two μM for all variants of *BCR-ABL1*1. Probes M3, M2, m, μ, JW, and JM were designed to capture and hybridise with target transcripts *BCR-ABL1* M-Bcr e14a2 (b3a2), M-Bcr e13a2 (b2a2), m-Bcr e1a2, micro-Bcr c3a2 (e19a2), *JAK2* wild-type, and *JAK2* V617F mutant, respectively.

Reverse Dot-Blot Hybridisation. Hybridisation protocol followed previous methods as described by Zhang et al. (1991) with some modification where a colorimetric instead of chemiluminescence method was used. Briefly, RT-PCR products were denatured at 95°C for 5 minutes, premixed with 500 μL of hybridisation solution, and hybridised with membranes for 15 minutes at 45°C. Washing was done twice with 800 μL post-hybridisation solutions. To visualise the presence of mutants, a 500 μL blocking solution was added for five minutes, and a 500 μL enzymatic conjugate solution for three minutes. Wash solution was then added twice followed by incubation with substrate solution for 3 minutes in the dark. A final wash solution of 1 ml was added, and membranes were dried at room temperature.

Sequencing. Direct DNA sequencing was performed to confirm the accuracy of the RDB method of *JAK2* genotyping using a 3500 Sequence Analyzer (Applied Biosystems).

3 RESULTS

3.1 *Design of Reverse Dot-Blot (RDB) method*

Sequences and RT-PCR protocols of multiplex primer set to amplify *BCR-ABL1* transcript variants were adopted from the previous study (Burmeister & Reinhardt, 2008). Choices of probes to be immobilised on the membrane were based on the frequency of *BCR-ABL1* variants that had been detected in 403 *BCR-ABL1* positive cDNA patients for routine clinical testing in the year 2014–2015. Proportion of transcript variants in *BCR-ABL1* positive samples was 31.39% M-Bcre13a2 (b2a2), 65.02% M-Bcre14a2 (b3a2), 1.79% m-Bcr e1a2, and 1.79% μ – Bcr c3a2 (e19a2). Among *BCR-ABL1* M-Bcr variants, the e14a2 frequency was higher than e13a2 in Indonesian patients, a pattern similar to other reports in the region (Hassan et al., 2008; Auewarakul et al., 2006).

Oligonucleotide probes were designed to bind four *BCR-ABL1* transcript variants and *JAK2* V617F mutation. The hybridisation process (RDB) was developed based on the previous report with several modifications such as finding optimal hybridisation temperatures (Zhang et al., 1991). Briefly, biotinylated PCR primers were used to amplify the cDNA template generated by reverse transcription of total RNA in blood samples. Biotinylated PCR products were then hybridised and retained on a nylon membrane containing oligonucleotide probes recognising four variants of *BCR-ABL1* and mutated *JAK2* V617F alleles. Oligonucleotide probes were spotted and organised as shown in Figure 1A. Naked eye visualisation of specific hybridisation was achieved as the result of the colorimetric development of streptavidin conjugated alkaline phosphatase binding to retained biotinylated PCR products.

RDB test results were considered conclusive when the positive signal was detected in a biotin probe position and an IC (internal control) probe position. Positive signals from the

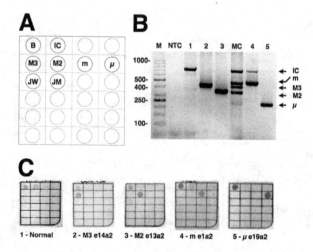

1 - Normal   2 - M3 e14a2   3 - M2 e13a2   4 - m e1a2   5 - μ e19a2

Figure 1. Validation of RT-PCR primers and oligonucleotide capture probes of RDB (Reverse dot-blot hybridisation) method.

biotin probe indicated a good visualisation reaction, and positive signals in IC probe suggested successful capture of a RT-PCR product of endogenous ABL gene expression within the sample. Four probes to detect *BCR-ABL1*, eighteen e13a2 positives, thirteen e14a2 positives, three e19a2 positives, and two e1a2 positive specimens.

3.2   *Qualitative BCR-ABL1 1 RDB test validation*

The limit of detection or analytical sensitivity of RDB was tested using serial dilution of K562 cDNA harbouring *BCR-ABL1* transcript variant e14a2 (b3a2) premixed with cDNA of *BCR-ABL1* negative HL60 cDNA. RDB was able to detect a *BCR-ABL1* transcript signal as low as 0.5% (Figure 2A). To determine the specificity of RDB in determining *BCR-ABL1* transcript variant, we tested a group of 41 archived cDNA patients whose *BCR-ABL1* had been previously characterised using gel electrophoresis. We had observed 100% concordance between the standard method and RDB in five specimens expressing no *BCR-ABL1*, eighteen e13a2 positives, thirteen e14a2 positives, three e19a2 positives, and two e1a2 positive specimens.

Recent guidelines suggest that CML patients should reach Major Molecular Response (MMR), whereby the level of detectable *BCR ABL1* transcripts is 0.1% IS or less within a year of imatinib mesylate treatment. Shown in Figure 2B, there were different hybridisation signals in samples having two different categories of *BCR-ABL1* (% IS), i.e., samples with expression levels being less or equal to 0.1% IS (MMR positive), and more than 0.1% IS (Non-MMR). One cDNA sample previously judged, contained undetected *BCR – ABL1* (0% IS) and showed a specific presence of minor *BCR-ABL1* transcript (Figure 2B, 0%IS*). Forty-nine archived cDNA specimens with known *BCR-ABL1* transcript levels were then collected and categorised according to 0.1% IS as cut off point of MMR. There were 28 specimens with equal to or higher than 0.1% IS (or MMR negative), and 20 specimens with less than 0.1% are (or MMR positive). All 20 MMR positive specimens were confirmed using RDB. In one MMR case, micro variant *BCR-ABL1* was detected because most quantitative *BCR ABL1* kits focus on major variant only. Out of 28 MMR negative specimens, RDB could only detect 24 specimens. Therefore, in comparison to quantitative real-time PCR methods, RDB diagnostic specificity, was 100%, and sensitivity was 85.7%.

3.3   *Qualitative JAK2 V617F mutation detection using RT-PCR RDB*

We performed dilution of JAK2 mutation alleles and compared analytical sensitivity between direct DNA sequencing and RDB. Our results showed that RDB was able to detect *JAK2*

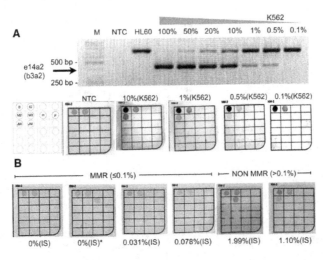

Figure 2. Analytical sensitivity of **RT-PCR RDB** to detect **BCR ABL** variants from cDNA specimens.

as little as 6.25% mutant allele, a level that was beyond direct DNA sequencing limit of detection (Figure 3). Twenty-nine cDNA specimens that had been previously tested for routine *JAK2* mutation using standard RT-PCR DNA sequencing were re-tested using RT-PCR RDB. Overall concordance between the two methods was 97% where 28 out of 29 patients showed the identical result. One patient (#25), previously tested negative for JAK2 mutation, was found to be positive using RDB, a method which had higher analytical sensitivity than direct DNA sequencing. Therefore, diagnostic sensitivity and specificity to detect JAK2 V617F was 100% and 92%.

3.4 *Concomitant BCR-ABL1 and JAK2 mutation in suspected MPN*

JAK2 V617F and *BCR-ABL1* mutations had been thought to be mutually exclusive, i.e., rarely occur within the same patient. We re-tested archived cDNAs of 36 consecutive cases of *JAK2* V617F mutation positive, which had been determined using direct DNA sequencing. Using both the standard method (gel electrophoreses to detect *BCR-ABL1*) and RDB, we found 22% or 8 of 36 JAK2 positive specimens were found to harbour *BCR-ABL1* transcripts (see Figure 4 for example in specimen #), constituting six major (b3a2 or b2a2) and two micro (e19a2) *BCR-ABL1* transcripts.

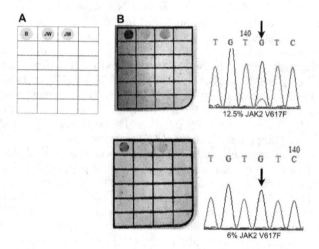

Figure 3. RT-PCR RDB JAK2 detection analytical sensitivity.

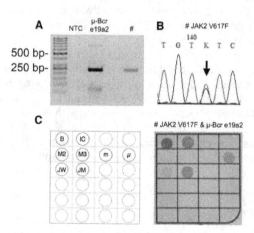

Figure 4. RT-PCR RDB multiplex JAK2 BCR ABL co-testing from cDNA specimen.

317

4   DISCUSSION

Current CML guideline suggests the use of RT-PCR for both qualitative and quantitative detection of *BCR-ABL1*, serving diagnostic and treatment monitoring purposes respectively (Foroni et al., 2011). Furthermore, JAK2 mutation testing has been recommended to follow up in the absence of *BCR-ABL1* in suspected MPN. Upfront testing of both *BCR-ABL1* and *JAK2* may be desirable in certain clinical case. We demonstrated a novel method of RTPCR RDB as a promising *BCR ABL1/JAK2* multiplex test. This principle of post PCR hybridisation has been demonstrated recently to detect multiple variants of leukaemic gene fusions in CML, ALL, and AML using DNA chip and electronic nano chip (Kang et al., 2012; Corradi et al., 2008) that are amenable to automation. However, to our knowledge, this is the first report showing the feasibility of RDB detecting both *BCR ABL1* transcript variants as well as *JAK2* together from the same cDNA. The use of cDNA to detect *JAK2* also has several advantages as described previously, which include higher sensitivity than genomic DNA, and direct analyses of transcript levels in platelets (Merker et al., 2010).

Multiplex RDB may also be used to screen or diagnose suspected MPN patients for the presence of *BCR ABL1* and *JAK2*, because it has higher analytical sensitivity than any of the many widely used qualitative screening methods using conventional multiplex RT-PCR gel electrophoreses (Lam et al., 2013) and direct DNA sequencing (Didone et al., 2016; Bench et al., 2013) respectively. We demonstrated in the K562 serial dilution experiment, that RT-PCR RDB was able to detect *BCR-ABL1* when its presence was as low as 0.5%. This level of analytical sensitivity is in line with previous observations describing transcripts level at diagnosis around 16.24–184.4% *BCR-ABL1* (IS) (Bonecker et al., 2015), with the median being 69.3% *BCR-ABL1*(IS) (range: 25.0–121.0%) (Huet et al., 2014). RDB sensitivity limit to detect as low as 6% JAK2 V617F transcripts may be sufficient to help diagnose new cases of PV and ET having average expression mutant *JAK2* V617F relative to normal *JAK2* alleles being 62% (median 61% range 8% – 98%) and 20% (median 19%; range 3% – 50%) (Lippert et al., 2016). *JAK2* mutation and *BCR-ABL1* translocation have been thought to be mutually exclusive. On rare occasion, both *JAK2* mutation and *BCR-ABL1* translocation may occur or coexist in the same patient reflecting the dynamics of the disease at baseline or progression (Zhou et al., 2015; Carranza et al., 2014). Within our small cohort of 36 JAK2 V617F mutation positive cases, 8 (or 22%) harboured *BCR-ABL1* positive transcripts. Our approach of finding *BCR-ABL1* in *JAK2* V617F positive cases was different than previous reports that describe the prevalence of concomitant JAK2 and BCR-ABL1 in cohorts of total MPN, CML, or non-CML (individual PV, ET, or MF) cases (Cambier et al., 2008; Qin et al., 2014; Hussein et al., 2008). For example, retrospective studies showed the concomitant rate being 2.6% out of 314 CML cases (Pieri et al., 2011), 12.7% out of 142 treatment naïve MPN cases (Trejo et al., 2012), 44% out of 25 Pakistani CML (Tabassum et al., 2014), and 0.2% out of total 10,875 MPN cases (Martin-Cabrera et al., 2016).

Nevertheless, there will be instances where clinicians would prefer to order both *BCR-ABL1* and *JAK2* testing from peripheral blood at the same time [10]. For instance, patients with some 'isolated' thrombocythemia may benefit from having both *BCR-ABL1* and *JAK2* V617F to be tested (Tefferi et al., 2009). Also, simultaneous screening for both *JAK2* and *BCR-ABL1* may be useful because some patients with *BCR-ABL1* positive or CML may progress to PMF due to the pre-existing presence of *the JAK2* mutation (Yamada et al., 2014). Clinicians may also consider JAK2 mutation testing in established CML cases who develop myeloproliferation and disease progression despite remission (Pastore et al., 2013).

ACKNOWLEDGEMENT

The authors are grateful to PT Kalbe Farma for funding this research.

Compliance with Ethical Standards:

Funding: This study was funded by an internal research grant from PT Kalbe Farma Tbk.

Ethical approval: This study was performed to the ethical standards of the local institutional research committee Stem-Cell and Cancer Institute (SCI) and with the 1964 Helsinki declaration and its later amendments.

REFERENCES

Auewarakul, C.U., Huang, S., Yimyam, M. & Boonmoh, S. (2006). Natural history of Southeast Asian chronic myeloid leukemia patients with different BCR-ABL gene variants. *Acta Haematologica, 116,* 114–119. doi: 10.1159/000093641.

Bench, A.J., White, H.E., Foroni, L, et al. (2013). Molecular diagnosis of the myeloproliferative neoplasms: UK guidelines for the detection of JAK2 V617F and other relevant mutations. *British Journal of Haematology, 160,* 25–34. doi: 10.1111/bjh.12075.

Bonecker, S., Magnago, M., Kaeda, J., et al. (2015). Is the BCR-ABL/GUSB transcript level at diagnosis an early predictive marker for chronic myeloid leukemia patients treated with imatinib? *Brazilian Journal of Hematology and Hemotherapy, 37,* 142–143. doi: 10.1016/j.bjhh.2014.08.003.

Burmeister, T., Maurer, J., Aivado, M., et al. (2000). Quality assurance in RT-PCR-based BCR/ABL diagnostics—results of an interlaboratory test and a standardization approach. *Journal of Leukemia, 14,* 1850–1856. doi: 10.1038/sj.leu.2401899.

Burmeister, T. & Reinhardt, R. (2008). A multiplex PCR for improved detection of typical and atypical BCR–ABL fusion transcripts. *Leukemia Research, 32,* 579–585. doi: 10.1016/j.leukres.2007.08.017.

Cambier, N., Renneville, A., Cazaentre, T., et al. (2008). JAK2V617F-positive polycythemia vera and Philadelphia chromosome-positive chronic myeloid leukemia: one patient with two distinct myeloproliferative disorders. *Journal of Leukemia, 22,* 1454–1455. doi: 10.1038/sj.leu.2405088.

Cankovic, M., Whiteley, L., Hawley, R.C., et al. (2009). Clinical performance of JAK2 V617F mutation detection assays in a molecular diagnostics laboratory: evaluation of screening and quantitation methods. *American Journal of Clinical Pathology, 132,* 713–721. doi: 10.1309/AJCPFHUQZ9 AGUEKA.

Carranza, C., Tinti, D., Herrera, M. & Rosales, L. (2014). Detection of Jak2 V617f Mutation, secondary to the presence of Bcr-Abl1 translocation in a patient with chronic myeloid leukemia: Report of a case and review of the literature. *International Journal of Genomic Medicine, 2,* 1–5. doi: 10.4172/2332-0672.1000116.

Corradi, B., Fazio, G., Palmi, C., et al. (2008). Efficient detection of leukaemia-related fusion transcripts by multiplex PCR applied on a microelectronic platform. *Journal of Leukemia, 22,* 294–302. doi: 10.1038/sj.leu.2404987.

Didone, A., Nardinelli, L., Marchiani, M., et al. (2016). Comparative study of different methodologies to detect the JAK2 V617F mutation in chronic BCR-ABL1 negative myeloproliferative neoplasms. *Practical Laboratory Medicine, 4,* 30–37. doi: 10.1016/j.plabm.2015.12.004.

Foroni, L., Wilson, G., Gerrard, G., et al. (2011). Guidelines for the measurement of BCR-ABL1 transcripts in chronic myeloid leukemia. *British Journal of Haematology, 153,* 179–190. doi: 10.1111/j.1365–2141.2011.08603.x.

Gong, J.Z., Cook, J.R., Greiner, T.C., et al. (2013). Laboratory practice guidelines for detecting and reporting JAK2 and MPL mutations in myeloproliferative neoplasms: a report of the Association for Molecular Pathology. *Journal of Molecular Diagnostics, 15,* 733–744. doi: 10.1016/j.jmoldx.2013.07.002.

Gonzalez, M.S., De Brasi, C.D., Bianchini, M., et al. (2014). Improved diagnosis of the transition to JAK2 (V617F) homozygosity: the key feature for predicting the evolution of myeloproliferative neoplasms. *PLOS ONE, 9,* e86401. doi: 10.1371/journal.pone.0086401.

Gutiérrez, M.I, Timson, G, Siraj, A.K, et al. (2010). Single monochrome real-time RT-PCR assay for identification, quantification, and breakpoint cluster region determination of t(9;22) transcripts. *Journal of Molecular Diagnostics, 7,* 40–47. doi: 10.1016/S1525-1578(10)60007-4.

Hassan, R., Ramli, M. & Zaidah, W. (2008). One-step multiplex RT-PCR for detection of BCR/ABL gene in Malay patients with chronic myeloid leukaemia. *Asia Pacific Journal of Molecular Biology and Biotechnology.*

Huet, S., Cony-Makhoul, P., Heiblig, M., et al. (2014). Major molecular response achievement in CML patients can be predicted by BCR-ABL1/ABL1 or BCR-ABL1/GUS ratio at an earlier time point of follow-up than currently recommended. *PLOS ONE, 9,* e106250–9. doi: 10.1371/journal.pone.0106250.

Hussein, K., Bock, O., Theophile, K., et al. (2008). Chronic myeloproliferative diseases with concurrent BCR–ABL junction and JAK2 V617F mutation. *Journal of Leukemia, 22*, 1059–1062. doi: 10.1038/sj.leu.2404993.

Järås, M., Johnels, P., Hansen, N., et al. (2010). Isolation and killing of candidate chronic myeloid leukemia stem cells by antibody targeting of IL-1 receptor accessory protein. *Proceedings of the National Academy of Sciences of the United States of America, 107*, 16280–16285. doi: 10.1073/pnas.1004408107.

Kang, J.H., Goh, H.G., Chae, S.H., et al. (2012). Genotyping of chimerical BCR-ABL1 RNA in chronic myeloid leukemia by integrated DNA chip. *Journal of Molecular Diagnostics, 14*, 487–493. doi: 10.1016/j.jmoldx.2012.04.003.

Lam, E.P.-T., Chan, C.M.-L., Tsui, N.B.-Y., et al. (2013). Clinical applications of molecular technologies in hematology. *Journal of Medical Diagnostic Methods.* doi: 10.4172/2168-9784.1000130.

Lippert, E., Boissinot, M., Kralovics, R., et al. (2006). The JAK2-V617F mutation is frequently present at diagnosis in patients with essential thrombocythemia and polycythemia vera. *Blood, 108*, 1865–1867. doi: 10.1182/blood-2006–01–013540.

Martin-Cabrera, P., Haferlach, C., Kern, W., et al. (2016). BCR BL1 positive and JAK2 V617F positive clones in 23 patients with both aberrations reveal biologic and clinical importance. *British Journal of Haematology.* doi: 10.1111/bjh.13932.

McCarron, S.L., Haslam, K., Crampe, M. & Langabeer, S.E. (2012). The incidence of co-existing BCR-ABL1 and JAK2 V617F rearrangements: implications for molecular diagnostics. *Laboratory Hematology, 18*, 20–21. doi: 10.1532/LH96.12009.

Merker, J.D., Jones, C.D., Oh, S.T., et al. (2010). Design and evaluation of a real-time PCR assay for quantification of JAK2 V617F and wild-type JAK2 transcript levels in the clinical laboratory. *Journal of Molecular Diagnostics, 12*, 58–64. doi: 10.2353/jmoldx.2010.090068.

Pastore, F., Schneider, S., Christ, O., et al. (2013). Impressive thrombocytosis evolving in a patient with a BCR-ABL positive CML in major molecular response during dasatinib treatment unmasks an additional JAK2 V617F. *Experimental Hematology and Oncology, 2*, 24. doi: 10.1186/2162-3619-2-2.

Pieri, L., Spolverini, A., Scappini, B., et al. (2011). Concomitant occurrence of BCR-ABL and JAK2V617F mutation. *Blood, 118*, 3445–3446. doi: 10.1182/blood-2011-07-365007.

Qin, Y.-W., Yang, Y.-N., Li, S. & Wang, C. (2014). Coexistence of JAK2V617F mutation and BCR–ABL translocation in a pregnant woman with essential thrombocythemia. *Indian Journal of Hematology and Blood Transfusion, 30*, 331–334. doi: 10.1007/s12288-014-0385-1.

Tabassum, N., Saboor, M., Ghani, R. & Moinuddin, M. (2014). Frequency of JAK2 V617F mutation in patients with Philadelphia positive chronic myeloid leukemia in Pakistan. *Pakistan Journal of Medical Sciences, 30*, 185–188. doi: 10.12669/pjms.301.3906.

Tefferi, A., Skoda, R.& Vardiman, J.W. (2009). Myeloproliferative neoplasms: contemporary diagnosis using histology and genetics. Nature Reviews Clinical Oncology, 1–11. doi: 10.1038/nrclinonc.2009.149.

Tefferi, A. & Vardiman, J.W. (2008). Classification and diagnosis of myeloproliferative neoplasms: the 2008 World Health Organization criteria and point-of-care diagnostic algorithms. *Journal of Leukemia, 22*, 14–22. doi: 10.1038/sj.leu.2404955.

Trejo, R.M.A., Gonzalez, V.A., Saldivar, I., et al. (2012). High frequency of concurrent JAK2 V617F mutation and BCR/ABL fusion gene in a cohort (18/142) of Mexican patients with MPD. *Blood, 120*, 1766–1766.

Vannucchi, A.M., Pieri, L. & Guglielmelli, P. (2010). JAK2 allele burden in the myeloproliferative neoplasms: effects on phenotype, prognosis, and change with treatment. *Therapeutic Advances in Hematology, 2*, 2040620710394474–32. doi: 10.1177/2040620710394474.

Yamada, O., Mahfoudhi, E., Plo I., et al. (2014). The emergence of a BCR-ABL translocation in a patient with the JAK2V617F mutation: evidence for secondary acquisition of BCR-ABL in the JAK2 V617F clone. *Journal of Clinical Oncology, 32*, e76–9. doi: 10.1200/JCO.2012.47.8669.

Zhang, Y., Coyne, M.Y., Will, S.G., et al. (1991). Single-base mutational analysis of cancer and genetic diseases using membrane bound modified oligonucleotides. *Nucleic Acids Research, 19*, 3929–3933. doi: 10.1093/nar/19.14.3929.

Zhou, A., Knoche, E.M., Engle, E.K. & Fisher, D. (2015). Concomitant JAK2 V617F-positive polycythemia vera and BCR-ABL-positive chronic myelogenous leukemia treated with ruxolitinib and dasatinib. *Blood Cancer Journal, 5*, e351–3. doi: 10.1038/bcj.2015.77.

Stem Cell Oncology – Adella (Ed.)
© 2018 Taylor & Francis Group, London, ISBN 978-0-8153-9272-9

Effect of zinc supplementation on linear growth velocity of children with short stature

I.T. Pujiastuti, M. Deliana, E. Mutiara & M. Lubis
Department of Child Health, Faculty of Medicine, Universitas Sumatera Utara, Medan, North Sumatera, Indonesia

ABSTRACT: Short stature is still a burden in many parts of the world, and can be a result of long-standing malnutrition. By increasing the availability of zinc, zinc supplementation can facilitate growth in children. This study aims to determine the effect of zinc supplementation on linear growth velocity in children with short stature. An open label randomised placebo-controlled trial was conducted in Singkuang Village, Mandailing Natal Regency, North Sumatera from March to September 2016. Children aged 7–10 years were screened for short stature. Subjects were divided into two groups; the intervention group received zinc supplementation of 10 mg/day, six days a week, and the control group received a placebo. After six months of zinc supplementation, there was no statistically significant increase in height (p = 0.493) and linear growth velocity (p = 0.365). Conclusion: There is no significant increase in height and linear growth velocity after zinc supplementation for six months in children with short stature.

Keywords: zinc supplementation, linear growth velocity, children with short stature

1   INTRODUCTION

In the last decade, some malnutrition problems have tended to show an improvement. However, these changes were not significant, one of them is on short stature issues (WHO, 2014). According to the National Basic Health Survey (RISKESDAS) by the Ministry of Health of the Republic of Indonesia in 2013, the incidence of stunted growth in Indonesia amounted to 37.2% (8 million children). In a preliminary study in Singkuang Village, Muara Batang Gadis District, Mandailing Natal Regency, North Sumatra, there was a prevalence of children with short stature of 40% (Hutasuhut et al., 2014).

Short stature can result from prolonged malnutrition. Macronutrients and micronutrients are needed for growth, including zinc which is one of the essential micronutrients. Zinc deficiency can affect many organ systems including the immune, gastrointestinal, skeletal, reproductive, and central nervous systems. Even a slight zinc deficiency can lead to immune dysfunction and restriction of physical development (UNICEF, 2015; WHO, 2014; Benoist, 2007). In one study there was an increase in growth velocity in children with zinc supplementation by 30% (Nakamura et al., 1993).

According to a review of 80 studies, zinc supplementation is associated with increased stature which was small but significant (Mayo-Wilson et al., 2014). The World Health Organization (WHO) recommended zinc supplementation for children with diarrhoea because it is proven to reduce the duration and severity. However, the provision of zinc supplements to improve child growth is still controversial (Vakili et al., 2015; Sjarif et al., 2014; Soetjiningih, 2008).

The aim of this study was to determine the effect of zinc supplementation on the growth velocity in children with short stature.

2 METHODS

The study protocol and the informed-consent process were approved by the Research Ethics Committee of the Faculty of Medicine, Universitas Sumatera Utara, Indonesia. This was a descriptive study with a cross sectional approach.

The research was conducted at SDN 382 and SDN 395, Singkuang, Muara Batang Gadis District, Mandailing Natal Regency, North Sumatra from March to September 2016. Samples were selected by simple random sampling, which included children aged 7–10 years, with height below the 3rd percentile on the CDC 2000 growth chart. Children with a chronic systemic disease including those with syndrome, protein energy malnutrition, and who had a history of dietary supplements during the three months before the study were excluded.

This study was analysed by SPSS software, using an independent t test, where $p > 0.05$ was considered significant.

3 RESULT

From a total of 173 children, the number of children with short stature in SDN 382 Singkuang was 23, and in SDN 395 was 37. Two children from SDN 382 were excluded because

Table 1. Baseline characteristics.

Characteristics	Intervention (n = 17)	Control (n = 16)	P
Sex, n			0.393*
Male	6	8	
Female	11	8	
Parent's occupation, n			0.980*
Fisherman	4	1	
Farmer	4	8	
Labourer	2	0	
Entrepreneur	7	7	
Parent's earning, n			0.533*
<IDR 500.000	1	2	
IDR 500.000–1.000.000	12	7	
>IDR 1.000.000	4	7	
Parental education, n			0.183*
Elementary school	12	10	
Junior high school	4	0	
Senior high school	1	6	
Age, mean (SD)	8.6	8.6	1.000**
Height (cm), mean (SD)	115.9	116.2	0.857***
Weight (kg), mean (SD)	17.8	19.6	0.063***

*Chi Square, **Mann-Whitney, ***Independent t test.

Table 2. Height before and after zinc supplementation.

	Height (cm)	Mean (SD)	t	CI 95%	p
Intervention	Before	115.9 (4.59)	−16.73	2.37–3.71	< 0.001*
	After	118.9 (4.60)			
Control	Before	116.3 (5.76)	−20.44	2.51–3.09	< 0.001*
	After	119.1 (5.95)			

*Independent t test.

Table 3. Height difference before and after zinc supplementation.

	Zinc supplementation			
	Yes	No	T	p
Height difference (SD)	3.0 (1.3)	2.8	0.697	0.493*

*Dependent t test.

Table 4. Difference in linear growth velocity.

	Zinc supplementation			
	Yes	No	T	p
Linear growth velocity (cm/month), mean (SD)	0.5 (0.20)	0.4 (0.09)	0.925	0.365*

of severe malnutrition. Seven children did not get parental consent for the study. Fifty-one children were randomised, 28 children were admitted to the intervention group and 23 children to the control group. At the end of the sixth month, nine children in the intervention group refused to continue the study, and two children moved out of school. Six children from the control group refused to continue the study. No child showed signs of puberty until the end of the study. No side effects were found in this study.

Based on statistical analysis, there was no significant increase in height and growth velocity after zinc supplementation in children with short stature.

4 DISCUSSION

Zinc supplementation is the only effective intervention strategy for treating zinc deficiency compared to other alternatives such as fortified foods, complimentary food and diet modifications. Research in Iran in 2013 showed zinc supplementation of 5 mg for 4 months in healthy children aged 9–18 years without zinc deficiency increase linear growth rate (Kaseb & Fallah, 2013). Research in Vietnam in 1999, in children aged 6–24 months who were given zinc supplementation for 11 mg per day for 3 months, found a significant increase in body length (Nasution, 2016).

In this study, it was found that the six-month difference of height in the intervention group was greater than in the control group. However, the results are not statistically significant. The rate of linear growth, which is a better indicator for assessing a child's linear growth, also showed similar results. The same was also observed in a randomised placebo-controlled trial study in Burkina Faso in 2003 with a larger sample, suggesting that there was no significant difference in height before and after zinc supplementation for six months in children with short stature (Muller, 2003).

This is proof that linear growth is influenced by many factors, including growth hormone and thyroid hormone that are not assessed in this study. In addition, multivitamin deficiency conditions play a greater role in linear growth, compared to zinc alone (Nasution, 2016).

5 CONCLUSION

There was no significant difference in height gain and linear growth rate after zinc supplementation for six months in children with short stature compared to the control group.

REFERENCES

Badan Penelitian dan Pengembangan Kesehatan Republik Indonesia. Riset kesehatan dasar. Jakarta: Kementerian Kesehatan RI. 2013.

de Benoist, B., Darnton-Hill. I., Davidsson, L., Fontaine, O. & Hotz, C. (2007) *Conclusions of the joint WHO/UNICEF/IAEA/IZiNCG interagency meeting on zinc status indicators secretariat.* Geneva: The United Nations.

Braun, L. & Marino, R. (2017). Disorders of growth and stature. *Pediatrics in Review, 38*(7), 293–304.

Brook, C.D.G. (2005). *Clinical practice of pediatric endocrinology* (pp. 34–5). Cambridge, England: Blackwell.

Cousminer, D.L., Berry, D.J., Timpson, N.J., Ang, W., Thiering, M., Byrne, E.M. et al. (2013). Genome-wide association and longitudinal analyses reveal genetic loci linking pubertal height growth, pubertal timing and childhood adiposity. *Human Molecular Genetics, 1–13.*

Ghaemmaghami, P., Ayatollahi, S., Alinejad, V. & Haem, E (2015). Longitudinal standards for growth velocity of infants from birth to 4 years born in West Azerbaijan Province of northwest Iran. *Epidemiology and Health, 37,* e2015029. 10.4178/epih/e2015029.

Haymond, M., Kappelgaard, A.M., Zernichow, P., Biller, B.M.K., Takano, K. & Kiess, W. (2013). Early recognition of growth abnormalities permitting early intervention. *Acta Pædiatrica, 102,* 787–96.

Hutasuhut, S.M., Deliana, M., Effendy, E. & Lubis, M. (2106). Hubungan Perawakan Pendek dengan Kesehatan Mental pada Anak usia 11–17 Tahun. Unpublished.

IDAI. (2010). Buku ajar endokrinologi anak. Jakarta: EGC, 19–23.

Kaseb, F. & Fallah, R. (2013). Efficacy of zinc supplementation on improvement of weight and height growth of healthy 9–18 year old children. *WAJS, 26,*189–93.

Kelly, A., Winer, K., Kalkwarf, H., Oberfield, S., Lappe, J., Gilsanz, V., et al. (2014). Age-based reference ranges for Annual Height Velocity in US children. *The Journal of Clinical Endocrinology and Metabolism, 99*(6), 2104–2112.

Kementerian, P. (2008). Pemberlakuan Standar Nasional Indonesia (SNI) tepung terigu sebagai bahan makanan secara wajib. Dalam: Peraturan Menteri Perindustrian Nomor 49/M-IND/PER/7/2008.

Kleinman, R.E. (2013). *Pediatric nutrition handbook* (8th Ed.). American Academy of Pediatrics, 423–6.

Kliegman, R.M. (2015). *Nelson textbook of pediatrics* (20th Ed.). Philadelphia: Elsevier.

Larsen, P.R. (2003). *Williams textbook of endocrinology* (10th Ed.). Boston: Elsevier.

Lifshitz, F. (2013). *Pediatric Endocrinology* (5th Ed.). Hoboken: Taylor and Francis.

Locks, L.M., Manji, K.P., McDonald, C.M., Kupka, R., Kisenge, R., Aboud, S., et al. (2016). Effect of zinc and multivitamin supplementation on the growth of Tanzanian children aged 6–84 weeks: a randomized, placebo-controlled, double-blind trial. *The American Journal of Clinical Nutrition, 1–9.*

Mayo-Wilson, E., Junior, J.A., Imdad, A., Dean, S., Chan, X.H.S., Chan, E.S., Jaswal, A. & Bhutta, Z.A. (2014). Zinc supplementation for preventing mortality, morbidity, and growth failure in children aged 6 months to 12 years of age (Review). The Cochrane Collaboration.

Nakamura, T., Nishiyama, S., Futagoishi-Suginohara, T., Matsuda, I. & Higashi, A. (1990). Mild to moderate zinc deficiency in short children: Effect of zinc supplementation on linear growth velocity. *Journal of Pediatrics, 123,* 65–9.

Nasution, E. (2004). Efek suplementasi zinc dan besi pada pertumbuhan anak. Medan. USU digital library. Diunduh dari library.usu.ac.id pada 03/02/2016.

Oxford University. (2009). *Mother and child nutrition in the tropics and subtropics.* Oxford: Oxford University Press.

Sjarif, D.R., Lestari, E.D., Mexitalia, M. & Nasar, S.S. (Eds). (2014). Buku Ajar Nutrisi Pediatrik dan Penyakit Metabolik. Jilid I. Jakarta: IDAI, 182–9.

Soetjiningsih. (2008). Tumbuh kembang anak. Surabaya: EGC, 11–8.

Thu, B.D., Schultink, W., Dillon, D., Gross, R., Leswara, N.D. & Khoi, H.H. (1999). Effect of daily and weekly micronutrient supplementation on micronutrient deficiencies and growth in young Vietnamese children. *American Journal of Clinical Nutrition, 69,* 80–6.

UNICEF. (2015). Levels and trends in child malnutrition. UNICEF.

Vakili, R., Bhakhs, M.Y., Vahedian, M., Mahmoudi, M., Saeidi, M., et al. (2015). The effect of zinc supplementation on linear growth and growth factors in primary school children in the suburbs Mashhad, Iran. *International Journal of Pediatrics, 1–7.*

Wardlaw, G.M. & Jeffrey, S. (2002). Perspective in nutrition (5th Ed). Boston: McGraw-Hill, 478–80.

World Health Organization. (2014). *Comprehensive implementation plan on maternal, infant, and young child nutrition.* Geneva: World Health Organization. World Health Organization. (1999). *Trace elements in human nutrition and health.* Geneva: World Health Organization. 72–100.

Stem Cell Oncology – Adella (Ed.)
© 2018 Taylor & Francis Group, London, ISBN 978-0-8153-9272-9

The outcomes of tibial fracture patients who underwent ORIF compared to MIPO

R. Oktavia & H. Hanafiah

Department of Orthopaedics and Traumatology, Faculty of Medicine, Universitas Sumatera Utara, Medan, North Sumatera, Indonesia

ABSTRACT: Minimal Invasive Plate Osteosynthesis (MIPO) is a new technique of internal fixation that is aimed to fix the weaknesses of conventional techniques. In this study, we researched the outcome of patients with a tibial fracture who underwent Open Reduction Internal Fixation (ORIF) compared to MIPO. We found 30 patients, of which 15 had conventional internal fixation surgery (ORIP) and 15 had minimally invasive internal fixation surgery (MIPO). The chi-square test for length of hospital stay resulted in a p value = 0.043 (p <0.05), showing there was a difference in length of stay between the ORIP group and the MIPO group. From all the postoperative complications studied, the chi-square test resulted in p >0.05 which meant there was no difference in the variables between the ORIF group and the MIPO group. Meanwhile, for postoperative complications, there were no differences between the ORIF group and the MIPO group.

Keywords: Tibial fracture, Open Reduction Internal Fixation, Minimal Invasive Plate Osteosynthesis

1   INTRODUCTION

Trauma is the most common cause of death in the 16–44 years old age group worldwide. The largest proportion of mortality (1.2 million per year) is traffic accidents. The World Health Organization (WHO) predicted that by 2020, traffic injury would rank third for cause of death.

Tibial fracture is the long bone fracture that frequently occurs and is the lower extremity fracture that most commonly occurs. Tibial fracture is a complication caused by traffic accidents or other traumas. The incidence of long bone fracture is 11.5/100,000 people/year, and 40% occur on the lower extremities. There are various surgery choices which may be performed for the management of tibial fracture, including ORIF (Open Reduction Internal Fixation), intramedullary fixation, and external fixation. ORIF is the most common technique used for the majority of fracture cases. Minimal Invasive Plate Osteosynthesis (MIPO) is a new technique of internal fixation published by Christian Krettek et al. in 1997 that is aimed to fix the weaknesses of conventional techniques.

ORIF is an operation to look at the fracture directly by surgery techniques including the installation of plate, screw, metal or prosthesis to mobilise the fracture during healing. In the MIPO technique, the potential for healing is considerable, because it can avoid tissue damage to cutaneous and subcutaneous skin, muscles and the vascularisation system around the fracture site. In this study, we researched the outcome of patients with tibial fracture who underwent ORIF compared to MIPO.

2   METHOD

This study is a comparative-analytic study with a cross-sectional design to search secondary data from medical records of patients diagnosed with a tibial fracture who underwent ORIF

Table 1. The difference of Internal Fixation Surgery Group and Minimally invasive surgery group based on characteristics

Characteristic	Internal fixation surgery group	Minimally invasive surgery group
Mean Age	35	28
Male	12	11
Female	3	4

Table 2. The difference of Internal Fixation Surgery Group and Minimally invasive surgery group based on length of stay.

Length of stay (days)	Internal fixation surgery group	Minimally invasive surgery group
> 7	2	9
7–14	8	4
> 14	5	2

or internal fixation minimally invasive at H. Adam Malik General Hospital in Medan during the period January 2015–December 2016. The exclusion criteria were patients with blood clotting disorders, previous kidney disorders, diabetes mellitus, and chronic obstructive pulmonary disease. The outcomes assessed in this study were length of stay and postoperative complications, including pain (VAS score 0–10), bleeding, postoperative infection, sepsis, compartment syndrome, and death. Bivariate data analysis was carried out on secondary data using statistical (Chi-Square test) and parametric measurements (T-test).

3 RESULTS

We found 30 patients, whom 15 were in the conventional internal fixation surgery group (ORIF) and 15 were in the internal fixation surgery minimally invasive group (MIPO). In the ORIF group, the mean age was 19 (14–38 years old), comprising ten men and five women. In the MIPO group, the mean age was 17 (13–42 years old) comprising 12 men and three women.

For the length of stay, the chi-square test resulted in a p value = 0.043 ($p < 0.05$), showing there was a difference in length of stay between the ORIF group and the MIPO group.

From the postoperative complications studied, the chi-square test resulted in $p > 0.05$. These complications were pain intensity/VAS score (p = 0.067), amount of bleeding (p + 0.056), postoperative infection (p + 0.73), the presence of sepsis (p + 0.084), the presence of compartment syndrome (p + 0.062), and the occurrence of death (p + 0.062), which indicated there were no differences in the variables between the ORIF group and the MIPO group.

4 DISCUSSION

In this study, the majority of patients involved were men (24 patients). The mean age of the patients that underwent internal fixation surgery was 35 years old and that for minimally invasive surgery was 28. The length of stay for patients who underwent internal fixation surgery compared to those who underwent minimally invasive surgery was different ($p < 0.05$). There have been a lot of studies that support that the MIPO technique accelerates the healing process, such as by Ahmed Rizk in Egypt (2015), Devendra in India (2015), Zeng et al. in China (2014) and Gulabi in Turkey (2016). In the H. Adam Malik General Hospital, the MIPO technique had been performed since the beginning of 2015.

The intensity of pain for patients who underwent internal fixation surgery compared to those who underwent minimally invasive surgery was not much different ($p > 0.05$). The amount of bleeding for patients who underwent internal fixation surgery compared to those who underwent minimally invasive surgery was not much different ($p > 0.05$). Postoperative infection in patients who underwent internal fixation surgery compared to those who had minimally invasive surgery were not much different ($p > 0.05$). The presence of sepsis in patients who underwent internal fixation surgery compared to those who underwent minimally invasive surgery was not much different ($p > 0.05$). The presence of compartment syndrome in patients who underwent internal fixation surgery compared to those who underwent minimally invasive surgery was not much different ($p > 0.05$). The occurrence of death in patients who underwent internal fixation surgery compared to those who underwent minimally invasive surgery was not much different ($p > 0.05$).

5 CONCLUSION

From the bivariate analysis, the outcome using chi-square test, there was a difference in length of stay between the ORIF group and the MIPO group. Meanwhile, for postoperative complications, there were no differences between the ORIF group and the MIPO group.

REFERENCES

Gulabi, D. (2016). Surgical treatment of distal tibia fractures: Open versus MIPO. *Turkish Journal of Trauma and Emergency Surgery, 22*(1).

Rizk, A. (2015). Minimally invasive plate osteosynthesis for the treatment of high energy tibial shaft fractures. *Egyptian Orthopaedic Journal, 50*, 36–44.

World Health Organization. (2011). *Road traffic injury prevention*. Geneva: WHO.

Zeng. (2014). Limited open reduction is better for simple distal tibial shaft fractures than minimally invasive plate osteosynthesis. *Genetic and Molecular Research, 13*(3), 5361–5368.

Stem Cell Oncology – Adella (Ed.)
© 2018 Taylor & Francis Group, London, ISBN 978-0-8153-9272-9

Association of ascariasis with IL-10 enzyme gene polymorphism in diabetes mellitus patients with tuberculosis

N.K. Arrasyid

Department of Parasitology, Faculty of Medicine, Universitas Sumatera Utara, Medan, North Sumatera, Indonesia

Y.S. Pane

Department of Pharmacology and Therapeutics, Faculty of Medicine, Universitas Sumatera Utara, Medan, North Sumatera, Indonesia

M.R.Z. Tala

Department of Obstetrics and Gynaecology, Faculty of Medicine, Universitas Sumatera Utara, Medan, North Sumatera, Indonesia

M.I. Sari

Department of Biochemistry, Faculty of Medicine, Universitas Sumatera Utara, Medan, North Sumatera, Indonesia

D.K. Sari

Department of Nutrition, Faculty of Medicine, Universitas Sumatera Utara, Medan, North Sumatera, Indonesia

ABSTRACT: Hyperglycaemia causes a phagocytic injection of Polymorphonuclear Leukocyte (PMN), which is associated with an increased frequency of infection. Impaired function of PMN phagocytosis is associated with an increased risk of infection that stimulates the formation of proinflammatory cytokines. In chronic worm infections, Treg cell activation results in IL-10 production, which plays a role in class switching antibody response in which IgE-producing cells switch to produce IgG4 which inhibits effector effranulation. This study aims to examine the correlation between Soil-Transmitted Helminth (STH) infection and IL-10 enzyme gene polymorphism among patients with both Diabetes Mellitus (DM) and Tuberculosis (Tb). The results showed that negative significant correlation between STH infection and IL-10 enzyme gene polymorphism among DM and Tb patients.

Keywords: soil-transmitted helminth, IL-10, diabetes mellitus, tuberculosis

1   INTRODUCTION

Diabetes Mellitus (DM) is a metabolic disorder in the body characterised by elevated blood glucose levels. A global survey in 2008 conducted by the World Health Organization (WHO) shows that there are 347 million people with DM, and this continues to increase. Based on the pattern of population growth, it is estimated that by 2030 there will be 194 million Indonesians aged over 20 years suffering from DM (Riskesdas, 2013; WHO, 2011).

Since the beginning of the 20th century, clinicians have observed an association between DM and Tuberculosis (Tb). Some hypotheses about the role of cytokines in DM patients as important molecules in the human defence mechanism against Tb. Hyperglycaemia causes a phagocytic injection of polymorphonuclear leukocyte (PMN), which is associated with an increased frequency of infection. Impaired function of PMN phagocytosis is associated with an increased risk of infection that stimulates the formation of proinflammatory cytokines. Several studies have shown that there is an increased expression of cytokines in vitro in people with diabetes one IL-10. The production of IL-10 cytokines is controlled at the transcriptional level depending on the regulatory factor bond with the introduction of a specific sequence on the promoter (Almeras & Print, 2006; Beamen, 2008; Oh et al., 2007; Sharma & Bose, 2001).

As a tropical country, the spread of infectious diseases in Indonesia is still a public health problem and one of these is Soil-Transmitted Helminth (STH) infection. The disease is chronic with the absence of clear clinical symptoms, and its effects are only seen in the long term. Such effects include increasing susceptibility to other infectious diseases such as Tb (Bethony et al., 2006; Kurniawan, 2010; Markell et al., 1996).

Based on the background presented above, this study aims to determine the relationship of IL-10 enzyme gene polymorphism in patients with DM and Tb with STH infection.

2 METHODS

Ethical approval was received from the Health Research Ethical Committee, Faculty of Medicine, Universitas Sumatera Utara, Medan, Indonesia. The research was conducted during the period of June 2017 to September 2017 at the Tuberculosis Disease Centre and recruited 40 consecutive samples from patients diagnosed with both DM and Tb. Exclusion criteria in this study included DM without Tb.

Informed consent was gained from the patients (or their legal representative if the patient could not give consent) before collection of 3 ml of venous blood samples. Determining the level of IL-10 was carried out using the ELISA technique (Oh et al., 2007). Stool examination was by the Kato method.

Data were collected and calculated using Fischer's exact test on more than 40 study samples.

3 RESULTS

This study obtained the results of STH infection suffered by one person (2.5%) male patients with DM+Tb in the age range 41–45 years. Variable characteristics of the patients are shown in Table 1.

Table 2 shows no correlation of ascariasis with IL-10 enzyme gene polymorphism among DM patients with Tb.

Table 1. Characteristics of the 40 DM+Tb patients with ascariasis.

| | Soil-transmitted helminth | | | | | |
| | Negative | | Positive | | Total | |
Parameter	n	%	n	%	n	%
Gender						
Male	28	70.0	1	2.5	29	72.5
Female	11	27.5	0	0	11	27.5
Age						
30–40	9	22.5	0	0	9	22.5
41–45	12	30	1	2.5	13	32.5
46–50	6	15.0	0	0	6	15.0
51–55	6	15.0	0	0	6	15.0
56–60	4	10.0	0	0	4	10.0
>60	2	5.0	0	0	0	5.0

Table 2. The genotype and allele frequency of IL-10 polymorphism in DM+Tb patients with ascariasis.

| Polymorphism | Soil-transmitted helminth | | | | | | |
| | Negative | | Positive | | Total | | |
	n	%	n	%	n	%	P
IL-10-592A/C							
CC	4	10.0	0	0.0	4	10.0	>0.05
AA	21	52.5	1	2.5	22	55.0	
AC	14	35.0	0	35.0	14	35.0	

Table 3. Association between IL-10 and ascariasis.

| | | STH infection | | |
		Positive	Negative	p-value
IL-10	High	1	5	0,23
	Low	–	34	

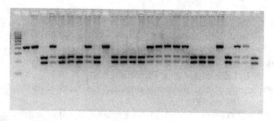

Figure 1. PCR-RFLP assay of DM+Tb patients.

Of the 40 DM patients with Tb who were examined, one person suffered from ascariasis with high levels of IL-10.

Of the 40 patients with DM+Tb who were examined, one person suffering from STH infection and had high levels of IL-10 (Table 3).

Polymorphism of DM+Tb patients can be seen in Figure 1 dominated by a genotype AA of 52.5%.

4 DISCUSSION

The results of this study found one person (2.5%) male respondents with DM+Tb suffering from ascariasis. This is in line with Bethony et al.'s (2006) statement which says worm infections can increase susceptibility to other important diseases such as Tb, diarrhoea and anaemia. However, Rusjdi's (2009) study did not find correlation between STH infection and IL-10 levels among DM+Tb patients.

5 CONCLUSION

In conclusion, our results suggest that there is no correlation between STH infection and IL-10-592A/C genotype among DM+Tb patients.

ACKNOWLEDGEMENTS

This research was supported by grants from the Universitas Sumatra Utara (USU) Research Institute.

REFERENCES

Almeras, L. & Prin, L. (2006). Genetic polymorphism of IL-10 and relevance to immune function. In F.M. Marincola (Ed.), *Interleukin-10* (pp. 1–10). Texas: Landes Bioscience.

American Diabetes Association. (2014). Position Statement: Diagnosis and classification of diabetes mellitus. *Diabetes Care, 37*(SUPPL.1), 81–90. https://doi.org/10.2337/dc14-S081.

Beamen, G.I. (2008). Interleukin-10 promotor Mycobacterium tuberculosis disease progression in CBA/a mice. *The Journal of Immunology.*

Bethony, J., Brooker, S., Albonico, M., Geiger, S.M., Loukas A, et al. (2006). Soil-transmitted helminth infections: Ascariasis trichuriasis, and hookworm. *Lancet, 367*, 1521–32.

Jeon, C.Y. & Murray, M.B. (2008). Diabetes mellitus increases the risk of active tuberculosis: a systematic review of 13 observational studies. *PLOS Medicine, 5*(7), 11p.

Kurniawan, A. (2010). Infeksi Parasit: Dulu dan Masa Kini. Maj Kedokt Indon, *60*(11), 487–88.

Maj. Ked. Andalas: 33(2), 94–100.

Markell, E.K., Voge, M. & Jhon, D.T. (1996). *Medical Parasitology* (6th Ed.). Philadelphia, USA: W.B. Sounders Company.

O'Leary, S., O'Sullivan, M.P. & Keane, J. (2011). IL-10 blocks Phagosome maturation in Mycobacterium tuberculosis-infected human macrophages. *American Journal of Respiratory Cell and Molecular Biology, 45*, 172–80.

Oh, J.H., Yang, C.S., Noh, Y.K., Kweon, Y.M., Jung, S.G., Son, J.W., Kong, S.J., et al. (2007). Polymorphisms of interleukin-10 and tumour necrosis factor-α genes are associated with newly diagnosed and recurrent pulmonary tuberculosis. *Respirology, 12*, 594–8.

Perkumpulan Endokrinologi Indonesia-PERKENI. (2011). Konsensus pengelolaan dan pencegahan diabetes melitus tipe 2 di Indonesia. Jakarta: PB PERKENI.

Ramamurti, T. (1999). Pathology of mycobacterial infection in diabetes. *International Journal of Diabetes in Developing Countries, 19*, 56–60.

Redford, P.S., Murray, P.J. & O'Garra, A. (2011). The role of IL-10 in immune regulation during M. tuberculosis infection. *Mucosal Immunology, 4*, 260–6.

Riskesdas. (2013). Kementerian kesehatan. Riset kesehatan Dasar.

Rusjdi, S.R. (2009). Respon Th2 pada infeksi cacing usus. *Maj. Ked. Andalas: 33*(2), 94–100.

Sharma, S. & Bose, M. (2001). Role of cytokines in immune response to pulmonary tuberculosis. *Asian Pacific Journal of Allergy and Immunology.*

Sheikhpour, R. (2013). Diabetes and oxidative stress: The mechanism and action. *Iranian Journal of Diabetes and Obesity, 5*(1), 40–45.

World Health Organization. (2011). Non communicable disease report. [Cited 2017 Mar19]. Available from http://www.who.int/nmh/publications/ncd_report_chapter1.pdf.

Stem Cell Oncology – Adella (Ed.)
© *2018 Taylor & Francis Group, London, ISBN 978-0-8153-9272-9*

Acetyl salicylic acid resistance and inhibition to platelet aggregation

D.M. Amoryna, Z. Mukthar & H. Hariman
Department of Clinical Pathology, Faculty of Medicine, Universitas Sumatera Utara, Medan, North Sumatera, Indonesia

ABSTRACT: The adverse side-effects of Acetyl Salicylic Acid (ASA) are mainly gastro-intestinal bleeding. The objective is to determine if 50 mg ASA is as effective as 100 mg when used in normal healthy subjects. The 18 normal subjects had a normal platelet count of mean $301 \pm 72.3 \times 10^9$/L. Significant ($P = <0.001$) platelet inhibition was seen in 15 subjects ingesting 50 mg ASA (mean $50.3 \pm 21.9\%$) and 100 mg ASA (mean $75.7 \pm 19.3\%$). Further significantly enhanced ($P = <0.001$) inhibition was seen in 100 mg ASA compared to 50 mg. Three subjects were non-responders to 50 mg ASA (16.7%) and two to 100 mg (11.1%). The study showed that a 100 mg ASA dose is better suited for antiplatelet therapy compared with 50 mg. Significantly greater platelet inhibition was seen with 100 mg ASA with no gastro-intestinal bleeding or other side-effects reported. ASA resistance was seen in 16.7% of subjects ingesting 50 mg ASA and 11.1% ingesting the 100 mg dose.

Keywords: Acetyl Salicylic Acid (ASA), inhibition in normal subjects, resistance

1 INTRODUCTION

Platelets play an important role in the pathogenesis of arterial thrombosis, activated platelet initiate thrombus formation and antiplatelet therapy modifies these properties involving aspirin (acetyl salicylic acid, ASA) (Oesman, 2009; Setiabudi, 2009). ASA is widely used as an antiplatelet agent to reduce the risk of non-fatal stroke, non-fatal myocardial infarction and vascular death in patients at high risk of arterial thrombosis. It was reported to reduce mortality in acute coronary syndrome (ACS) and to improve the condition (Setiabudi, 2006). However, ASA failed to inhibit platelet aggregation in acute myocardial infarction (AMI) (Poulsen et al., 2007) and their use in AMI is of little or no use (Borna et al., 2005). ASA resistance is of unknown etiological phenomenon describing decreased platelet activation by ASA. The existence of ASA resistance affects more than 50% of patients with cardiovascular disease (Oesman, 2009; Setiabudi, 2009) and 25.8% in severe symptomatic Peripheral Artery Disease (PAD) (Chen et al., 2007). In stable Coronary Artery Disease (CAD), it has been reported that 36% of Asian Indian patients were non-responders to ASA (Chadha et al., 2016). Abnormal platelet aggregation studies due to aspirin-like defect were seen in up to 9% of platelet donors (Stohlawerz et al., 2001). The adverse effects of ASA are mainly gastro-intestinal bleeding, and this effect is greater with daily 300 mg ASA use (Taneja et al., 2004). Very low doses of ASA spare prostacyclin formation and reduce gastro-intestinal side-effects but are less effective in inhibiting platelet aggregation. Doses of 100 mg and 162.5 mg ASA had shown greater inhibition than lower doses (Maree et al., 2005). For doses higher than 162 mg ASA, only 6% did not show any response in another study (Dengo et al., 2016). Aspirin resistance is associated with an increased risk of severe stroke, and a large infarct volume in patients taking aspirin before stroke onset (Oh et al., 2016) and between 5% to 65% was seen in patients with ischaemic stroke (Ozben et al., 2011).

Platelet aggregation is performed to identify and quantify platelet response and monitor platelet inhibition by drug therapy. It is based on the addition of a platelet agonist to a blood sample (usually platelet-rich plasma). It may be assessed using various agonists such as adenosine di-phosphate (ADP), collagen and others. Arachidonic acid (AA), a precursor of thromboxane A_2 and hydroxyl fatty acids liberated from human platelets on activation, converts the enzyme cyclooxygenase-1 (COX-1) into a potent inducer of platelet aggregation. Ingestion of ASA inhibits COX-1 thus inhibits platelet aggregation. The aggregation of platelets is an essential physiologic life-saving process of blood coagulation. The role of platelets in haemostasis involves adherence to sites of injury, activation of internal signalling pathways, aggregation to form plugs and the acceleration of the coagulation reactions to form thrombin. Platelet aggregation, particularly at the site of plaque rupture, results in thrombus formation blocking normal blood circulation in the heart musculature in ACS (Fuster et al., 1996). Platelet function may be impaired if any of the pathways mediated by the activation process by agonists are defective. The objective of this small cohort study is to determine whether an ASA of 50 mg dose is as effective as a 100 mg dose in normal healthy subjects.

2 METHODS

The study received ethical approval from the Health Research Ethical Committee of North Sumatera (No: 357/KOMET/FK USU2013), Medical School, University of Sumatera Utara, Medan, Indonesia. It was conducted at the Department of Clinical Pathology, Faculty of Medicine, University of North Sumatera/Haj Adam Malik Hospital. The inclusion criteria for the study: age above 18 years old, not on any medication for the past ten days, and agreed to give informed consent. The exclusion criteria: body mass index (BMI) > 30, known medical disorders.

Subjects: Initially, 46 subjects gave their informed consent, but 12 failed to turn up for the study. Of the remaining 34 subjects, only 18 completed the protocol study whilst the remainder failed to turn up for the 100 mg ASA protocol and therefore were excluded from the analysis. Data from the 18 subjects (female n = 15, male n = 3) who completed the 50 mg and 100 mg ASA protocol were therefore analysed. Their mean age was 41.7 ± 7.4 years ranging between 31 years and 50 years old. The study subjects were healthy individuals recruited from within the institution, they had no known medical history and had given written informed consent to participate in the study.

Blood sampling: After having fasted overnight, a clean venepuncture was performed and blood collected into EDTA anticoagulant (2 mL, BD Vacutainer) for platelets and 3.6 mL blood into 0.4 mL 3.8% sodium citrate for preparation of Platelet-Rich Plasma (PRP). Blood sampling was performed pre-ASA ingestion and three days later after daily ingestion of 50 mg ASA. A wash-out period of 7 days was instituted before another blood sampling was performed after daily ingestion of 100 mg ASA for three days. Citrated blood was centrifuged at room temperature at 150 g for 10 mins for PRP and again centrifuged at 2000 g for 15 minutes to obtain poor platelet plasma (PPP). Platelet aggregation was performed within two to three hours from blood sampling.

Laboratory analysis: Platelets (EDTA blood) and PRP were determined in the automatic cell counter Sysmex XT 4000 (Kobe, Japan). The ex-vivo platelet aggregation studies were performed using arachidonic acid (AA, PT Helena Laboratories (Australia) Pte Ltd, product 5364) as an agonist at a final concentration of 500 μg/mL to the PRP in the platelet aggregometer, Aggregation Remote Analyzer (Helena Laboratories, model SUF52001). PPP was calibrated as maximum transmission at 100%.

Statistical analysis: The Statistical Package for Social Sciences (SPSS 22 IBM Corp. USA) was used to perform statistical analysis. On paired samples a t-test was performed to compare differences in platelet aggregation inhibition with 50 mg and 100 mg. Three subjects were considered non-responders to 50 mg ASA and remaining two to both 50 mg and 100 mg ASA. They were excluded from the final analysis. A P value of less than 0.05 was considered statistically significant.

3 RESULT

3.1 *Platelets and platelet-rich plasma*

Platelet numbers of the 18 normal subjects were a mean of $301 \pm 72.3 \times 10^9$/L and ranged between 204 and 448×10^9/L. The mean platelet number in PRP was $240 \pm 56.3 \times 10^9$/L and ranged between 185 and 360×10^9/L. For platelet aggregation studies, the platelet numbers in the PRP sample should be in the region of 150 to 400×10^9/L.

Platelet aggregation (T max%) and inhibition to 50 mg and 100 mg acetyl salicylic acid (ASA) in normal healthy subjects was compared with that pre-ASA (excluding three non-responders to ASA).

Significant inhibition (P = <0.001) of ex-vivo platelet aggregation to 50 mg ASA (mean 50.3%, ranged from 10.6% to 85.5%) and 100 mg dose (mean 75.7%, ranged from 11.8% to 93.6%) compared with pre-ASA state in the 15 normal subjects was seen. Further enhanced inhibition (P = <0.001) with the 100 mg dose compared to the 50 mg dose was also seen (Table 1).

Non-responders or resistance to 50 mg ASA (16.7%) was seen in 3 normal subjects. One subject was resistant to 50 mg ASA only but responded to the 100 mg dose (77.4% inhibition). With 100 mg ASA, the resistance rate is 11.1% (2/18) in this small cohort study. Their results (T max%) are shown in Table 2.

4 DISCUSSION

Aspirin (ASA) is widely used as an antiplatelet agent to reduce the risk of non-fatal stroke, non-fatal myocardial infarction and vascular death in patients at high risk of arterial thrombosis. It was reported to reduce mortality in ACS and improve the condition (Setiabudi, 2006). However, ASA failed to inhibit platelet aggregation in AMI (Poulsen et al., 2007) and its use in AMI is of little or no use (Borna et al., 2005). ASA resistance has been shown to be associated with an increased risk of severe stroke and large infarct volume in patients taking aspirin before stroke onset (Oh et al., 2016). High platelet activity contributes to poor prognosis, but the mechanism of ASA resistance describing decreased platelet activation remains unclear (Hankey & Eikelboom, 2006). Ingestion of ASA inhibits COX-1 activity thus inhibits platelet aggregation. Abnormal platelet aggregation studies due to an aspirin-like defect were seen in up to 9% of platelet donors (Taneja et al., 2004). The adverse effects of ASA are mainly gastro-intestinal bleeding, and this effect is greater with daily 300 mg ASA use (Taneja et al., 2004). In our small study, the subjects had normal platelet counts and had no known medical history to report, but only 88.9% responded to 100 mg ASA and 83.3% to 50 mg ASA. Greater inhibition of platelet aggregation was seen at 100 mg compared to 50 mg ASA suggesting 100 mg ASA is better suited for therapy as an antiplatelet agent. We report here that 11.1% of normal subjects are ASA resistance to 100 mg ASA and 16.7% to 50 mg ASA dose which is much higher than reported for platelet donors, up to 9% in one study (Stohlawerz et al., 2001) and 6% in another study with 162 mg ASA (Dengo et al., 2016). In stable coronary artery disease in Asian Indian patients it has been reported that 36% were non-responders to ASA therapy (Chadha et al., 2016). There were no reports of gastro-intestinal bleeding or other side-effects in the study subjects probably due to the short duration of ASA use.

In conclusion, the study showed that a 100 mg ASA dose is better suited for antiplatelet therapy compared to a 50 mg dose. Significantly greater platelet inhibition was seen with 100 mg ASA use, with no gastro-intestinal bleeding or other side-effects reported. ASA resistance was seen in 16.7% of subjects ingesting 50 mg ASA and 11.1% in 100 mg ASA in this short duration study.

ACKNOWLEDGEMENT

The authors wish to express their sincere gratitude to the subjects who were volunteers within the institution for participating in the study.

REFERENCES

Borna, C., E. Lazaruski, C.V. Heusden, H. Olhlin, and D. Erling. (2005). Resistance to aspirin is increased by ST-elevation myocardial infarction and correlates with adenosine diphosphate levels. *Thrombosis Journal, 26, 3–10.*. http://doi.org/10.1186/1477.9560.3.10 26 pp.3: 10.

Chadha, B. Sumana, G. Karthekeyan, V. Jayaprasad, S.S. Arun. (2016). Prevalence of aspirin resistance in Asian-Indian patients with stable coronary artery disease. Catherization and Cardiovascular *Interventions, 88*(4), E126-E131. doi10.1002/ccd.25420.

Chen, X., Cheng, P.Y., Lee, Ng W., J.Y. Kwik et al. 2007. Aspirin resistance and adverse clinical events in patients with coronary artery disease. *American Journal of Medicine, 120*(7), 631–5. doi: 10.1016.

Dengo, E.S., Westphsl, M.M. Rainka. (2016). Platelet response to increased aspirin dose in patients with persistent platelet aggregation while treated with 81 mg. *Journal of Clinical Pharmacology, 56*, 414–21.

Fuster, J., Badimon, J.H., Chesebro, J.T. Fallon. (1996). Plaque rupture, thrombosis and therapeutic implications. *Haemostasis, 26*, 269–84.

Hankey, J.W. Eikelboom. (2006). Aspirin resistance. *Lancet, 357* (9510), 606–17.

Maree, R.J., Curtin, M., Dooley, R.M., Conroy, P. Crean. (2005). Platelet response to low-dose enteric-coated aspirin in patients with stable cardio vascular diseases. *Journal of the American College of Cardiology, 47*(7), 1258–1262.

Oesman, R.D. Setiabudi. (2009). Fisiologi Hemostasis Dan Thrombosis., keempat ed. Jakarta; Balai Penerbit FKUI.

Oh, K.-H. Yu, J.-H. Lee. (2016). Aspirin resistance is associated with increased stroke severity and infarct volume. *Neurology*, April 6. doi.org/10.1212/WNL.

Ozben, B., Ozben, A.M., Tanrikulu, F., Ozer, T. Ozben. (2011). Aspirin resistance in patients with acute ischemic stroke. *Journal of Neurology, 258*, 1979–86.

Poulsen, Bo., Jorgensen, L. Kursholm, P.B. Licht, T. Hughfall, and H. Mickey. (2007). Prevalence of aspirin resistance in patients with an evolving acute myocardial infarction. *Thrombosis Research, 119*(5), 555–562. Retrieved from www.thrombosisresearch.com/article/500049-3848(06)00154.

Setiabudi. (2006). Disfungsi trombosit: klasifikasi dan diagnosa. In: M. Suryaatmadja, ed. Pendidikan berkesinambungan Patologi Klinik 2006. Jakarta; Continuing Medical Education dana Profesional development departemen patologi klinik. Fakutas Kedokteran Uniersitas Indonesia., 12–14.

Stohlawerz, N., Hergovich, M. Homoncik. (2001). Impaired platelet function among platelet donors. *Journal of Thrombosis and Haemostasis, 86*, 880–6.

Taneja, U. Mallich, and M.D. Flather. (2004). Anti platelet agent. In D.L. Bhatt, D.L. & M.D. Flather, M.D. (Eds), *Handbook of Acute Coronary Syndromes* (pp. 84) London-Chicago: British Library Cataloguing.

Author index